The Role of the Mitochondria in Human Aging and Disease

The Role of the Mitochondria in Human Aging and Disease

Edited by John Binnington

New York

Hayle Medical,
750 Third Avenue, 9th Floor,
New York, NY 10017, USA

Visit us on the World Wide Web at:
www.haylemedical.com

ISBN: 978-1-64647-528-5

Cataloging-in-Publication Data

The role of the mitochondria in human aging and disease / edited by John Binnington.
   p. cm.
Includes bibliographical references and index.
ISBN 978-1-64647-528-5
1. Mitochondrial pathology. 2. Mitochondrial DNA. 3. Mitochondria.
4. Aging. 5. Metabolism--Disorders. I. Binnington, John.
RB147.5 .R65 2023
616.07--dc23

Table of Contents

Preface

Mitochondria are membrane-bound cell organelles, which are considered to be key factors involved in the aging process. They are involved in energy production by oxidative phosphorylation. They also play a significant role in maintaining calcium balance, intracellular homeostasis, and the metabolism and inter-conversion of dietary substrates. They play a crucial function in signaling their metabolic state to the nucleus and other cells. Mitochondria possess a protein synthetic apparatus and can self-replicate. These apparatuses can be easily disrupted in aging and disease. Mitochondria are continuously involved in the processes of fission and fusion, which is essential for the proper functioning of cells. Mitochondria play an important metabolic role in all organ systems; therefore, they are specifically influenced by diseases which contribute in the process of aging. This book unravels the recent studies related to the role of the mitochondria in human aging and disease. It provides the readers with a thorough understanding of the subject.

This book is the end result of constructive efforts and intensive research done by experts in this field. The aim of this book is to enlighten the readers with recent information in this area of research. The information provided in this profound book would serve as a valuable reference to students and researchers in this field.

At the end, I would like to thank all the authors for devoting their precious time and providing their valuable contribution to this book. I would also like to express my gratitude to my fellow colleagues who encouraged me throughout the process.

Editor

Mitochondria as the Linchpin of General Intelligence and the Link between *g*, Health and Aging

David C. Geary⦿

Department of Psychological Sciences, Interdisciplinary Neuroscience, University of Missouri, Columbia, MO 65211-2500, USA; GearyD@Missouri.edu.

Abstract: In a recent theoretical article, I proposed that the efficiency of mitochondrial functioning is the most fundamental biological mechanism contributing to individual differences in general intelligence (*g*; Geary, 2018). The hypothesis accommodates other contributing mechanisms at higher levels of analysis (e.g., brain networks), and is attractive because mitochondrial energy production undergirds the developmental, maintenance, and expression of these other mechanisms and provides a means to link individual differences in *g* to individual differences in health and successful aging in adulthood. I provide a brief summation here and a few clarifications to the original article.

Keywords: general intelligence; mitochondria; cognitive aging; health

It has been well over a century since Spearman discovered that individuals who perform well in one cognitive or academic domain generally perform well in all other domains, leading him to conclude "that all branches of intellectual activity have in common one fundamental function (or group of functions)" [1] (p. 285), which he termed general intelligence, or *g*. Statistically, about 50% of the covariance among cognitive and academic measures is captured by this function or functions [2], making the concept of *g* (whatever it is indexing) of substantial theoretical and practical importance. The ensuing search for the basis of *g* has led to myriad theories and research traditions at multiple levels of analysis including complex (e.g., working memory) to more basic (e.g., speed of processing) cognitive systems [3,4]; complex (large-scale networks) to more basic (e.g., speed of neural conduction) neural systems [5]; aspects of cellular functioning (e.g., control of oxidative stress; [6,7]); and, g as an illusionary construct resulting from the mathematics underlying factor analyses [8,9].

In a recent proposal, I suggested that *g* is best conceptualized as a group of cognitive and neural functions that are all undergirded by one evolutionarily old, fundamental function [10]; specifically, the efficiency of various mitochondrial processes, especially the production of cellular energy. The group of functions means that multiple cognitive and brain systems contribute to *g* in a nested fashion, as shown in Figure 1. The outer level is represented by the engagement of the cognitive systems, such as working memory, and problem-solving approaches, such as analogical reasoning (e.g., [11]), that manifest in the real world as intelligent decision making and behavior. It is now well established that these competencies are supported by distributed and dynamically interacting networks of brain systems (the intermodular ring in Figure 1), although the engaged networks likely depend on task demands and the individuals' level of expertise in the area ([5,12,13]). The efficiency of these complex intermodular systems will necessarily be modulated by the efficiency of the intramodular systems that compose them [14], and these in turn are dependent on the functioning of the constituent neurons and supporting cells (glia; [15]). At the core are mitochondria and their many functions, including the bulk of cellular energy production [16]. Genetic, neuroimaging, and neuropsychological studies can be marshalled to support each of these mechanisms as contributing to *g* [17–19], but none of them in and of itself will likely provide a full explanation.

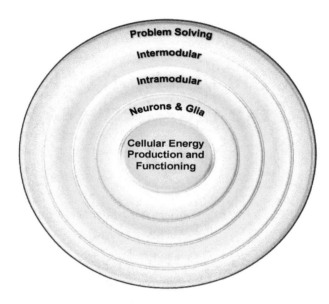

Figure 1. Individual differences in *g* are likely to be influenced by the functioning of multiple cognitive and brain systems, the optimal functioning of which is dependent on systems below it. Cellular energy is the lowest common currency driving the development and expression of all biological systems and thus places upper-limit constraints on the development and expression of all other systems.

A core implication of the nested structure shown in Figure 1 is that deficits or inefficiencies at lower levels will ripple through all higher levels but deficits at higher levels (e.g., resulting from traumatic brain injury) need not have broad influences at lower levels. In other words, the full expression of the competencies supported at higher levels, within the genetic and experiential constraints of the individual, will be limited by the efficiency of systems at all lower levels. On this view, subtle variation—either due to genetics [20] or experiences (e.g., toxin exposure, chronic stress; [21])—in mitochondrial energy production or the mechanisms that protect mitochondria from degradation will manifest as variation in the development and expression of all of the brain and cognitive systems that have been linked to *g*.

Critically, mitochondria produce the majority of energy consumed by all biological systems, not just the brain, and the initial tranche of mitochondria within all of these systems comes from the same limited pool. As a result, variation in the efficiency (e.g., in energy production, control of oxidative stress) of the initial pool of mitochondria will be expressed throughout the body and will contribute to individual differences in resilience to disease and stressors—factors that can degrade mitochondrial functioning—and can influence the rate of aging in adulthood [22–24]. Variation in the initial pool of mitochondria also provides a straightforward explanation of the well-documented relations among *g*, general health, and successful aging in adulthood [25–27].

As just one example of these relations, there is a single statistical factor that explains individual differences in rate of age-related declines across cognitive domains (e.g., reasoning, speed of processing; [28]). As people age, individuals who show sharp performance declines in one area, such as fluid intelligence, also show parallel declines in other cognitive domains, such as speed of processing. The implication is there is a single mechanism (or group of related mechanisms) that supports cognition and declines as a natural consequence of biological aging. The statistical factor that captures this common age-related decline is moderately correlated (*r* ~0.5) with an estimate of *g* [29]. In other words, there is overlap in the mechanisms that contribute to *g* and to natural age-related declines in cognition. These types of studies, however, are not evidence that the overlap is the result of a single mechanism, as this is unlikely.

Normal age-related declines in mitochondrial energy production is a very plausible contributing mechanism, even if it is not the whole story. Age-related decrements in energy production will occur, at least to some extent, in parallel across biological systems and individual differences in the rate of change will result in correlations across cognitive and health measures. Moreover, the relative importance of mitochondrial functions in relation to other factors might increase with aging in adulthood. The increasing importance of mitochondria follows from its role as a limiting mechanism on the functioning of more complex systems. With normal age-related declines in energy production, an increasing number of individuals will have energy-production levels that approach or drop below the thresholds needed to maintain and express higher-level systems at their optimal; that is, optimal for the individual depending on the genetic and experiential factors that contribute to the construction of these systems, given sufficient energy levels.

Stated somewhat differently, the capacity for mitochondria to produce energy places a ceiling on the performance of higher-level systems. With normal aging in adulthood that ceiling slowly descends and reduces the capacity for higher-level systems to operate at levels they once did. These declines would be related to reductions in the ability to maintain the complex brain systems that support intelligence and in the ability to use them as effectively during periods of high-energy demand, such as maintaining focus during a novel and complex problem-solving task. During development individual differences in mitochondrial energy production are likely to place constraints on the construction of these systems in addition to constraints on optimal functioning. In this latter case, the overall ceiling is higher and thus variation in g might be more strongly related to variation in higher-level than lower-level systems, but this remains to be determined.

References

1. Spearman, C. General Intelligence, Objectively Determined and Measured. *Am. J. Psychol.* **1904**, *15*, 201–292. [CrossRef]
2. Warne, R.T.; Burningham, C. Spearman's g found in 31 non-Western nations: Strong Evidence that g is a Universal Phenomenon. *Psychol. Bull.* **2019**, *145*, 237–272. [CrossRef] [PubMed]
3. Engle, R.W.; Kane, M.J.; Tuholski, S.W. Individual differences in working memory capacity and what they tell us about controlled attention, General Fluid Intelligence, and Functions of the Prefrontal Cortex. In *Models of Working Memory: Mechanisms of Active Maintenance and Executive*; Miyake, A., Shah, P., Eds.; Cambridge University Press: Cambridge, UK, 1999; pp. 102–134.
4. Kranzler, J.H.; Jensen, A.R. The nature of psychometric g: Unitary Process or A Number of Independent Processes? *Intelligence* **1991**, *15*, 397–422. [CrossRef]
5. Jung, R.E.; Haier, R.J. The Parieto-Frontal Integration Theory (P-FIT) of intelligence: Converging Neuroimaging Evidence. *Behav. Brain Sci.* **2007**, *30*, 135–154. [CrossRef] [PubMed]
6. Gottfredson, L.S.; Deary, I.J. Intelligence Predicts Health and Longevity, but why? *Curr. Dir. Psychol. Sci.* **2004**, *13*, 1–4. [CrossRef]
7. Hendrickson, D.E.; Hendrickson, A.E. The Biological Basis of Individual Differences in Intelligence. *Personal. Individ. Differ.* **1980**, *1*, 3–33. [CrossRef]
8. Kovacs, K.; Conway, A.R. Process overlap theory: A Unified Account of the General Factor of Intelligence. *Psychol. Inq.* **2016**, *27*, 151–177. [CrossRef]
9. Krijnen, W.P. Positive Loadings and Factor Correlations from Positive Covariance Matrices. *Psychometrika* **2004**, *69*, 655–660. [CrossRef]
10. Geary, D.C. Efficiency of Mitochondrial Functioning as the Fundamental Biological Mechanism of General Intelligence (g). *Psychol. Rev.* **2018**, *125*, 1028–1050. [CrossRef]
11. Holyoak, K.J.; Thagard, P. The Analogical Mind. *Am. Psychol.* **1997**, *52*, 35–44. [CrossRef]
12. Neubauer, A.C.; Fink, A. Intelligence and Neural Efficiency. *Neurosci. Biobehav. Rev.* **2009**, *33*, 1004–1023. [CrossRef] [PubMed]
13. Santarnecchi, E.; Emmendorfer, A.; Pascual-Leone, A. Dissecting the parieto-frontal correlates of fluid intelligence: A Comprehensive ALE Meta-Analysis Study. *Intelligence* **2017**, *63*, 9–28. [CrossRef]
14. Bullmore, E.; Sporns, O. The Economy of Brain Network Organization. *Nat. Rev. Neurosci.* **2012**, *13*, 336–349. [CrossRef] [PubMed]
15. Tseng, P.Y.; Lee, I.H.; Chen, K.C.; Chen, P.S.; Chiu, N.T.; Yao, W.J.; Chu, C.L.; Yeh, T.L.; Yang, Y.K. The Correlation between Mid-Brain Serotonin Transporter Availability and Intelligence Quotient in Healthy Volunteers. *Eur. Psychiatry* **2015**, *30*, 193–197. [CrossRef] [PubMed]

16. Lane, N. Mitonuclear match: Optimizing Fitness and Fertility over Generations Drives Ageing within Generations. *Bioessays* **2011**, *33*, 860–869. [CrossRef]

17. Barbey, A.K.; Colom, R.; Solomon, J.; Krueger, F.; Forbes, C.; Grafman, J. An Integrative Architecture for General Intelligence and Executive Function Revealed by Lesion Mapping. *Brain* **2012**, *135*, 1154–1164. [CrossRef]

18. Lee, J.J.; McGue, M.; Iacono, W.G.; Michael, A.M.; Chabris, C.F. The causal influence of brain size on human intelligence: Evidence from Within–Family Phenotypic Associations and GWAS Modeling. *Intelligence* **2019**, *75*, 48–58. [CrossRef]

19. Savage, J.E.; Jansen, P.R.; Stringer, S.; Watanabe, K.; Bryois, J.; De Leeuw, C.A.; Nagel, M.; Awasthi, S.; Barr, P.B.; Coleman, J.R.; et al. Genome-Wide Association Meta-Analysis in 269,867 Individuals Identifies New Genetic and Functional links to Intelligence. *Nat. Genet.* **2018**, *50*, 912–919. [CrossRef]

20. Latorre-Pellicer, A.; Moreno-Loshuertos, R.; Lechuga-Vieco, A.V.; Sánchez-Cabo, F.; Torroja, C.; Acín-Pérez, R.; Calvo, E.; Aix, E.; González–Guerra, A.; Bernad-Miana, M.L.; et al. Mitochondrial and Nuclear DNA Matching Shapes Metabolism and Healthy Ageing. *Nature* **2016**, *535*, 561–565. [CrossRef]

21. Caito, S.W.; Aschner, M. Mitochondrial Redox Dysfunction and Environmental Exposures. *Antioxid. Redox Signal.* **2015**, *23*, 578–595. [CrossRef]

22. Harman, D. The biologic clock: The Mitochondria? *J. Am. Geriatr. Soc.* **1972**, *20*, 145–147. [CrossRef] [PubMed]

23. Koch, R.E.; Josefson, C.C.; Hill, G.E. Mitochondrial Function, Ornamentation, and Immunocompetence. *Biol. Rev.* **2017**, *92*, 1459–1474. [CrossRef] [PubMed]

24. Stewart, J.B.; Freyer, C.; Elson, J.L.; Larsson, N.G. Purifying Selection of mtDNA and its Implications for Understanding Evolution and Mitochondrial Disease. *Nat. Rev. Genet.* **2008**, *9*, 657–662. [CrossRef] [PubMed]

25. Deary, I.J.; Weiss, A.; Batty, G.D. Intelligence and personality as predictors of illness and death: How Researchers in Differential Psychology and Chronic Disease Epidemiology are Collaborating to Understand and Address Health Inequalities. *Psychol. Sci. Public Interest* **2010**, *11*, 53–79. [CrossRef] [PubMed]

26. Lindenberger, U.; Baltes, P.B. Sensory functioning and intelligence in old age: A Strong Connection. *Psychol. Aging* **1994**, *9*, 339–355. [CrossRef] [PubMed]

27. Lubinski, D.; Humphreys, L.G. Some Bodily and Medical Correlates of Mathematical Giftedness and Commensurate Levels of Socioeconomic Status. *Intelligence* **1992**, *16*, 99–115. [CrossRef]

28. Salthouse, T.A. How Many Causes are there of Aging-Related Decrements in Cognitive Functioning? *Dev. Rev.* **1994**, *14*, 413–437. [CrossRef]

29. Tucker-Drob, E.M.; Brandmaier, A.M.; Lindenberger, U. Coupled cognitive changes in adulthood: A Meta-Analysis. *Psychol. Bull.* **2019**, *145*, 273–301. [CrossRef]

Melatonin/Nrf2/NLRP3 Connection in Mouse Heart Mitochondria during Aging

Marisol Fernández-Ortiz [1][iD], Ramy K. A. Sayed [1,2][iD], José Fernández-Martínez [1],
Antonia Cionfrini [1], Paula Aranda-Martínez [1], Germaine Escames [1,3][iD], Tomás de Haro [4]
and Darío Acuña-Castroviejo [1,3,4,*][iD]

[1] Centro de Investigación Biomédica, Departamento de Fisiología, Facultad de Medicina,
Instituto de Biotecnología, Parque Tecnológico de Ciencias de la Salud, Universidad de Granada,
18016 Granada, Spain; sol92@correo.ugr.es (M.F.-O.); ramy.kamal@vet.sohag.edu.eg (R.K.A.S.);
josefermar@ugr.es (J.F.-M.); acionfrini@correo.ugr.es (A.C.); ampaula@correo.ugr.es (P.A.-M.);
gescames@ugr.es (G.E.)

[2] Department of Anatomy and Embryology, Faculty of Veterinary Medicine, Sohag University,
Sohag 82524, Egypt

[3] CIBERfes, Ibs. Granada, 18016 Granada, Spain

[4] UGC de Laboratorios Clínicos, Hospital Universitario San Cecilio, 18016 Granada, Spain;
tomas.haro.sspa@juntadeandalucia.es

[*] Correspondence: dacuna@ugr.es.

Abstract: Aging is a major risk for cardiovascular diseases (CVD). Age-related disorders include oxidative stress, mitochondria dysfunction, and exacerbation of the NF-κB/NLRP3 innate immune response pathways. Some of the molecular mechanisms underlying these processes, however, remain unclear. This study tested the hypothesis that NLRP3 inflammasome plays a role in cardiac aging and melatonin is able to counteract its effects. With the aim of investigating the impact of NLRP3 inflammasome and the actions and target of melatonin in aged myocardium, we analyzed the expression of proteins implied in mitochondria dynamics, autophagy, apoptosis, Nrf2-dependent antioxidant response and mitochondria ultrastructure in heart of wild-type and NLRP3-knockout mice of 3, 12, and 24 months-old, with and without melatonin treatment. Our results showed that the absence of NLRP3 prevented age-related mitochondrial dynamic alterations in cardiac muscle with minimal effects in cardiac autophagy during aging. The deficiency of the inflammasome affected Bax/Bcl2 ratio, but not p53 or caspase 9. The Nrf2-antioxidant pathway was also unaffected by the absence of NLRP3. Furthermore, NLRP3-deficiency prevented the drop in autophagy and mice showed less mitochondrial damage than wild-type animals. Interestingly, melatonin treatment recovered mitochondrial dynamics altered by aging and had few effects on cardiac autophagy. Melatonin supplementation also had an anti-apoptotic action in addition to restoring Nrf2-antioxidant capacity and improving mitochondria ultrastructure altered by aging.

Keywords: melatonin; mitochondria; NLRP3 inflammasome; Nrf2; heart ultrastructure; apoptosis; mitochondrial dynamics

1. Introduction

Cardiovascular diseases (CVD) constitute the leading cause of death in the world, especially in industrialized countries [1]. Genetics, hypertension, diabetes, obesity, smoking, and physical inactivity have been identified as risk factors for these diseases [2]. However, aging is by far the major risk factor for cardiac dysfunction, since its prevalence increases dramatically in aged people.

The connection between aging and these cardiac pathologies have been widely reported [3–5]. Cardiac aging correlates with hemodynamic and metabolic alterations together, with changes in the structure and function of cardiovascular tissues. Furthermore, the increase in reactive oxygen species (ROS) and the activation of inflammation-related pathways have also been documented [6–8]. Aging is characterized by an increase in oxidative damage and persistent activation of innate immunity resulting in immunosenescence. This immune dysregulation results in a state of age-associated chronic inflammation termed 'inflammaging', which plays an important role in the onset and progression of cardiovascular diseases, in addition to other age-related disorders [9–12].

The main components of the innate immunity include NF-kB and NLRP3 inflammasome. Focusing on the NLRP3 inflammasome, it consists of the scaffold protein NLRP3, the adaptor protein ASC and caspase-1, forming a multiprotein complex [13]. The NLRP3 inflammasome is induced upon different signs of cellular 'danger' and is responsible for the maturation of the NF-kB-dependent pro-inflammatory cytokines including interleukin-1β (IL-1β), potentiating the inflammatory response [14]. Some of these danger signals, such as ROS and mitochondrial DNA (mtDNA), come from impaired mitochondria during inflammation [15]. Additionally, age-related alterations in processes that maintain mitochondrial homeostasis, including fusion, fission, autophagy (mitophagy), and mitochondrial biogenesis, have been described. The resulting accumulation of dysfunctional mitochondria enhances ROS production and mtDNA release [16,17]. Another fact that could contribute to NLRP3 inflammasome activation is the reduced endogenous antioxidant defense capacity, which occurs during aging, in particular, the decline of transcription factor Nrf2 [18,19]. Thus, there seems to be a close relationship between aging, NF-kB/NLRP3 inflammasome response, cardiac and mitochondrial dysfunction, ROS formation, and decrease in Nrf2.

Melatonin (N-acetyl-5-methoxytryptamine, aMT) is an ubiquitous molecule that, aside from the pineal gland [20], is synthesized by most body organs and tissues, including the heart [21,22]. In addition to its chronobiotic effects, this indoleamine presents important anti-oxidative and anti-inflammatory properties that depend on the high levels of extrapineal melatonin [23–25]. Within the cell, melatonin acts on its main target, the mitochondria, boosting their bioenergetic properties, enhancing the ATP levels and reducing the formation of free radicals [26–30]. In multiple experimental conditions including acute and chronic inflammation, and aging in mouse heart, melatonin consistently prevented oxidative stress, reduced the innate immunity activation, and boosted cardiac mitochondria function [12,23,25,31].

The mechanisms by which NLRP3 contributes to cardiovascular disorders are still unclear [32]. We hypothesized that NLPR3 inflammasome has a role in aged cardiac muscle and we considered it worthwhile to evaluate its association with molecular mechanisms underlying the development of cardiovascular diseases with age. Moreover, we also hypothesized that melatonin is able to counteract the age-related changes in the myocardium and we investigated where it exerts its action. For this purpose, we assessed age-associated disturbances regarding mitochondrial dynamics (fusion/fission), autophagy (mitophagy), apoptosis, Nrf2-dependent antioxidant response, and mitochondrial ultrastructure in the heart of the wild-type and NLRP3-knockout mice at 3, 12, and 24 months of age, with and without melatonin treatment.

2. Materials and Methods

2.1. Animals and Treatment

Wild-type C57BL/6J and NLRP3-knockout mice NLRP3$^{-/-}$ (B6.129S6-NLRP3tm1Bhk/J) on the wild-type C57BL/6J background (>10 backcrosses) aged 3 weeks were purchased from Charles River (Barcelona, Spain) and The Jackson Laboratory (Bar Harbor, ME, USA), respectively. Mice were housed in the animal facility of the University of Granada under a specific pathogen-free barrier and were kept under controlled temperature (22 °C ± 1 °C). Room illumination was on automated 12 h light/dark cycle (lights on at 08:00 h). Animals had ad libitum access to tap water and pelleted rodent chow.

This study was carried out in accordance with the National Institutes of Health Guide for the Care and Use of Laboratory Animals (National Research Council, National Academy of Sciences, Bethesda, MD, USA), the European Convention for the Protection of Vertebrate Animals used for Experimental and Other Scientific Purposes (CETS #123), and the Spanish law for animal experimentation (R.D. 53/2013). The protocol was approved by the Andalusian's Ethical Committee (05/07/2016/130).

Wild-type (WT) and NLRP3$^{-/-}$ mice were divided into five experimental groups ($n = 7$ animals per group) (Figure 1): (I) young (Y, 3-months old), (II) early-aged (EA, 12-months old), (III) early-aged plus melatonin (EA + aMT), (IV) old-aged (OA, 24-months old), and (V) old-aged plus melatonin (OA + aMT) mice. Melatonin (aMT) was orally administered at 10 mg/kg/day in the chow during the last two months before early and old-aged treated mice were sacrificed (EA + aMT at the age of 10 months and OA + aMT at the age of 22 months). The other groups of animals (Y, EA and OA) were fed with normal chow without melatonin. The melatonin pelleted chow was prepared by the Diet Production Unit facility of the University of Granada. The amount of melatonin in the pellets was calculated according to the average daily food intake, number, weight and age of mice [33]. The use of 10 mg/kg/day was selected on the basis of previous studies that demonstrated the effectiveness of this dose on the aging process [11,34] and mitochondrial function [35,36]. C57/BL6A was reported to be a strain of mice that responds well to melatonin therapy [37,38]. Therefore, we deemed them suitable for the purpose of this study.

Figure 1. Study design summary: experimental groups and melatonin treatment.

Animals were killed by cervical dislocation after ketamine plus xylazine anesthesia, and hearts were collected. The left ventricle was dissected and divided into two parts. One part was washed in saline, and rapidly fixed in 2.5% glutaraldehyde for transmission electron microscopy analysis, while the other part was stored at −80 °C for further western blot analysis.

2.2. Western Blot Analysis

Pure cytosolic subcellular fraction was isolated from heart tissue according to Dimauro et al. [39] with some adjustments described in Rahim et al. [30]. Briefly, heart tissue was homogenized on ice at 800 rpm in 500 μL of STM buffer containing 250 mM sucrose, 50 mM Tris-HCl pH 7.4, 5 mM MgCl$_2$, 0.5 mM DTT, 5% phosphatase inhibitor buffer (125 mM NaF, 250 mM β-glycerophosphate, 250 mM p-nitrophenyl phosphate, and 25 mM NaVO3), and a protease inhibitor cocktail (Cat. 78429, Thermo Fisher Scientific, Waltham, MA, USA) with a Teflon pestle. The homogenate was maintained on ice for 30 min, then centrifuged at 800 g for 15 min at 4 °C. The supernatant was labeled as S0 and used for subsequent isolation of cytosolic fractions. S0 was centrifuged at 800× g for 10 min at 4 °C and the supernatant S1 was centrifuged at 11,000× g for 10 min. The resulting supernatant S2, containing cytosol and microsomal fraction, was precipitated in cold 100% acetone at −20 °C for 1 h followed by centrifugation at 12,000× g for 5 min. The pellet was then resuspended in 300 μL STM buffer and labeled as cytosolic fraction.

Western blot analysis was performed on cytosolic fractions of mice hearts. Denatured protein samples (40 µg/fraction) were separated by sodium dodecyl sulfate polyacrylamide gel electrophoresis (SDS-PAGE) using 12% or 15% acrylamide/bis-acrylamide gels. Proteins were then wet transferred to a polyvinylidene difluoride (PVDF) membrane (Merck Life Science S.L.U., Madrid, Spain). The membrane was blocked in 5% bovine serum albumin (BSA) in PBST (PBS with 0.1% Tween-20) at room temperature and then incubated overnight at 4°C with the primary antibodies (Table S1) diluted in blocking buffer as per manufacturer's specification. Membranes were washed with PBST 3 × 10 min and incubated for 1 h at room temperature with anti-mouse (BD Biosciences Pharmigen, San Jose, CA, USA) or anti-rabbit (Thermo Scientific, Madrid, Spain) IgG-horseradish peroxidase conjugated secondary antibodies diluted according to the manufacturer's instructions. After washing with PBST, immunoreaction was detected using ClarityTM Western ECL Substrate (Bio-Rad, Madrid, Spain) and revealed in Kodak Image Station 4000MM PRO (Carestream Health, Rochester, NY, USA). Bands were analyzed and quantified using Kodak Molecular Imaging Software v. 4.5.1 (Carestream Health, Rochester, NY, USA). GAPDH protein content was used to normalize the cytosolic subcellular fraction. Data obtained from early and old-aged mice were always compared to young mice of the same group. The value of WT Y mice group was defined as 100%. Full images of western blots are available in Figure S1.

2.3. Transmission Electron Microscopy (TEM)

Small pieces from the left ventricle of the heart were rapidly immersed in a 2.5% glutaraldehyde in 0.1M cacodylate buffer (pH 7.4) for fixation, then post-fixed in 0.1 M cacodylate buffer-with 1% osmium tetroxide and 1% potassium ferrocyanide for 1 h. The specimens were then immersed in 0.15% tannic acid for 50 s, incubated in 1% uranyl acetate for 1.5 h, dehydrated in ethanol, and embedded in resin. Ultrathin sections of 65 nm thickness were cut using a Reichert-Jung Ultracut E ultramicrotome. These sections were double stained with uranyl acetate and lead citrate [40], and examined by a Carl Zeiss Leo 906E electron microscope and digital electron micrographs were acquired.

2.4. Morphometric Analyses

Using electron micrographs, mitochondrial number and percentage of the mitochondrial damage (as number of damaged mitochondria/total mitochondrial number 100) were analyzed in areas with a width and height of 5.24 µm and 3.99 µm, respectively. Moreover, some morphometric analyses, including cross-sectional area (CSA) and Feret's diameter of the intermyofibrillar mitochondria of cardiac muscle fibers were performed on images of electron microscopy using Image J processing software.

2.5. Statistical Analyses

Data are expressed as mean ± standard error of the mean (SEM) of $n = 7$ animals per group. All statistical analyses were carried out using GraphPad Prism 6.0 software (GraphPad Software, San Diego, CA, USA). One-way ANOVA with a Tukey's post hoc test was used to compare the differences between experimental groups. The values were found to be significantly different when $p < 0.05$.

3. Results

3.1. NLRP3 Deficiency Prevents, and Melatonin Treatment Restores Cardiac Muscle Mitochondrial Dynamics Altered by Aging

Anomalies in mitochondrial dynamics (fusion/fission) are typical of aged cardiac muscle [16]. Here, we showed that aging induced a decrease in the levels of proteins involved in mitochondrial dynamics, including Mfn2, Opa1, and Drp1, in WT mice, an effect absent in NLRP3$^{-/-}$ mice (Figure 2A–C). Melatonin supplementation counteracted the decline of Mfn2, Opa1, and Drp1 caused by aging in WT mice. Interestingly, no significant effect of melatonin was observed in fusion proteins Mfn2 and Opa1 in NLRP3$^{-/-}$ mice at the age of 12 and 24 months (Figure 2A,B). A slight, but not significant enhancement in fission protein Drp1 was noted in EA and OA NLRP3$^{-/-}$ mice with melatonin supplementation (Figure 2C).

Figure 2. Changes in mitochondrial dynamics (fusion/fission) in WT and NLRP3$^{-/-}$ mice during aging and melatonin treatment. (**A**) Protein levels of Mfn2. (**B**) Protein levels of Opa1. (**C**) Protein levels of Drp1. Experiments were performed in hearts of young (Y), early-aged (EA), early-aged with melatonin (EA + aMT), old-aged (OA), and old-aged with melatonin (OA + aMT) wild type and NLRP3$^{-/-}$ mice. Data are expressed as means ± SEM ($n = 7$ animals/group). * $p < 0.05$, ** $p < 0.01$ vs. Y; $^{\#}$ $p < 0.05$, $^{\#\#}$ $p < 0.01$ vs. group without melatonin treatment.

3.2. NLRP3 Deficiency and Melatonin Therapy Had Minimal Effects in Autophagy in Cardiac Muscle during Aging

A drop in the autophagic capacity observed in cardiac aging is associated with the accumulation of dysfunctional mitochondria, exaggerated ROS production, and mtDNA release [16,17]. Unsurprisingly, the conversion of LC3I to LC3II, a hallmark of autophagy [41], was significantly reduced in WT mice during aging, as reflected in the decrease in the LC3II/LC3I ratio in WT EA and OA mice (Figure 3). LC3II/LC3I ratio trends to increase in NLRP3$^{-/-}$ EA and OA mice, which may explain the attempt to restore autophagy events. Melatonin administration had minimal effects on the LC3II/LC3I ratio in all cases.

Figure 3. Changes in autophagy in WT and NLRP3$^{-/-}$ mice during aging and melatonin treatment. LC3II/LC3I ratio. Experiments were performed in hearts of young (Y), early-aged (EA), early-aged with melatonin (EA + aMT), old-aged (OA), and old-aged with melatonin (OA + aMT) wild type and NLRP3$^{-/-}$ mice. Data are expressed as means ± SEM ($n = 7$ animals/group). * $p < 0.05$ vs. Y.

3.3. Melatonin Treatment and, to a Lesser Extent NLRP3 Deficiency, Reduced Apoptosis in Cardiac Muscle during Aging

Despite being intensively studied over the past three decades, many of the mechanisms of apoptotic cell death remain unknown. Although the relationship between aging and apoptosis have been a subject of controversy in scientific community, there seems to be consensus that apoptosis plays a significant role in cardiac aging [42]. Here, we showed that aging induced a rise in the levels of some proteins involved in apoptotic processes, including p53 and caspase 9 in both WT and NLRP3$^{-/-}$ mice. Melatonin treatment significantly diminished the levels of p53 and caspase 9 in EA WT mice and in EA and OA mutant mice (Figure 4A,B). The pro-apoptotic protein Bax and the anti-apoptotic Bcl2 were significantly enhanced by aging in WT mice. Mutant mice only showed Bcl2 increased in OA animal's group (Figure 4C,D). We observed a slight rise in Bax/Bcl2 ratio in EA and a significantly increase in WT OA mice (Figure 4E). The absence of NLRP3, however, prevented the apoptotic process associated with aging since Bax/Bcl2 ratio remained at similar levels as that of Y mutant mice. Melatonin supplementation significantly decreased the Bax/Bcl2 ratio in EA and OA WT mice, but had no effect in NLRP3$^{-/-}$ mice.

Figure 4. Changes in apoptosis in WT and NLRP3$^{-/-}$ mice during aging and melatonin treatment. (**A**) Protein levels of p53. (**B**) Protein levels of caspase 9. (**C**) Protein levels of Bax. (**D**) Protein levels of Bcl2. (**E**) Bax/Bcl2 ratio. Experiments were performed in hearts of young (Y), early-aged (EA), early-aged with melatonin (EA + aMT), old-aged (OA), and old-aged with melatonin (OA + aMT) wild type and NLRP3$^{-/-}$ mice. Data are expressed as means ± SEM (n = 7 animals/group). * $p < 0.05$, ** $p < 0.01$ vs. Y; # $p < 0.05$, ## $p < 0.01$ vs. group without melatonin treatment.

3.4. Melatonin Treatment, but not NLRP3 Deficiency, Recovered the Nrf2-Dependent Antioxidant Capacity in Cardiac Muscle Declined by Aging

In recent years, emerging evidence has indicated that aging leads to a gradual reduction of the Nrf2-dependent antioxidant response, which in turn contributes to the accumulation of oxidative stress [18,19]. Our results showed a significant decrease in the protein levels of Nrf2 and its active form pNrf2 (Ser40) in WT and NLRP3$^{-/-}$ mice with age, suggesting that NLRP3 deficiency was unable to ameliorate the age-related decline of Nrf2 and pNrf2 (Ser40) in these animals (Figure 5A,B). Melatonin supplementation markedly recovered the levels of Nrf2 and pNrf2 (Ser40) in both WT and mutant EA and OA mice. Aging and melatonin therapy did not significantly modify the levels of the Nrf2 inhibitor, Keap1, in either mouse strain (Figure 5C). Hmox1, Nqo1, and γGclc, three cytoprotective enzymes transcriptionally regulated by Nrf2, also remarkably decreased in WT OA mice (Figure 5D–F). The levels of Hmox1 and γGclc significantly dropped in NLRP3$^{-/-}$ EA and OA mice (Figure 5D,F). Protein content of Nqo1 enzyme was not modified by aging in mutant animals (Figure 5E). Again, melatonin treatment greatly enhanced the levels of Hmox1, Nqo1, and γGclc in WT and NLRP3$^{-/-}$ mice.

Figure 5. Changes in the Nrf2-dependent antioxidant pathway in WT and NLRP3$^{-/-}$ mice during aging and melatonin treatment. (**A**) Protein levels of Nrf2. (**B**) Protein levels of pNrf2 (Ser40). (**C**) Protein levels of Keap1. (**D**) Protein levels of Hmox1. (**E**) Protein levels of Nqo1. (**F**) Protein levels of γGclc. Experiments were performed in hearts of young (Y), early-aged (EA), early-aged with melatonin (EA + aMT), old-aged (OA), and old-aged with melatonin (OA + aMT) wild type and NLRP3$^{-/-}$ mice. Data are expressed as means ± SEM (n = 7 animals/group). * $p < 0.05$, ** $p < 0.01$, *** $p < 0.001$ vs. Y; # $p < 0.05$, ## $p < 0.01$, ### $p < 0.001$ vs. group without melatonin treatment.

3.5. NLRP3 Deficiency and Melatonin Therapy Improved Mitochondria Ultrastructure Altered by Age in Cardiac Muscle

Transmission electron microscopy of the cardiac muscles of Y WT mice revealed the presence of normally intact and compacted mitochondria with clearly organized cristae distributed in the intermyofibrillar spaces (Figure 6A,B). At the age of 12 months (EA), most of these mitochondria were found normally; however, a few showed cristae damage (Figure 6C,D). These changes were exacerbated and numerous mitochondria were severely damaged, hypertrophied, and vacuolated with completely destroyed cristae in WT OA mice (Figure 6G,H). Melatonin supplementation, however, preserved the normal ultrastructure of the cardiac mitochondria in EA (Figure 6E,F) and OA WT mice (Figure 6I,J), maintaining their healthy and compact appearance.

Cardiac muscle fibers of NLRP3$^{-/-}$ Y mice presented normal highly compacted mitochondria with densely packed cristae (Figure 7A,B). Mitochondrial structure did not change in EA mice, except one that showed damage in peripheral cristae (Figure 7C,D). The mitochondrial damage was less prevalent at 24 months in comparison with WT OA mice. Mitochondria were characterized by their widely-separated and organized cristae, with the presence of small-sized membranous vacuoles of possibly autophagic nature (Figure 7G,H). Melatonin treatment exhibited an obvious protective effect at the age of 12 (Figure 7E,F) and 24 months (Figure 7I,J), where it kept normal mitochondrial architecture with aging, in addition to formation of multivesicular bodies, which reflect the induction of the autophagic processes.

Figure 6. Age-associated ultrastructural changes of mitochondria in cardiac muscle fibers of WT mice and melatonin treatment. (**A,B**) Electron micrographs of cardiac muscle fibers of Y WT mice revealing the presence of normally intact and compacted mitochondria (M) distributed among myofibrils (Mf). (**C,D**) Electron micrographs of cardiac muscle fibers of EA WT mice demonstrating the presence of normal mitochondria (M) with few demonstrating cristae damage (asterisk). (**E,F**) Electron micrographs of cardiac muscle fibers of EA + aMT WT mice showing the protective effect of melatonin supplementation in preserving normal mitochondrial structure (M) with the presence of lipid droplets (L), N; nucleus. (**G,H**) Electron micrographs of cardiac muscle fibers of OA WT mice clarifying the presence of numerous severely damaged hypertrophied vacuolated mitochondria with completely destructed cristae (asterisk). (**I,J**) Electron micrographs of cardiac muscle fibers of OA + aMT WT mice exhibiting the beneficial effect of melatonin supplementation in keeping normal mitochondrial architecture (M). (**A,C,E,G,I**): bar = 2 μm and (**B,D,F,H,J**): bar = 1 μm.

Figure 7. Age-related ultrastructural changes of mitochondria in cardiac muscle fibers of NLRP3$^{-/-}$ mice and melatonin treatment. (**A,B**) Electron micrographs of cardiac muscle fibers of Y NLRP3$^{-/-}$ mice showing the presence of normally highly compacted mitochondria with densely packed cristae (M) distributed among myofibrils (Mf). (**C,D**) Electron micrographs of cardiac muscle fibers of EA NLRP3$^{-/-}$ mice demonstrating intact mitochondria (M) with individual ones depicting damaged peripherally cristae (asterisk). (**E,F**) Electron micrographs of cardiac muscle fibers of EA + aMT NLRP3$^{-/-}$ mice revealing the clearly apparent prophylactic effect of melatonin supplementation in keeping normal mitochondrial architecture (M) with aging. (**G,H**) Electron micrographs of cardiac muscle fibers of OA NLRP3$^{-/-}$ mice indicating less detectable mitochondrial damage compared with WT mice, with the presence of numerous mitochondria showing widely-separated organized cristae (asterisk) and small-sized membranous vacuoles of possibly autophagic nature (V). (**I,J**) Electron micrographs of cardiac muscle fibers of OA + aMT NLRP3$^{-/-}$ mice showing the protective effect of melatonin supplementation in preserving normal mitochondrial structure (M), with formation of multivesicular bodies (MVB), which reflect the induction of the autophagic processes, N; nucleus. (**A,C,E,G,I**): bar = 2 μm and (**B,D,F,H,J**): bar = 1 μm.

3.6. Lack of NLRP3 Reduced Mitochondria Number Loss and Mitochondrial Damage, an Effect Shared by Melatonin

Morphometric analysis of cardiac mitochondria revealed that mitochondrial number exhibited initial non-significant decline in cardiac muscles of WT and NLRP3$^{-/-}$ EA mice. Nevertheless, mitochondrial number was significantly decreased in OA, being more pronounced in WT mice than NLRP3$^{-/-}$ one, an effect significantly counteracted after melatonin therapy (Figure 8A). Furthermore, the percentage of the mitochondrial damage was significantly increased in aged mice, especially in WT animals, and it was counteracted by melatonin supplementation (Figure 8B). Morphometrical analysis of the mitochondrial CSA illustrated a non-significant increase in cardiac muscle of WT and NLRP3$^{-/-}$ EA mice, whereas the former increased in aged animals (Figure 8C). Mitochondrial diameter showed non-significant increase in WT EA mice, increasing in OA animals. NLRP3$^{-/-}$ mice revealed non-significant changes in mitochondrial diameter among all experimental groups (Figure 8D).

Figure 8. Age-associated morphometrical changes of intermyofibrillar mitochondria in cardiac muscle fibers of WT and NLRP3$^{-/-}$ mice and melatonin treatment. (**A**) Analysis of mitochondrial number. (**B**) Analysis of mitochondrial damage percentage. (**C**) Analysis of cross-section area (CSA, μm^2). (**D**) Analysis of mitochondrial Feret's diameter (μm). Data are expressed as means ± SEM ($n = 7$ animals/group). * $p < 0.05$, ** $p < 0.01$, *** $p < 0.001$ vs. Y; # $p < 0.05$, ## $p < 0.01$ vs. group without melatonin treatment.

4. Discussion

Immunosenescence and inflammaging are caused by persistent activation of NF-κB/NLRP3 inflammasome pathways generates chronic low-grade inflammation, which leads to, among other detriments, accumulation of cardiac mitochondrial dysfunction, characterized by dysregulation of mitochondrial dynamics, autophagy, apoptosis, Nrf2 antioxidant pathway, and maintenance of ultrastructure of mitochondria [43]. Another hallmark of aging is a decline in melatonin levels and its protective roles [44]. This brings about increased oxidative damage, chronodisruption, upregulation of pro-inflammatory cytokines, and downregulation of anti-oxidant/-inflammatory processes that contribute to inflammaging by facilitating mitochondrial disruption [45]. The role of the NLRP3 inflammasome and melatonin levels in regulation of mitochondrial dysfunction, associated with cardiac aging, is not fully understood. Our results suggest direct involvement of this inflammasome by marked amelioration of some mitochondrial dysfunctions with NLRP3 ablation both involved with, and independent of, melatonin supplementation in EA and OA mice (Figures 9 and 10).

Figure 9. Proposed mechanism of melatonin in mitochondria of WT mice during cardiac aging. (**A**) Mitochondrial dynamics: aging led to a decline in fusion (Mfn2 and Opa1) and fission proteins (Opa1). Melatonin treatment counteracted this decrease. (**B**) Autophagy (mitophagy): autophagic capacity dropped in aged myocardium. Melatonin therapy had minimal impact on this pathway. (**C**) Intrinsic and (**D**) extrinsic apoptosis: WT mice have intrinsic and extrinsic pathways mediated by p53 and caspase 9. Those apoptotic markers, as well as Bax/Bcl2 ratio, increased with aging and are related with NLRP3 activation. This inflammasome seemed to have a regulatory effect on the intrinsic apoptotic pathway, which depends on mitochondria cytochrome c release. Melatonin supplementation had an anti-apoptotic effect in both intrinsic and extrinsic apoptosis. (**E**) Nrf2-dependent antioxidant response: Nrf2 and pNrf2 (Ser40) were reduced with aging. This loss was linked to the decrease of the cytoprotective enzyme transcriptionally regulated by Nrf2: Hmox1, Nqo1 and γGclc. Melatonin recovered this antioxidant pathway. No changes in Keap1 were reported. Red-purple arrow: impact of aging. Green-blue arrow: effect of melatonin treatment.

Figure 10. Proposed mechanism of melatonin in mitochondria of NLRP3$^{-/-}$ mice during cardiac aging. Lack of NLRP3 inflammasome reduced mitochondria dysfunction. (**A**) Mitochondrial dynamics: the absence of NLRP3 prevented the decline in fusion (Mfn2 and Opa1) and fission proteins (Opa1) with aging. Melatonin treatment had no effect on these mice. (**B**) Autophagy (mitophagy): autophagic capacity was restored by NLRP3 deficiency. Melatonin therapy had minimal impact on autophagic capacity. (**C**) Intrinsic and (**D**) extrinsic apoptosis: loss of NLRP3 had an anti-apoptotic effect in Bax/Blc2 ratio, but not in p53 or caspase 9. The ablation of this inflammasome could trigger extrinsic apoptosis mediated by TNFα binding to death receptor. Melatonin supplementation had an anti-apoptotic effect in p53 and caspase 9. (**E**) Nrf2-dependent antioxidant response: lack of NLRP3 did not recover the decrease of this antioxidant pathway with aging. Only Nqo1 were not diminished in mutant mice. Melatonin improved this antioxidant pathway. No changes in Keap1 were reported. Red-purple arrow: impact of aging. Green-blue arrow: effect of melatonin treatment.

Mitochondria fusion (Mfn2 and Opa1) and fission (Drp1) proteins decrease naturally with aging, as seen in WT mice (Figure 9A). Findings in the literature link declines in regulatory proteins of mitochondrial dynamics and age-related development of cardiovascular disease [46–49]. Cardiomyocytes of Mfn2-deficient mice showed cardiac hypertrophy [50]. Low levels of Opa1 have been reported in failing human heart [51]. Loss of Drp1 in adult mice results in lethal dilated cardiomyopathy [52]. Our study also concluded that the absence of NLRP3 prevented the decrease in fusion and fission processes associated with aging that were observed in WT mice (Figure 10A). This cardioprotective effect observed in NLRP3$^{-/-}$ mice supports the existence of a close relationship between mitochondrial dynamics and inflammaging. Our results are in line with scientific evidence that connects impaired mitochondria dynamics, stimulation of innate immune response and inflammasome activation [53–58]. On the other hand, melatonin's mechanism of action in mitochondria dynamics and aging remains unclear. We indicate herein that melatonin promotes fusion by increasing the expression of the Mfn2 and Opa1 proteins in WT EA and OA mice (Figure 9A).

Most investigations agree that this indolamine stimulates mitochondria fusion, contributing to the survival of cardiomyocytes and reducing mitochondria damage [59–61]. Moreover, numerous studies remark a melatonin-induced reduction of mitochondria fission with stressful stimuli [62–65], showing a protective effect in cardiac function against ischemia/reperfusion injury and post-traumatic cardiac dysfunction in vitro and in vivo models, respectively [66–68]. Conversely, we found that melatonin supplementation increased the levels of the Drp1 protein in EA and OA WT mice. Supporting our results, recent findings showed that increasement in Drp1 levels enhanced regulation of mitochondria homeostasis through mitophagy [69]. Additionally, Drp1 overexpression in flies reversed age-related mitochondria dysfunction and age-onset pathologies [70]. Taken together, our data suggests that melatonin enhances the response of mitochondria dynamics to maintain homeostasis during age-related metabolic stressors like inflammasome activation. It should be noted that melatonin did not trigger significant changes in EA and OA NLRP3$^{-/-}$ mice either (Figure 10A). This effect of melatonin has previously been related to its cytoprotective activity, since its effect will be greater the more cellular damage there is, while in situations of low damage or physiological conditions its response is minimal [71].

The LC3II/LC3I ratio showed a significant decrease in autophagy in EA and OA WT mice compared to Y WT mice (Figure 9B). Numerous findings indicate a loss of autophagy with aging in most organisms and tissues, including the heart [72–76]. Changes in the expression of autophagic proteins such as Atg9, LAMP-1, and LC3II in aged mice and rats resulted in cardiac dysfunction [77–79]. The consequent accumulation of altered organelles, mutated mtDNA, cristae disarray, and ROS, have been shown to propagate different age-related cardiac pathologies [74,75,80–82] and produce risk-associated molecular pattern derived from mitochondria (DAMP) that activate NLRP3 inflammasome [83]. Our results showed that the absence of NLRP3 prevented the drop in LC3II/LC3I ratio in mice during aging (Figure 10B). Ablation of the NLRP3 inflammasome in old NLRP3$^{-/-}$ mice has been reported to improve the quality of autophagy by increasing the levels of ATG12, beclin 1 and LC3II and decreasing p62/SQSTM1 [84]. Several studies have demonstrated the protective influence of melatonin by both increasing and decreasing autophagic capacity, in response to sterile and non-sterile inflammation [85–92]. Interestingly, in our results, it is implied that melatonin had no effect on EA and OA WT mice compared to their corresponding controls (Figure 9B). Similar results were obtained in the brain of SAMP8 mice, where melatonin did not cause changes in autophagy [93]. However, it is noteworthy that melatonin was able to increase autophagy of OA WT mice, thereby restoring levels like Y WT mice, but not in EA mice. This action suggests that melatonin and autophagy operate synergistically to increase cell survival, delay immunosenescence, and decrease oxidative stress. Thus, melatonin could act selectively, increasing autophagy only when antioxidant activity is severely impaired, or when sufficient loss of cellular homeostasis results in abnormal mitochondrial morphology and death receptor pathway activation [94–98]. Melatonin did not cause significant changes in the LC3II/LC3I ratio in NLRP3$^{-/-}$ mice (Figure 10B), possibly due to the protective effect resulting from ablation of the inflammasome.

Apoptotic proteins p53 and caspase 9 were found to be increased in EA and OA vs. Y mice in both WT and NLP3$^{-/-}$ mice (Figure 9C,D and Figure 10C,D). Oxidative stress that occurs during aging has been shown to induce apoptosis, mitochondria dysfunction in cardiomyocytes, and ultimately heart failure [99–102]. The Bax/Bcl2 ratio confirmed the increase in apoptosis with aging in WT mice. Interestingly, no changes were observed between ages in mutant mice. The ablation of NLRP3 had an anti-apoptotic protective effect during cardiac aging in Bax/Bcl2 ratio, but not in p53 or caspase 9. This finding suggests that NLRP3 is a direct regulator of the intrinsic apoptotic pathway in cardiac aging, which is dependent on the balance between Bax and Bcl2 and cytochrome c release (Figure 10C). The absence of this inflammasome could trigger activation of extrinsic apoptosis with ligand-induced activation of several death receptors since the participation of p53 and caspase 9 in this pathway has been reported in various tissues and cell models [103–105]. In support of our hypothesis, recent studies revealed an increase in TNFα in the serum of old NLRP3$^{-/-}$ mice compared to young mice [106].

This cytokine is linked to inflammaging [107] and induces extrinsic apoptotic pathway by binding to the cell death receptor TNFR1. On the other hand, findings have showed that caspase 8, which is key in extrinsic apoptosis, plays a role in NLRP3 inflammasome priming and cytochrome c independent caspase 9 activation [108–110]. Without NLRP3, cardiac aging-induced inflammation is favored and could start with extrinsic TNFα apoptosis pathway preceding activation of caspase 8, which in turn activates caspase 9 (Figure 10D). Further investigations centered on the impact of aging on the heart are required to elucidate the extent of the complex interactions between NLRP3 and apoptosis. In most cases, melatonin counteracted the high levels of p53 and caspase 9 associated with aging in WT and mutant mice and Bax/Bcl2 ratio in WT. This anti-apoptotic effect of melatonin during cardiac aging was evident in both extrinsic and intrinsic pathways (Figure 9C,D and Figure 10C,D) and can be explained due to its ability to restore the redox potential of the mitochondria membrane and reduce oxidative stress. These actions increase ATP production and decrease mitochondrial outer membrane permeabilization (MOMP) following release of cytochrome c [111].

Mitochondrial theory of aging [112,113] postulates that an alteration in the redox state of the mitochondria, the main source of free radicals in the cell, causes oxidative damage that results in senescence, the primary driver of the aging process. In this sense, Nrf2 is defined as a 'guardian of health span' and a 'master regulator of aging' giving it enormous importance in the control of numerous antioxidant enzymes [114,115]. It is well stablished that Nrf2 improves mitochondria function by balancing reduction and oxidation processes and influencing ATP production, membrane potential, fatty acid oxidation, and structural integrity [116]. However, changes in the levels of this protein during aging, as well as the antioxidant enzymes it regulates, have been the subject of debate in recent years. Controversial and even opposite results appear in many studies, which seem to depend on the species, strain, tissue, sex and experimental design. Our results in cardiac muscle indicate that cytosolic levels of Nrf2 and pNrf2 (Ser40) decrease with aging, both in WT and in NLRP3$^{-/-}$ mice at EA and OA (Figures 9E and 10E). This may suggest translocation to the nucleus to activate transcription, to mediate age-related increases in ROS, decreasing cytosolic levels. The presence of pNrf2 in the cytosol could also be due to phosphorylation of Nrf2 by GSK-3β which translocates pNrf2 out of the nucleus [117]. Our data agree with investigations showing that mice deficient in Nrf2 have a higher susceptibility to inflammation and oxidative stress [118]. This alteration in the Nrf2 pathway is associated with cardiovascular diseases [119,120]. Nrf2$^{-/-}$ mice were more prone to heart failure and their mortality increased ten days after suffering a myocardial infarction [121,122]. Although most studies point to a decrease in Nrf2 in heart tissue with aging, the causes are unknown. Surprisingly, our results discarded Keap1 as the responsible of this declining since there were no changes in its levels between the different ages and experimental groups. In line with our findings, levels of Nrf2 and its mRNA were found to be reduced in the liver of 10-month-old SAMP8 mice compared to SAMR1 mice, while Keap1 mRNA and its protein levels remained unchanged with age [117]. The decrease in the antioxidant enzymes Hmox1, Nqo1, and γGclc during aging is possibly due to a less efficient Nrf2 signaling [123,124]. Similar results using aortas of 24-month-old rats, whose Nrf2 levels were lower compared to 3-month-old young rats, resulted in a drop in the enzymes Hmox1, Nqo1 and γGclc [125]. However, the same group demonstrated that oxidative stress associated with aging did not induce significant changes in Nrf2 levels of carotid arteries in aged Rhesus macaques (20 years) compared to young individuals (10 years), and their respective antioxidant enzymes were not induced either [126]. Together, these data confirm that the expression of these antioxidant enzymes is linked to Nrf2. It also suggests the activation of this signaling pathway in the cardiovascular system during aging depends not only on the animal model but on the degree of oxidative stress as well. In this light, recent works described that there is a shift in Nrf2 target to Klf9 instead of Hmox1, Nqo1, and γGclc at excessive oxidative damage [127,128]. This could explain the fact that Hmox1 and γGclc were decreased to a greater degree than WT by showing decline in EA while WT decreased only at OA. Interestingly, Nqo1 expression levels were not reduced in NLRP3$^{-/-}$ mice but were still upregulated by melatonin supplementation. Several studies show that Nqo1 is the prototype gene target for Nrf2 activation. In BV2 cells after cerebral ischemia reperfusion, Nrf2 ROS response was linked to Nqo1 expression [129]. This could illuminate the limited decrease in cytosolic Nqo1 by being preferentially targeted by the ever-shrinking pool of Nrf2 and pNrf2 as aging ensues. This study also proved that scavenging of ROS by Nqo1 restrained NLRP3 inflammasome activation and IL-1β expression. Except for Keap1 expression levels, which remained unchanged during aging, treatment with melatonin counteracted the age-associated decline in expression of all the parameters of the Nrf2 signaling pathway, both in WT and NLRP3$^{-/-}$ mice (Figures 9E and 10E). Melatonin has been shown to have a protective effect on the mitochondria by acting as a powerful antioxidant in a direct way, as a scavenger of free radicals, detoxifying reactive oxygen and nitrogen species, and indirectly, increasing the rest of the Nrf2-dependent and independent antioxidant systems [130–133].

Studies in animal models confirm that the ultrastructure of cardiac mitochondria changes with aging [134]. Our study supported these results. A small number of isolated mitochondria had damaged cristae in EA mice, and severe mitochondrial damage, with destroyed, separated, vacuolated and hypertrophied cristae in OA mice. This mitochondrial impairment was more remarkable in WT mice than in mutants. These findings reveal age-induced cellular senescence and mitochondrial dysfunction [135], as well as the cardioprotective effect linked to the ablation of the NLRP3 inflammasome [32]. Melatonin treatment maintained normal mitochondrial ultrastructure in all experimental groups. Multivesicular bodies increased in treated OA NLRP3$^{-/-}$ mice, which indicate autophagy induction. These results, once again, highlight the protective role of melatonin against age-mediated mitochondria impairment and its ability to restore altered autophagic processes during cardiac aging [34].

Various morphometric analyses show that the size and number of mitochondria per cell is impacted during cardiac aging [136]. Our results showed an increase in CSA and Feret's diameter in the mitochondria of OA WT mice, accompanied by a decrease in number of mitochondria. This mitochondrial hypertrophy has been related to a systemic demand from overload stress on the heart [137,138], and our results suggest that it could also be an adaptive mechanism to compensate for the decrease in the amount of this organelle. The ablation of the NLRP3 inflammasome reduced cardiac hypertrophy, as there were no changes in Feret's diameter with age and less significant increase in CSA and decline in mitochondria number. To our knowledge, this is the first time that these morphometrical parameters are studied specifically in IMF during cardiac aging using a mice model. In line with our findings, CSA of cardiomyocytes from the left ventricle of male Fischer 344 rats increased with aging, while the number of cardiomyocytes decreased [139]. In Wistar rats, mitochondria volume fraction and mean size both in left and right ventricle were decreased in 2 years old vs. 6 weeks old animals [140]. Our results showed that melatonin significantly increased the number of mitochondria in WT and NLRP3$^{-/-}$ mice, with no effect on CSA or Feret's diameter. It is possible that in this case, two-month treatment is not enough to counter the age-related changes in CSA and Feret's diameter in the heart, one of the most energy-demanding organs of our body [141]. This 'cardiac sarcopenia' has hardly been investigated since most studies focus on skeletal muscle. Indeed, our group previously performed the same analyses in gastrocnemius and morphometric alterations were observed earlier, in EA mice and protected in NLRP3 deficient mice [142]. Our findings suggest that cardiac muscle and its mitochondria are physiologically more protected from age-related sarcopenia than skeletal muscle. Its ability to make a metabolic switch in favor of glycolysis instead of fatty acid oxidation during aging [143,144], being one of the organs where the NLRP3 inflammasome is expressed less [145,146], or the presence of resident macrophages with tissue protective function [147] are some of the many possible adaptations of the heart that could explain its greater resistance to sarcopenia.

5. Conclusions

The results of this study clarify the impact of NLRP3 inflammasome and melatonin treatment in the mitochondria during cardiac aging. The main findings can be summarized as (1) NLRP3 knocking out and melatonin supplementation avoided mitochondrial dynamics changes of heart with aging; (2) loss of NLRP3 and melatonin treatment revealed few impacts on cardiac autophagy during aging; (3) NLRP3 absence had a less role on cardiac apoptosis during aging compared to melatonin therapy; (4) melatonin restored aged-related Nrf2-dependent antioxidant capacity while NLRP3 inflammasome showed no effect on this pathway; (5) lack of NLRP3 as well as melatonin treatment enhanced mitochondria ultrastructure alterations in aged myocardium.

Author Contributions: Conceptualization, D.A.-C.; methodology, M.F.-O., R.K.A.S., and A.C.; formal analysis, J.F.-M.; data curation, P.A.-M.; writing—original draft preparation, M.F.O. and G.E.; writing—review and editing, D.A.-C.; project administration, T.d.H.; funding acquisition, D.A.-C. All authors have read and agreed to the published version of the manuscript.

Acknowledgments: We are thankful to members of the Electron Microscopy Unit (Assiut University, Egypt) for their technical support with transmission electron microscopy.

References

1. Chiao, Y.A.; Rabinovitch, P.S. The Aging Heart. *Cold Spring Harb. Perspect. Med.* **2015**, *5*, a025148. [CrossRef]
2. Gómez-Pardo, E.; Fernández-Alvira, J.M.; Vilanova, M.; Haro, D.; Martínez, R.; Carvajal, I.; Carral, V.; Rodríguez, C.; de Miguel, M.; Bodega, P.; et al. A Comprehensive Lifestyle Peer Group-Based Intervention on Cardiovascular Risk Factors: The Randomized Controlled Fifty-Fifty Program. *J. Am. Coll. Cardiol.* **2016**, *67*, 476–485. [CrossRef] [PubMed]
3. Li, S.-Y.; Du, M.; Dolence, E.K.; Fang, C.X.; Mayer, G.E.; Ceylan-Isik, A.F.; LaCour, K.H.; Yang, X.; Wilbert, C.J.; Sreejayan, N.; et al. Aging induces cardiac diastolic dysfunction, oxidative stress, accumulation of advanced glycation endproducts and protein modification. *Aging Cell* **2005**, *4*, 57–64. [CrossRef] [PubMed]
4. Go, A.S.; Mozaffarian, D.; Roger, V.L.; Benjamin, E.J.; Berry, J.D.; Blaha, M.J.; Dai, S.; Ford, E.S.; Fox, C.S.; Franco, S.; et al. Heart disease and stroke statistics—2014 update: A report from the American Heart Association. *Circulation* **2014**, *129*, e28–e292. [CrossRef] [PubMed]
5. Lakatta, E.G. Cardiovascular ageing in health sets the stage for cardiovascular disease. *Heart Lung Circ.* **2002**, *11*, 76–91. [CrossRef]
6. Forman, K.; Vara, E.; García, C.; Kireev, R.; Cuesta, S.; Acuña-Castroviejo, D.; Tresguerres, J.A.F. Influence of aging and growth hormone on different members of the NFkB family and IkB expression in the heart from a murine model of senescence-accelerated aging. *Exp. Gerontol.* **2016**, *73*, 114–120. [CrossRef]
7. Csiszar, A.; Wang, M.; Lakatta, E.G.; Ungvari, Z. Inflammation and endothelial dysfunction during aging: Role of NF-kappaB. *J. Appl. Physiol.* **2008**, *105*, 1333–1341. [CrossRef]
8. Shi, Y.; Camici, G.G.; Lüscher, T.F. Cardiovascular determinants of life span. *Pflugers Arch.* **2010**, *459*, 315–324. [CrossRef]
9. Ferrucci, L.; Fabbri, E. Inflammageing: Chronic inflammation in ageing, cardiovascular disease, and frailty. *Nat. Rev. Cardiol.* **2018**, *15*, 505–522. [CrossRef]
10. Franceschi, C.; Campisi, J. Chronic inflammation (inflammaging) and its potential contribution to age-associated diseases. *J. Gerontol. Ser. A Biol. Sci. Med. Sci.* **2014**, *69* (Suppl. 1), S4–S9. [CrossRef]
11. Rodríguez, M.I.; Carretero, M.; Escames, G.; López, L.C.; Maldonado, M.D.; Tan, D.-X.; Reiter, R.J.; Acuña-Castroviejo, D. Chronic melatonin treatment prevents age-dependent cardiac mitochondrial dysfunction in senescence-accelerated mice. *Free Radic. Res.* **2007**, *41*, 15–24. [CrossRef] [PubMed]
12. Rodriguez, M.I.; Escames, G.; López, L.C.; García, J.A.; Ortiz, F.; López, A.; Acuña-Castroviejo, D. Melatonin administration prevents cardiac and diaphragmatic mitochondrial oxidative damage in senescence-accelerated mice. *J. Endocrinol.* **2007**, *194*, 637–643. [CrossRef] [PubMed]
13. Schroder, K.; Tschopp, J. The inflammasomes. *Cell* **2010**, *140*, 821–832. [CrossRef] [PubMed]
14. Zhou, R.; Tardivel, A.; Thorens, B.; Choi, I.; Tschopp, J. Thioredoxin-interacting protein links oxidative stress to inflammasome activation. *Nat. Immunol.* **2010**, *11*, 136–140. [CrossRef]
15. Escames, G.; López, L.C.; García, J.A.; García-Corzo, L.; Ortiz, F.; Acuña-Castroviejo, D. Mitochondrial DNA and inflammatory diseases. *Hum. Genet.* **2012**, *131*, 161–173. [CrossRef] [PubMed]
16. Wu, N.N.; Zhang, Y.; Ren, J. Mitophagy, Mitochondrial Dynamics, and Homeostasis in Cardiovascular Aging. *Oxid. Med. Cell. Longev.* **2019**, *2019*, 9825061. [CrossRef]
17. Zhou, R.; Yazdi, A.S.; Menu, P.; Tschopp, J. A role for mitochondria in NLRP3 inflammasome activation. *Nature* **2011**, *469*, 221–225. [CrossRef]

18. Schmidlin, C.J.; Dodson, M.B.; Madhavan, L.; Zhang, D.D. Redox regulation by NRF2 in aging and disease. *Free Radic. Biol. Med.* **2019**, *134*, 702–707. [CrossRef]

19. Zhang, H.; Davies, K.J.A.; Forman, H.J. Oxidative stress response and Nrf2 signaling in aging. *Free Radic. Biol. Med.* **2015**, *88*, 314–336. [CrossRef]

20. Reiter, R.J. Melatonin: The chemical expression of darkness. *Mol. Cell. Endocrinol.* **1991**, *79*, C153–C158. [CrossRef]

21. Acuña-Castroviejo, D.; Escames, G.; Venegas, C.; Díaz-Casado, M.E.; Lima-Cabello, E.; López, L.C.; Rosales-Corral, S.; Tan, D.-X.; Reiter, R.J. Extrapineal melatonin: Sources, regulation, and potential functions. *Cell. Mol. Life Sci.* **2014**, *71*, 2997–3025. [CrossRef]

22. Acuña-Castroviejo, D.; Noguiera-Navarro, M.T.; Reiter, R.J.; Escames, G. Melatonin actions in the heart; more than a hormone. *Melatonin Res.* **2018**, *1*, 21–26. [CrossRef]

23. García, J.A.; Volt, H.; Venegas, C.; Doerrier, C.; Escames, G.; López, L.C.; Acuña-Castroviejo, D. Disruption of the NF-κB/NLRP3 connection by melatonin requires retinoid-related orphan receptor-α and blocks the septic response in mice. *FASEB J. Off. Publ. Fed. Am. Soc. Exp. Biol.* **2015**, *29*, 3863–3875. [CrossRef] [PubMed]

24. Reiter, R.J.; Mayo, J.C.; Tan, D.-X.; Sainz, R.M.; Alatorre-Jimenez, M.; Qin, L. Melatonin as an antioxidant: Under promises but over delivers. *J. Pineal Res.* **2016**, *61*, 253–278. [CrossRef] [PubMed]

25. Volt, H.; García, J.A.; Doerrier, C.; Díaz-Casado, M.E.; Guerra-Librero, A.; López, L.C.; Escames, G.; Tresguerres, J.A.; Acuña-Castroviejo, D. Same molecule but different expression: Aging and sepsis trigger NLRP3 inflammasome activation, a target of melatonin. *J. Pineal Res.* **2016**, *60*, 193–205. [CrossRef] [PubMed]

26. Escames, G.; León, J.; Macías, M.; Khaldy, H.; Acuña-Castroviejo, D. Melatonin counteracts lipopolysaccharide-induced expression and activity of mitochondrial nitric oxide synthase in rats. *FASEB J. Off. Publ. Fed. Am. Soc. Exp. Biol.* **2003**, *17*, 932–934. [CrossRef]

27. López, A.; García, J.A.; Escames, G.; Venegas, C.; Ortiz, F.; López, L.C.; Acuña-Castroviejo, D. Melatonin protects the mitochondria from oxidative damage reducing oxygen consumption, membrane potential, and superoxide anion production. *J. Pineal Res.* **2009**, *46*, 188–198. [CrossRef]

28. Martín, M.; Macías, M.; Escames, G.; León, J.; Acuña-Castroviejo, D. Melatonin but not vitamins C and E maintains glutathione homeostasis in t-butyl hydroperoxide-induced mitochondrial oxidative stress. *FASEB J. Off. Publ. Fed. Am. Soc. Exp. Biol.* **2000**, *14*, 1677–1679. [CrossRef]

29. Martín, M.; Macías, M.; León, J.; Escames, G.; Khaldy, H.; Acuña-Castroviejo, D. Melatonin increases the activity of the oxidative phosphorylation enzymes and the production of ATP in rat brain and liver mitochondria. *Int. J. Biochem. Cell Biol.* **2002**, *34*, 348–357. [CrossRef]

30. Rahim, I.; Djerdjouri, B.; Sayed, R.K.; Fernández-Ortiz, M.; Fernández-Gil, B.; Hidalgo-Gutiérrez, A.; López, L.C.; Escames, G.; Reiter, R.J.; Acuña-Castroviejo, D. Melatonin administration to wild-type mice and nontreated NLRP3 mutant mice share similar inhibition of the inflammatory response during sepsis. *J. Pineal Res.* **2017**, *63*. [CrossRef]

31. Forman, K.; Vara, E.; García, C.; Kireev, R.; Cuesta, S.; Acuña-Castroviejo, D.; Tresguerres, J.A.F. Beneficial effects of melatonin on cardiological alterations in a murine model of accelerated aging. *J. Pineal Res.* **2010**, *49*, 312–320. [CrossRef] [PubMed]

32. Wang, Z.; Hu, W.; Lu, C.; Ma, Z.; Jiang, S.; Gu, C.; Acuña-Castroviejo, D.; Yang, Y. Targeting NLRP3 (Nucleotide-Binding Domain, Leucine-Rich-Containing Family, Pyrin Domain-Containing-3) Inflammasome in Cardiovascular Disorders. *Arterioscler. Thromb. Vasc. Biol.* **2018**, *38*, 2765–2779. [CrossRef] [PubMed]

33. Bachmanov, A.A.; Reed, D.R.; Beauchamp, G.K.; Tordoff, M.G. Food intake, water intake, and drinking spout side preference of 28 mouse strains. *Behav. Genet.* **2002**, *32*, 435–443. [CrossRef] [PubMed]

34. Rodríguez, M.I.; Escames, G.; López, L.C.; López, A.; García, J.A.; Ortiz, F.; Sánchez, V.; Romeu, M.; Acuña-Castroviejo, D. Improved mitochondrial function and increased life span after chronic melatonin treatment in senescent prone mice. *Exp. Gerontol.* **2008**, *43*, 749–756. [CrossRef]

35. Carretero, M.; Escames, G.; López, L.C.; Venegas, C.; Dayoub, J.C.; García, L.; Acuña-Castroviejo, D. Long-term melatonin administration protects brain mitochondria from aging. *J. Pineal Res.* **2009**, *47*, 192–200. [CrossRef]

36. Martín, M.; Macías, M.; Escames, G.; Reiter, R.J.; Agapito, M.T.; Ortiz, G.G.; Acuña-Castroviejo, D. Melatonin-induced increased activity of the respiratory chain complexes I and IV can prevent mitochondrial damage induced by ruthenium red in vivo. *J. Pineal Res.* **2000**, *28*, 242–248. [CrossRef]

37. Khaldy, H.; León, J.; Escames, G.; Bikjdaouene, L.; García, J.J.; Acuña-Castroviejo, D. Circadian rhythms of dopamine and dihydroxyphenyl acetic acid in the mouse striatum: Effects of pinealectomy and of melatonin treatment. *Neuroendocrinology* **2002**, *75*, 201–208. [CrossRef]

38. López, A.; Ortiz, F.; Doerrier, C.; Venegas, C.; Fernández-Ortiz, M.; Aranda, P.; Díaz-Casado, M.E.; Fernández-Gil, B.; Barriocanal-Casado, E.; Escames, G.; et al. Mitochondrial impairment and melatonin protection in parkinsonian mice do not depend of inducible or neuronal nitric oxide synthases. *PLoS ONE* **2017**, *12*, e0183090. [CrossRef]

39. Dimauro, I.; Pearson, T.; Caporossi, D.; Jackson, M.J. A simple protocol for the subcellular fractionation of skeletal muscle cells and tissue. *BMC Res. Notes* **2012**, *5*, 513. [CrossRef]

40. Reynolds, E.S. The use of lead citrate at high pH as an electron-opaque stain in electron microscopy. *J. Cell Biol.* **1963**, *17*, 208–212. [CrossRef]

41. Lee, J.; Giordano, S.; Zhang, J. Autophagy, mitochondria and oxidative stress: Cross-talk and redox signalling. *Biochem. J.* **2012**, *441*, 523–540. [CrossRef] [PubMed]

42. Quarles, E.K.; Dai, D.-F.; Tocchi, A.; Basisty, N.; Gitari, L.; Rabinovitch, P.S. Quality control systems in cardiac aging. *Ageing Res. Rev.* **2015**, *23*, 101–115. [CrossRef] [PubMed]

43. Franceschi, C.; Bonafè, M.; Valensin, S.; Olivieri, F.; De Luca, M.; Ottaviani, E.; De Benedictis, G. Inflamm-aging. An evolutionary perspective on immunosenescence. *Ann. N. Y. Acad. Sci.* **2000**, *908*, 244–254. [CrossRef] [PubMed]

44. Reiter, R.J.; Guerrero, J.M.; Garcia, J.J.; Acuña-Castroviejo, D. Reactive oxygen intermediates, molecular damage, and aging. Relation to melatonin. *Ann. N. Y. Acad. Sci.* **1998**, *854*, 410–424. [CrossRef]

45. Hardeland, R. Aging, Melatonin, and the Pro- and Anti-Inflammatory Networks. *Int. J. Mol. Sci.* **2019**, *20*, 1223. [CrossRef] [PubMed]

46. Ahuja, P.; Wanagat, J.; Wang, Z.; Wang, Y.; Liem, D.A.; Ping, P.; Antoshechkin, I.A.; Margulies, K.B.; Maclellan, W.R. Divergent mitochondrial biogenesis responses in human cardiomyopathy. *Circulation* **2013**, *127*, 1957–1967. [CrossRef] [PubMed]

47. Zhao, L.; Zou, X.; Feng, Z.; Luo, C.; Liu, J.; Li, H.; Chang, L.; Wang, H.; Li, Y.; Long, J.; et al. Evidence for association of mitochondrial metabolism alteration with lipid accumulation in aging rats. *Exp. Gerontol.* **2014**, *56*, 3–12. [CrossRef]

48. Rosca, M.G.; Hoppel, C.L. Mitochondria in heart failure. *Cardiovasc. Res.* **2010**, *88*, 40–50. [CrossRef]

49. Stotland, A.; Gottlieb, R.A. α-MHC MitoTimer mouse: In vivo mitochondrial turnover model reveals remarkable mitochondrial heterogeneity in the heart. *J. Mol. Cell. Cardiol.* **2016**, *90*, 53–58. [CrossRef]

50. Papanicolaou, K.N.; Khairallah, R.J.; Ngoh, G.A.; Chikando, A.; Luptak, I.; O'Shea, K.M.; Riley, D.D.; Lugus, J.J.; Colucci, W.S.; Lederer, W.J.; et al. Mitofusin-2 maintains mitochondrial structure and contributes to stress-induced permeability transition in cardiac myocytes. *Mol. Cell. Biol.* **2011**, *31*, 1309–1328. [CrossRef]

51. Chen, L.; Gong, Q.; Stice, J.P.; Knowlton, A.A. Mitochondrial OPA1, apoptosis, and heart failure. *Cardiovasc. Res.* **2009**, *84*, 91–99. [CrossRef] [PubMed]

52. Song, M.; Mihara, K.; Chen, Y.; Scorrano, L.; Dorn, G.W. Mitochondrial Fission and Fusion Factors Reciprocally Orchestrate Mitophagic Culling in Mouse Hearts and Cultured Fibroblasts. *Cell Metab.* **2015**, *21*, 273–286. [CrossRef] [PubMed]

53. Yasukawa, K.; Oshiumi, H.; Takeda, M.; Ishihara, N.; Yanagi, Y.; Seya, T.; Kawabata, S.; Koshiba, T. Mitofusin 2 inhibits mitochondrial antiviral signaling. *Sci. Signal.* **2009**, *2*, ra47. [CrossRef] [PubMed]

54. Ichinohe, T.; Yamazaki, T.; Koshiba, T.; Yanagi, Y. Mitochondrial protein mitofusin 2 is required for NLRP3 inflammasome activation after RNA virus infection. *Proc. Natl. Acad. Sci. USA* **2013**, *110*, 17963–17968. [CrossRef] [PubMed]

55. Wang, X.; Jiang, W.; Yan, Y.; Gong, T.; Han, J.; Tian, Z.; Zhou, R. RNA viruses promote activation of the NLRP3 inflammasome through a RIP1-RIP3-DRP1 signaling pathway. *Nat. Immunol.* **2014**, *15*, 1126–1133. [CrossRef]

56. Park, S.; Won, J.-H.; Hwang, I.; Hong, S.; Lee, H.K.; Yu, J.-W. Defective mitochondrial fission augments NLRP3 inflammasome activation. *Sci. Rep.* **2015**, *5*, 15489. [CrossRef]

57. Szabadkai, G.; Simoni, A.M.; Chami, M.; Wieckowski, M.R.; Youle, R.J.; Rizzuto, R. Drp-1-dependent division of the mitochondrial network blocks intraorganellar Ca^{2+} waves and protects against Ca^{2+}-mediated apoptosis. *Mol. Cell* **2004**, *16*, 59–68. [CrossRef]

58. Horng, T. Calcium signaling and mitochondrial destabilization in the triggering of the NLRP3 inflammasome. *Trends Immunol.* **2014**, *35*, 253–261. [CrossRef]
59. Ma, S.; Dong, Z. Melatonin Attenuates Cardiac Reperfusion Stress by Improving OPA1-Related Mitochondrial Fusion in a Yap-Hippo Pathway-Dependent Manner. *J. Cardiovasc. Pharmacol.* **2019**, *73*, 27–39. [CrossRef]
60. Pei, H.; Du, J.; Song, X.; He, L.; Zhang, Y.; Li, X.; Qiu, C.; Zhang, Y.; Hou, J.; Feng, J.; et al. Melatonin prevents adverse myocardial infarction remodeling via Notch1/Mfn2 pathway. *Free Radic. Biol. Med.* **2016**, *97*, 408–417. [CrossRef]
61. Suwanjang, W.; Abramov, A.Y.; Charngkaew, K.; Govitrapong, P.; Chetsawang, B. Melatonin prevents cytosolic calcium overload, mitochondrial damage and cell death due to toxically high doses of dexamethasone-induced oxidative stress in human neuroblastoma SH-SY5Y cells. *Neurochem. Int.* **2016**, *97*, 34–41. [CrossRef] [PubMed]
62. Chuang, J.-I.; Pan, I.-L.; Hsieh, C.-Y.; Huang, C.-Y.; Chen, P.-C.; Shin, J.W. Melatonin prevents the dynamin-related protein 1-dependent mitochondrial fission and oxidative insult in the cortical neurons after 1-methyl-4-phenylpyridinium treatment. *J. Pineal Res.* **2016**, *61*, 230–240. [CrossRef] [PubMed]
63. Xu, S.; Pi, H.; Zhang, L.; Zhang, N.; Li, Y.; Zhang, H.; Tang, J.; Li, H.; Feng, M.; Deng, P.; et al. Melatonin prevents abnormal mitochondrial dynamics resulting from the neurotoxicity of cadmium by blocking calcium-dependent translocation of Drp1 to the mitochondria. *J. Pineal Res.* **2016**, *60*, 291–302. [CrossRef] [PubMed]
64. Parameyong, A.; Charngkaew, K.; Govitrapong, P.; Chetsawang, B. Melatonin attenuates methamphetamine-induced disturbances in mitochondrial dynamics and degeneration in neuroblastoma SH-SY5Y cells. *J. Pineal Res.* **2013**, *55*, 313–323. [CrossRef] [PubMed]
65. Parameyong, A.; Govitrapong, P.; Chetsawang, B. Melatonin attenuates the mitochondrial translocation of mitochondrial fission proteins and Bax, cytosolic calcium overload and cell death in methamphetamine-induced toxicity in neuroblastoma SH-SY5Y cells. *Mitochondrion* **2015**, *24*, 1–8. [CrossRef]
66. Ding, M.; Feng, N.; Tang, D.; Feng, J.; Li, Z.; Jia, M.; Liu, Z.; Gu, X.; Wang, Y.; Fu, F.; et al. Melatonin prevents Drp1-mediated mitochondrial fission in diabetic hearts through SIRT1-PGC1α pathway. *J. Pineal Res.* **2018**, *65*, e12491. [CrossRef]
67. Zhou, H.; Zhang, Y.; Hu, S.; Shi, C.; Zhu, P.; Ma, Q.; Jin, Q.; Cao, F.; Tian, F.; Chen, Y. Melatonin protects cardiac microvasculature against ischemia/reperfusion injury via suppression of mitochondrial fission-VDAC1-HK2-mPTP-mitophagy axis. *J. Pineal Res.* **2017**, *63*, e12413. [CrossRef]
68. Ding, M.; Ning, J.; Feng, N.; Li, Z.; Liu, Z.; Wang, Y.; Wang, Y.; Li, X.; Huo, C.; Jia, X.; et al. Dynamin-related protein 1-mediated mitochondrial fission contributes to post-traumatic cardiac dysfunction in rats and the protective effect of melatonin. *J. Pineal Res.* **2018**, *64*. [CrossRef]
69. Cho, H.M.; Ryu, J.R.; Jo, Y.; Seo, T.W.; Choi, Y.N.; Kim, J.H.; Chung, J.M.; Cho, B.; Kang, H.C.; Yu, S.-W.; et al. Drp1-Zip1 Interaction Regulates Mitochondrial Quality Surveillance System. *Mol. Cell* **2019**, *73*, 364–376.e8. [CrossRef] [PubMed]
70. Rana, A.; Oliveira, M.P.; Khamoui, A.V.; Aparicio, R.; Rera, M.; Rossiter, H.B.; Walker, D.W. Promoting Drp1-mediated mitochondrial fission in midlife prolongs healthy lifespan of Drosophila melanogaster. *Nat. Commun.* **2017**, *8*, 448. [CrossRef] [PubMed]
71. Acuña Castroviejo, D.; López, L.C.; Escames, G.; López, A.; García, J.A.; Reiter, R.J. Melatonin-mitochondria interplay in health and disease. *Curr. Top. Med. Chem.* **2011**, *11*, 221–240. [CrossRef] [PubMed]
72. Rubinsztein, D.C.; Mariño, G.; Kroemer, G. Autophagy and Aging. *Cell* **2011**, *146*, 682–695. [CrossRef] [PubMed]
73. Cuervo, A.M. Autophagy in neurons: It is not all about food. *Trends Mol. Med.* **2006**, *12*, 461–464. [CrossRef] [PubMed]
74. Zhou, J.; Chong, S.Y.; Lim, A.; Singh, B.K.; Sinha, R.A.; Salmon, A.B.; Yen, P.M. Changes in macroautophagy, chaperone-mediated autophagy, and mitochondrial metabolism in murine skeletal and cardiac muscle during aging. *Aging* **2017**, *9*, 583–599. [CrossRef]
75. Shirakabe, A.; Ikeda, Y.; Sciarretta, S.; Zablocki, D.K.; Sadoshima, J. Aging and Autophagy in the Heart. *Circ. Res.* **2016**, *118*, 1563–1576. [CrossRef]
76. Malicdan, M.C.; Noguchi, S.; Nishino, I. Chapter 19 Monitoring Autophagy in Muscle Diseases. *Methods Enzymol.* **2009**, *453*, 379–396. [CrossRef]

77. Taneike, M.; Yamaguchi, O.; Nakai, A.; Hikoso, S.; Takeda, T.; Mizote, I.; Oka, T.; Tamai, T.; Oyabu, J.; Murakawa, T.; et al. Inhibition of autophagy in the heart induces age-related cardiomyopathy. *Autophagy* **2010**, *6*, 600–606. [CrossRef]

78. Wohlgemuth, S.E.; Julian, D.; Akin, D.E.; Fried, J.; Toscano, K.; Leeuwenburgh, C.; Dunn, W.A., Jr. Autophagy in the Heart and Liver During Normal Aging and Calorie Restriction. *Rejuvenation Res.* **2007**, *10*, 281–292. [CrossRef]

79. Hua, Y.; Zhang, Y.; Ceylan-Isik, A.F.; Wold, L.E.; Nunn, J.M.; Ren, J. Chronic akt activation accentuates aging-induced cardiac hypertrophy and myocardial contractile dysfunction: Role of autophagy. *Basic Res. Cardiol.* **2011**, *106*, 1173–1191. [CrossRef]

80. Dai, D.-F.; Chiao, Y.A.; Marcinek, D.J.; Szeto, H.H.; Rabinovitch, P.S. Mitochondrial oxidative stress in aging and healthspan. *Longev. Healthspan* **2014**, *3*, 6. [CrossRef]

81. Boengler, K.; Schulz, R.; Heusch, G. Loss of cardioprotection with ageing. *Cardiovasc. Res.* **2009**, *83*, 247–261. [CrossRef] [PubMed]

82. Li, Y.; Ma, Y.; Song, L.; Yu, L.; Zhang, L.; Zhang, Y.; Xing, Y.; Yin, Y.; Ma, H. SIRT3 deficiency exacerbates p53/Parkin-mediated mitophagy inhibition and promotes mitochondrial dysfunction: Implication for aged hearts. *Int. J. Mol. Med.* **2018**, *41*, 3517–3526. [CrossRef] [PubMed]

83. Salminen, A.; Ojala, J.; Kaarniranta, K.; Kauppinen, A. Mitochondrial dysfunction and oxidative stress activate inflammasomes: Impact on the aging process and age-related diseases. *Cell. Mol. Life Sci.* **2012**, *69*, 2999–3013. [CrossRef]

84. Marín-Aguilar, F.; Lechuga-Vieco, A.V.; Alcocer-Gómez, E.; Castejón-Vega, B.; Lucas, J.; Garrido, C.; Peralta-Garcia, A.; Pérez-Pulido, A.J.; Varela-López, A.; Quiles, J.L.; et al. NLRP3 inflammasome suppression improves longevity and prevents cardiac aging in male mice. *Aging Cell* **2020**, *19*, e13050. [CrossRef]

85. Kang, J.-W.; Hong, J.-M.; Lee, S.-M. Melatonin enhances mitophagy and mitochondrial biogenesis in rats with carbon tetrachloride-induced liver fibrosis. *J. Pineal Res.* **2016**, *60*, 383–393. [CrossRef] [PubMed]

86. Lin, C.; Chao, H.; Li, Z.; Xu, X.; Liu, Y.; Hou, L.; Liu, N.; Ji, J. Melatonin attenuates traumatic brain injury-induced inflammation: A possible role for mitophagy. *J. Pineal Res.* **2016**, *61*, 177–186. [CrossRef] [PubMed]

87. Xie, S.; Deng, Y.; Pan, Y.-Y.; Wang, Z.-H.; Ren, J.; Guo, X.-L.; Yuan, X.; Shang, J.; Liu, H.-G. Melatonin protects against chronic intermittent hypoxia-induced cardiac hypertrophy by modulating autophagy through the 5′ adenosine monophosphate-activated protein kinase pathway. *Biochem. Biophys. Res. Commun.* **2015**, *464*, 975–981. [CrossRef] [PubMed]

88. Prieto-Domínguez, N.; Ordóñez, R.; Fernández, A.; Méndez-Blanco, C.; Baulies, A.; Garcia-Ruiz, C.; Fernández-Checa, J.C.; Mauriz, J.L.; González-Gallego, J. Melatonin-induced increase in sensitivity of human hepatocellular carcinoma cells to sorafenib is associated with reactive oxygen species production and mitophagy. *J. Pineal Res.* **2016**, *61*, 396–407. [CrossRef]

89. de Luxán-Delgado, B.; Potes, Y.; Rubio-González, A.; Caballero, B.; Solano, J.J.; Fernández-Fernández, M.; Bermúdez, M.; Rodrigues Moreira Guimarães, M.; Vega-Naredo, I.; Boga, J.A.; et al. Melatonin reduces endoplasmic reticulum stress and autophagy in liver of leptin-deficient mice. *J. Pineal Res.* **2016**, *61*, 108–123. [CrossRef]

90. San-Miguel, B.; Crespo, I.; Sánchez, D.I.; González-Fernández, B.; Ortiz de Urbina, J.J.; Tuñón, M.J.; González-Gallego, J. Melatonin inhibits autophagy and endoplasmic reticulum stress in mice with carbon tetrachloride-induced fibrosis. *J. Pineal Res.* **2015**, *59*, 151–162. [CrossRef]

91. Su, L.-Y.; Li, H.; Lv, L.; Feng, Y.-M.; Li, G.-D.; Luo, R.; Zhou, H.-J.; Lei, X.-G.; Ma, L.; Li, J.-L.; et al. Melatonin attenuates MPTP-induced neurotoxicity via preventing CDK5-mediated autophagy and SNCA/α-synuclein aggregation. *Autophagy* **2015**, *11*, 1745–1759. [CrossRef] [PubMed]

92. Ma, S.; Chen, J.; Feng, J.; Zhang, R.; Fan, M.; Han, D.; Li, X.; Li, C.; Ren, J.; Wang, Y.; et al. Melatonin Ameliorates the Progression of Atherosclerosis via Mitophagy Activation and NLRP3 Inflammasome Inhibition. *Oxid. Med. Cell. Longev.* **2018**, *2018*, 9286458. [CrossRef] [PubMed]

93. Caballero, B.; Vega-Naredo, I.; Sierra, V.; DeGonzalo-Calvo, D.; Medrano-Campillo, P.; Guerrero, J.M.; Tolivia, D.; Rodríguez-Colunga, M.J.; Coto-Montes, A. Autophagy upregulation and loss of NF-kappaB in oxidative stress-related immunodeficient SAMP8 mice. *Mech. Ageing Dev.* **2009**, *130*, 722–730. [CrossRef] [PubMed]

94. Moore, M.N. Autophagy as a second level protective process in conferring resistance to environmentally-induced oxidative stress. *Autophagy* **2008**, *4*, 254–256. [CrossRef]

95. Houtkooper, R.H.; Mouchiroud, L.; Ryu, D.; Moullan, N.; Katsyuba, E.; Knott, G.; Williams, R.W.; Auwerx, J. Mitonuclear protein imbalance as a conserved longevity mechanism. *Nature* **2013**, *497*, 451–457. [CrossRef]

96. Leduc-Gaudet, J.-P.; Picard, M.; St-Jean Pelletier, F.; Sgarioto, N.; Auger, M.-J.; Vallée, J.; Robitaille, R.; St-Pierre, D.H.; Gouspillou, G. Mitochondrial morphology is altered in atrophied skeletal muscle of aged mice. *Oncotarget* **2015**, *6*, 17923–17937. [CrossRef]

97. Moehle, E.A.; Shen, K.; Dillin, A. Mitochondrial proteostasis in the context of cellular and organismal health and aging. *J. Biol. Chem.* **2019**, *294*, 5396–5407. [CrossRef]

98. Sebastián, D.; Sorianello, E.; Segalés, J.; Irazoki, A.; Ruiz-Bonilla, V.; Sala, D.; Planet, E.; Berenguer-Llergo, A.; Muñoz, J.P.; Sánchez-Feutrie, M.; et al. Mfn2 deficiency links age-related sarcopenia and impaired autophagy to activation of an adaptive mitophagy pathway. *EMBO J.* **2016**, *35*, 1677–1693. [CrossRef]

99. Gustafsson, A.B.; Gottlieb, R.A. Mechanisms of apoptosis in the heart. *J. Clin. Immunol.* **2003**, *23*, 447–459. [CrossRef]

100. Kannan, K.; Jain, S.K. Oxidative stress and apoptosis. *Pathophysiology* **2000**, *7*, 153–163. [CrossRef]

101. Aggarwal, B.B. Apoptosis and nuclear factor-κb: A tale of association and dissociation. *Biochem. Pharmacol.* **2000**, *60*, 1033–1039. [CrossRef]

102. D'Oria, R.; Schipani, R.; Leonardini, A.; Natalicchio, A.; Perrini, S.; Cignarelli, A.; Laviola, L.; Giorgino, F. The Role of Oxidative Stress in Cardiac Disease: From Physiological Response to Injury Factor. *Oxid. Med. Cell. Longev.* **2020**, *2020*, 1–29. [CrossRef] [PubMed]

103. Haupt, S.; Berger, M.; Goldberg, Z.; Haupt, Y. Apoptosis—The p53 network. *J. Cell Sci.* **2003**, *116*, 4077–4085. [CrossRef] [PubMed]

104. McDonnell, M.A.; Wang, D.; Khan, S.M.; Vander Heiden, M.G.; Kelekar, A. Caspase-9 is activated in a cytochrome c-independent manner early during TNFalpha-induced apoptosis in murine cells. *Cell Death Differ.* **2003**, *10*, 1005–1015. [CrossRef] [PubMed]

105. D'Sa-Eipper, C.; Leonard, J.R.; Putcha, G.; Zheng, T.S.; Flavell, R.A.; Rakic, P.; Kuida, K.; Roth, K.A. DNA damage-induced neural precursor cell apoptosis requires p53 and caspase 9 but neither Bax nor caspase 3. *Development* **2001**, *128*, 137–146. [PubMed]

106. Cañadas-Lozano, D.; Marín-Aguilar, F.; Castejón-Vega, B.; Ryffel, B.; Navarro-Pando, J.M.; Ruiz-Cabello, J.; Alcocer-Gómez, E.; Bullón, P.; Cordero, M.D. Blockade of the NLRP3 inflammasome improves metabolic health and lifespan in obese mice. *GeroScience* **2020**, *42*, 715–725. [CrossRef] [PubMed]

107. López-Otín, C.; Galluzzi, L.; Freije, J.M.P.; Madeo, F.; Kroemer, G. Metabolic Control of Longevity. *Cell* **2016**, *166*, 802–821. [CrossRef]

108. Allam, R.; Lawlor, K.E.; Yu, E.C.-W.; Mildenhall, A.L.; Moujalled, D.M.; Lewis, R.S.; Ke, F.; Mason, K.D.; White, M.J.; Stacey, K.J.; et al. Mitochondrial apoptosis is dispensable for NLRP3 inflammasome activation but non-apoptotic caspase-8 is required for inflammasome priming. *EMBO Rep.* **2014**, *15*, 982–990. [CrossRef]

109. McDonnell, M.A.; Abedin, M.J.; Melendez, M.; Platikanova, T.N.; Ecklund, J.R.; Ahmed, K.; Kelekar, A. Phosphorylation of murine caspase-9 by the protein kinase casein kinase 2 regulates its cleavage by caspase-8. *J. Biol. Chem.* **2008**, *283*, 20149–20158. [CrossRef]

110. Vince, J.E.; De Nardo, D.; Gao, W.; Vince, A.J.; Hall, C.; McArthur, K.; Simpson, D.; Vijayaraj, S.; Lindqvist, L.M.; Bouillet, P.; et al. The Mitochondrial Apoptotic Effectors BAX/BAK Activate Caspase-3 and -7 to Trigger NLRP3 Inflammasome and Caspase-8 Driven IL-1β Activation. *Cell Rep.* **2018**, *25*, 2339–2353.e4. [CrossRef]

111. Acuna-Castroviejo, D.; Escames, G.; Rodriguez, M.I.; Lopez, L.C. Melatonin role in the mitochondrial function. *Front. Biosci.* **2007**, *12*, 947–963. [CrossRef] [PubMed]

112. Harman, D. The biologic clock: The mitochondria? *J. Am. Geriatr. Soc.* **1972**, *20*, 145–147. [CrossRef] [PubMed]

113. Miquel, J.; Economos, A.C.; Fleming, J.; Johnson, J.E. Mitochondrial role in cell aging. *Exp. Gerontol.* **1980**, *15*, 575–591. [CrossRef]

114. Lewis, K.N.; Mele, J.; Hayes, J.D.; Buffenstein, R. Nrf2, a guardian of healthspan and gatekeeper of species longevity. *Integr. Comp. Biol.* **2010**, *50*, 829–843. [CrossRef]

115. Bruns, D.R.; Drake, J.C.; Biela, L.M.; Peelor, F.F.; Miller, B.F.; Hamilton, K.L. Nrf2 Signaling and the Slowed Aging Phenotype: Evidence from Long-Lived Models. *Oxid. Med. Cell. Longev.* **2015**, *2015*, 732596. [CrossRef] [PubMed]

116. Dinkova-Kostova, A.T.; Abramov, A.Y. The emerging role of Nrf2 in mitochondrial function. *Free Radic. Biol. Med.* **2015**, *88*, 179–188. [CrossRef] [PubMed]

117. Tomobe, K.; Shinozuka, T.; Kuroiwa, M.; Nomura, Y. Age-related changes of Nrf2 and phosphorylated GSK-3β in a mouse model of accelerated aging (SAMP8). *Arch. Gerontol. Geriatr.* **2012**, *54*, e1–e7. [CrossRef]

118. Ma, Q.; Battelli, L.; Hubbs, A.F. Multiorgan Autoimmune Inflammation, Enhanced Lymphoproliferation, and Impaired Homeostasis of Reactive Oxygen Species in Mice Lacking the Antioxidant-Activated Transcription Factor Nrf2. *Am. J. Pathol.* **2006**, *168*, 1960–1974. [CrossRef]

119. Reuland, D.J.; McCord, J.M.; Hamilton, K.L. The role of Nrf2 in the attenuation of cardiovascular disease. *Exerc. Sport Sci. Rev.* **2013**, *41*, 162–168. [CrossRef]

120. Howden, R. Nrf2 and cardiovascular defense. *Oxid. Med. Cell. Longev.* **2013**, *2013*, 104308. [CrossRef]

121. Xu, B.; Zhang, J.; Strom, J.; Lee, S.; Chen, Q.M. Myocardial ischemic reperfusion induces de novo Nrf2 protein translation. *Biochim. Biophys. Acta BBA Mol. Basis Dis.* **2014**, *1842*, 1638–1647. [CrossRef] [PubMed]

122. Strom, J.; Chen, Q.M. Loss of Nrf2 promotes rapid progression to heart failure following myocardial infarction. *Toxicol. Appl. Pharmacol.* **2017**, *327*, 52–58. [CrossRef] [PubMed]

123. Suh, J.H.; Shenvi, S.V.; Dixon, B.M.; Liu, H.; Jaiswal, A.K.; Liu, R.-M.; Hagen, T.M. Decline in transcriptional activity of Nrf2 causes age-related loss of glutathione synthesis, which is reversible with lipoic acid. *Proc. Natl. Acad. Sci. USA* **2004**, *101*, 3381–3386. [CrossRef]

124. Shih, P.-H.; Yen, G.-C. Differential expressions of antioxidant status in aging rats: The role of transcriptional factor Nrf2 and MAPK signaling pathway. *Biogerontology* **2007**, *8*, 71–80. [CrossRef] [PubMed]

125. Ungvari, Z.; Bailey-Downs, L.; Sosnowska, D.; Gautam, T.; Koncz, P.; Losonczy, G.; Ballabh, P.; de Cabo, R.; Sonntag, W.E.; Csiszar, A. Vascular oxidative stress in aging: A homeostatic failure due to dysregulation of NRF2-mediated antioxidant response. *Am. J. Physiol. Heart Circ. Physiol.* **2011**, *301*, H363–H372. [CrossRef] [PubMed]

126. Ungvari, Z.; Bailey-Downs, L.; Gautam, T.; Sosnowska, D.; Wang, M.; Monticone, R.E.; Telljohann, R.; Pinto, J.T.; de Cabo, R.; Sonntag, W.E.; et al. Age-Associated Vascular Oxidative Stress, Nrf2 Dysfunction, and NF-κB Activation in the Nonhuman Primate Macaca mulatta. *J. Gerontol. Ser. A Biol. Sci. Med. Sci.* **2011**, *66A*, 866–875. [CrossRef]

127. Zucker, S.N.; Fink, E.E.; Bagati, A.; Mannava, S.; Bianchi-Smiraglia, A.; Bogner, P.N.; Wawrzyniak, J.A.; Foley, C.; Leonova, K.I.; Grimm, M.J.; et al. Nrf2 amplifies oxidative stress via induction of Klf9. *Mol. Cell* **2014**, *53*, 916–928. [CrossRef]

128. Chhunchha, B.; Kubo, E.; Singh, D.P. Sulforaphane-Induced Klf9/Prdx6 Axis Acts as a Molecular Switch to Control Redox Signaling and Determines Fate of Cells. *Cells* **2019**, *8*, 1159. [CrossRef]

129. Xu, X.; Zhang, L.; Ye, X.; Hao, Q.; Zhang, T.; Cui, G.; Yu, M. Nrf2/ARE pathway inhibits ROS-induced NLRP3 inflammasome activation in BV2 cells after cerebral ischemia reperfusion. *Inflamm. Res.* **2018**, *67*, 57–65. [CrossRef]

130. Reiter, R.J.; Tan, D.X.; Manchester, L.C.; Qi, W. Biochemical reactivity of melatonin with reactive oxygen and nitrogen species: A review of the evidence. *Cell Biochem. Biophys.* **2001**, *34*, 237–256. [CrossRef]

131. Rodriguez, C.; Mayo, J.C.; Sainz, R.M.; Antolín, I.; Herrera, F.; Martín, V.; Reiter, R.J. Regulation of antioxidant enzymes: A significant role for melatonin. *J. Pineal Res.* **2004**, *36*, 1–9. [CrossRef] [PubMed]

132. Tomás-Zapico, C.; Coto-Montes, A. A proposed mechanism to explain the stimulatory effect of melatonin on antioxidative enzymes. *J. Pineal Res.* **2005**, *39*, 99–104. [CrossRef] [PubMed]

133. Rahim, I.; Sayed, R.K.; Fernández-Ortiz, M.; Aranda-Martínez, P.; Guerra-Librero, A.; Fernández-Martínez, J.; Rusanova, I.; Escames, G.; Djerdjouri, B.; Acuña-Castroviejo, D. Melatonin alleviates sepsis-induced heart injury through activating the Nrf2 pathway and inhibiting the NLRP3 inflammasome. *Naunyn. Schmiedebergs Arch. Pharmacol.* **2020**. [CrossRef] [PubMed]

134. Corsetti, G.; Pasini, E.; D'Antona, G.; Nisoli, E.; Flati, V.; Assanelli, D.; Dioguardi, F.S.; Bianchi, R. Morphometric Changes Induced by Amino Acid Supplementation in Skeletal and Cardiac Muscles of Old Mice. *Am. J. Cardiol.* **2008**, *101*, S26–S34. [CrossRef] [PubMed]

135. Shigenaga, M.K.; Hagen, T.M.; Ames, B.N. Oxidative damage and mitochondrial decay in aging. *Proc. Natl. Acad. Sci. USA* **1994**, *91*, 10771–10778. [CrossRef] [PubMed]

136. El'darov, C.M.; Vays, V.B.; Vangeli, I.M.; Kolosova, N.G.; Bakeeva, L.E. Morphometric examination of mitochondrial ultrastructure in aging cardiomyocytes. *Biochemistry* **2015**, *80*, 604–609. [CrossRef] [PubMed]

137. Hefti, M.A.; Harder, B.A.; Eppenberger, H.M.; Schaub, M.C. Signaling pathways in cardiac myocyte hypertrophy. *J. Mol. Cell. Cardiol.* **1997**, *29*, 2873–2892. [CrossRef]

138. Dobaczewski, M.; Chen, W.; Frangogiannis, N.G. Transforming growth factor (TGF)-β signaling in cardiac remodeling. *J. Mol. Cell. Cardiol.* **2011**, *51*, 600–606. [CrossRef]

139. No, M.-H.; Choi, Y.; Cho, J.; Heo, J.-W.; Cho, E.-J.; Park, D.-H.; Kang, J.-H.; Kim, C.-J.; Seo, D.Y.; Han, J.; et al. Aging Promotes Mitochondria-Mediated Apoptosis in Rat Hearts. *Life* **2020**, *10*, 178. [CrossRef]

140. Frenzei, H.; Feimann, J. Age-dependent structural changes in the myocardium of rats. A quantitative light- and electron-microscopic study on the right and left chamber wall. *Mech. Ageing Dev.* **1984**, *27*, 29–41. [CrossRef]

141. Neubauer, S. The failing heart—An engine out of fuel. *N. Engl. J. Med.* **2007**, *356*, 1140–1151. [CrossRef] [PubMed]

142. Sayed, R.K.A.; Fernández-Ortiz, M.; Diaz-Casado, M.E.; Aranda-Martínez, P.; Fernández-Martínez, J.; Guerra-Librero, A.; Escames, G.; López, L.C.; Alsaadawy, R.M.; Acuña-Castroviejo, D. Lack of NLRP3 Inflammasome Activation Reduces Age-Dependent Sarcopenia and Mitochondrial Dysfunction, Favoring the Prophylactic Effect of Melatonin. *J. Gerontol. A. Biol. Sci. Med. Sci.* **2019**, *74*, 1699–1708. [CrossRef] [PubMed]

143. Kates, A.M.; Herrero, P.; Dence, C.; Soto, P.; Srinivasan, M.; Delano, D.G.; Ehsani, A.; Gropler, R.J. Impact of aging on substrate metabolism by the human heart. *J. Am. Coll. Cardiol.* **2003**, *41*, 293–299. [CrossRef]

144. Hyyti, O.M.; Ledee, D.; Ning, X.-H.; Ge, M.; Portman, M.A. Aging impairs myocardial fatty acid and ketone oxidation and modifies cardiac functional and metabolic responses to insulin in mice. *Am. J. Physiol. Heart Circ. Physiol.* **2010**, *299*, H868–H875. [CrossRef]

145. Ye, J.; Yu, M.; Zhang, K.; Liu, J.; Wang, Q.; Tao, P.; Jia, K.; Liao, M.; Ning, Z. Tissue-specific expression pattern and histological distribution of NLRP3 in Chinese yellow chicken. *Vet. Res. Commun.* **2015**, *39*, 171–177. [CrossRef]

146. Huang, Z.; Yu, M.; Tong, S.; Jia, K.; Liu, R.; Wang, H.; Li, S.; Ning, Z. Tissue-specific expression of the NOD-like receptor protein 3 in BALB/c mice. *J. Vet. Sci.* **2014**, *15*, 173–177. [CrossRef]

147. Pinto, A.R.; Paolicelli, R.; Salimova, E.; Gospocic, J.; Slonimsky, E.; Bilbao-Cortes, D.; Godwin, J.W.; Rosenthal, N.A. An Abundant Tissue Macrophage Population in the Adult Murine Heart with a Distinct Alternatively-Activated Macrophage Profile. *PLoS ONE* **2012**, *7*, e36814. [CrossRef]

Mitochondrial Dysfunction and Diabetes: Is Mitochondrial Transfer a Friend or Foe?

Magdalene K Montgomery

Department of Physiology, School of Biomedical Sciences, University of Melbourne, Melbourne 3010, Australia;
magdalene.montgomery@unimelb.edu.au

Abstract: Obesity, insulin resistance and type 2 diabetes are accompanied by a variety of systemic and tissue-specific metabolic defects, including inflammation, oxidative and endoplasmic reticulum stress, lipotoxicity, and mitochondrial dysfunction. Over the past 30 years, association studies and genetic manipulations, as well as lifestyle and pharmacological invention studies, have reported contrasting findings on the presence or physiological importance of mitochondrial dysfunction in the context of obesity and insulin resistance. It is still unclear if targeting mitochondrial function is a feasible therapeutic approach for the treatment of insulin resistance and glucose homeostasis. Interestingly, recent studies suggest that intact mitochondria, mitochondrial DNA, or other mitochondrial factors (proteins, lipids, miRNA) are found in the circulation, and that metabolic tissues secrete exosomes containing mitochondrial cargo. While this phenomenon has been investigated primarily in the context of cancer and a variety of inflammatory states, little is known about the importance of exosomal mitochondrial transfer in obesity and diabetes. We will discuss recent evidence suggesting that (1) tissues with mitochondrial dysfunction shed their mitochondria within exosomes, and that these exosomes impair the recipient's cell metabolic status, and that on the other hand, (2) physiologically healthy tissues can shed mitochondria to improve the metabolic status of recipient cells. In this context the determination of whether mitochondrial transfer in obesity and diabetes is a friend or foe requires further studies.

Keywords: mitochondrial dysfunction; insulin resistance; type 2 diabetes; mitochondrial transfer; exosomes

---

1. Introduction

The dysregulation of carbohydrate and lipid metabolism due to unbalanced diets (i.e., 'fast food') in western societies has led to a dramatic rise in the worldwide prevalence of obesity, with more than 1.9 billion adults worldwide considered overweight or obese in 2016 [1]. Undoubtedly, this number has increased even further within the last three years. Obesity is one of the most common causes of the development of insulin resistance, type 2 diabetes (T2D), and other related cardio-metabolic risk factors. As outlined by the National Institute for Diabetes and Digestive and Kidney Diseases (NIDDK), T2D is characterized by hyperglycaemia and is predominantly prevalent in middle-aged and older individuals (>45 years of age) [2]. Insulin resistance (i.e., pre-diabetes) and T2D are accompanied by a multitude of systemic and tissue-specific metabolic defects, including inflammation, oxidative and endoplasmic reticulum stress, and lipotoxicity (i.e ectopic lipid accumulation in peripheral tissues), as well as mitochondrial dysfunction [3]. Whether these metabolic aspects are a cause or consequence of insulin resistance remains a matter of debate, with studies pointing towards both scenarios, as reviewed in detail in [4–6]. This review will focus on mitochondrial dysfunction in T2D, with a special focus on the systemic implications of mitochondrial dysfunction occurring in peripheral metabolic tissues. Specifically, we will review evidence suggesting that dysfunctional mitochondria and/or mitochondrial

DNA can be packaged into extracellular vesicles, secreted from the respective tissue and can impact other tissues in a paracrine or endocrine manner.

2. Mitochondrial Function and Dysfunction

Mitochondria have a multitude of roles, with the most prominent one being the generation of ATP for the maintenance of cellular processes. In addition, mitochondria play a role in reactive oxygen species (ROS)-mediated signalling [7–10], apoptosis [11,12], calcium signalling [8,13], and haem [14,15] and steroid synthesis [16], just to name a few. Due to the importance of mitochondria in cellular energy metabolism, defects in the processes mentioned above have significant outcomes on tissue and systemic level. In this respect, the term 'mitochondrial dysfunction' was firstly mentioned in 1975 in the context of glucose intolerance [17]. While the term 'mitochondrial dysfunction' is nowadays commonly used in the scientific literature, the definitions and methods of assessment vary between studies. Mitochondrial dysfunction has been assessed as changes in gene expression of mitochondrial markers [18,19], protein content, or enzymatic activities of mitochondrial proteins [18,20], changes in mitochondrial size and shape [20,21], as well as functional assessment of mitochondrial oxidative capacity [22] and ROS generation [23]. For details on these studies and for mechanistic insights into possible causes of mitochondrial dysfunction, please refer to our recent review on 'mitochondrial dysfunction and insulin resistance' [24].

3. Mitochondrial Dysfunction in Obesity and Type 2 Diabetes

Since the first mention of mitochondrial dysfunction in the context of glucose intolerance in 1975 [17], the importance of mitochondrial function/dysfunction in insulin resistance has been disputed for many years. While some studies in both humans and rodents describe a decrease in mitochondrial function (decreased mitochondrial enzyme activities, decreased lipid metabolism, reduced mitochondrial size and number) in obese and insulin resistant individuals [25,26], others show no correlation [27,28] or even a compensatory increase in mitochondrial capacity with lipid oversupply [29,30], with most studies focusing on skeletal muscle (reviewed in detail in [24]). The discrepancies between studies in both rodents and humans suggest that mitochondrial dysfunction is not a requisite feature of insulin resistance and T2D, and that study outcomes (i.e., if mitochondrial dysfunction is present) are likely dependent on methodological approaches, the model system examined (human or rodent) and the definition of the term mitochondrial dysfunction in the context of each study. In addition, differences in mitochondrial defects between metabolic tissues need to be considered. While skeletal muscle is the most common tissue examined in the context of T2D and mitochondrial function [31], the importance of mitochondrial function in other tissues, such as heart, liver and pancreas, and the impact on systemic homeostasis, should not be underestimated.

4. Tissue-Specific Effects of Mitochondrial Function and T2D

Skeletal muscle is packed with mitochondria, which are required for ATP generation during muscle contraction. With the number of mitochondria in a cell being proportional to the energy demand of the cell, it is not surprising that skeletal muscle and heart are the two tissues with the highest mitochondrial abundance [32]. We have reviewed changes in mitochondrial function in skeletal muscle in the presence of insulin resistance and T2D in detail previously [24], with the major 'conclusion' being that skeletal muscle-related investigations into changes in mitochondrial function in the presence of insulin resistance or T2D have been 'inconclusive' (i.e., decreased, unchanged, or compensatory increased in mitochondrial function in insulin resistance have been suggested). Here we briefly describe changes in mitochondrial function and capacity in the heart, due to the hearts high rate of ATP production and turnover, and its reliance on mitochondrial metabolism to produce energy.

A large number of studies points towards mitochondrial defects being present in the heart in individuals with insulin resistance and diabetes [33–37] as well as in rodent models [38–43]. Markers examined in these studies included mitochondrial oxygen consumption, ROS and ATP generation, changes in mitochondrial size, and structure and calcium handling, as well as mRNA, protein, or enzymatic activity levels of markers of mitochondrial biogenesis, content, and oxidative capacity. Of note, whereas studies in humans are of an associative nature and limit investigations of cause-or-consequence scenarios, a majority of rodent models investigating cardiac function in the presence of diabetes use streptozotocin, a compound that shows high toxicity towards the pancreas and destruction of insulin-producing beta cells, and that is used for the generation of type 1 diabetes phenotypes [44]. The use of dietary interventions that more closely mimic human obesity and insulin resistance, as well as rapid improvements in generation and accessibility to transgenic rodent models are crucial for delineating cause-and-consequence relationships. For example, Turkieh and colleagues showed recently that apolipoprotein O (APOO) is overexpressed in diabetic hearts, and, using transgenic APOO mice, show that APOO links impaired mitochondrial function and the onset of cardiomyopathy [45]. Furthermore, using genetic approaches a recent study showed that myocardial function depends on balanced mitochondrial fusion and fission, and defined a critical regulator of cardiomyocyte survival, the mitochondrial metalloendopeptidase OMA1 [46]. In addition, expression of extracellular signal-regulated protein kinase 5 (Erk5) was shown to be lost in diabetic hearts, and cardiac-specific deletion of Erk5 in mice substantiated mitochondrial abnormalities and decreased fuel oxidation [47]. Lastly, epigenetic regulation of metabolic functions was shown to be important in the preservation of cardiac function. Specifically, an N-terminal proteolytically derived fragment of histone deacetylase 4 (HDAC4) was shown to be decreased in failing mouse hearts and that overexpression of this HDAC4 fragment improved calcium handling and contractile function [48].

While diving into the topic of cardiac dysfunction, I noticed that alterations in mitochondrial energy metabolism are a common feature of various forms of heart disease [49,50]. Most predominantly, diabetic cardiomyopathies (ventricular dysfunction in patients with diabetes mellitus) are associated with dysregulated oxidative substrate selection. In humans and rodents, obesity and insulin resistance are associated with increased myocardial fatty acid uptake and fatty acid oxidation [51,52], with a simultaneous decrease in glucose oxidation [53,54]. As fatty acid oxidation produces less ATP (per mol oxygen consumed), this scenario makes the heart less energy efficient [52]. In addition, increased fatty acid supply to the heart is also associated with oxidative stress [55] and accumulation of bioactive lipid intermediates that directly interfere with insulin signalling [56], and lead to a greater decline in heart function with age [57]. Of interest, therapeutic approaches to increase glucose utilization of the diabetic heart, either actively through activation of pyruvate dehydrogenase [58–60] or passively by inhibiting fatty acid oxidation [61,62], were shown to improve heart function.

5. Can Mitochondrial Dysfunction be Reversed?—Insight into Genetic and Pharmacological Interventions

Targeting mitochondrial oxidative capacity as a means to improve insulin sensitivity is questionable with contradicting findings in various genetic mouse models. For example, inhibition of mitochondrial fatty acid uptake (through inhibition of CPT1) improves insulin sensitivity in muscle of diet-induced obese mice, healthy male subjects and in primary human myotubes [63,64]. In addition, activating heat shock protein 72 (HSP72) in skeletal muscle was found to improve mitochondrial oxidative capacity and insulin sensitivity in the setting of lipotoxicity [65], whereas cardiac-specific overexpression showed no metabolic improvements [66]. Furthermore, increasing the capacity of fatty acid transport protein (FATP) 1 in skeletal muscle resulted in increased channelling of fatty acids into oxidative pathways, however without changes in muscle or systemic insulin sensitivity [67].

Similarly, contradicting findings come from lifestyle or pharmacological intervention studies. The major lifestyle interventions are diet and exercise, with both dietary restriction and physical activity shown to reduce the risk of developing insulin resistance and T2D [68,69], and to improve/restore muscle mitochondrial function [70,71]. While the impact of exercise on mitochondrial biogenesis and oxidative capacity is well accepted (as recently reviewed in [72]), the picture is not that clear in respect to mitochondrial improvements after dietary interventions. In addition to the studies above, other reports suggest that caloric restriction improves insulin sensitivity without changes (or even with decreases) in skeletal muscle mitochondrial oxidative capacity [73,74].

Although exercise and dietary interventions represent a good and some might say 'easy' way to improveinsulin sensitivity, long-term adherence to these lifestyle interventions is problematic and remains a public health challenge. In this respect, finding an ideal pharmacological agent that improves metabolic health, by improving mitochondrial function, has shown some promise in rodent models and in the clinic. One of the most well described modulators of oxidative metabolism are peroxisome proliferator-activated receptors (PPARs). For example, PPAR agonists were shown to increase mitochondrial content and oxidative capacity, in the livers of pre-diabetic mice [75], in adipose tissue [76] and skeletal muscle of insulin resistant and T2D patients [76,77] and mice [78], and these mitochondrial adaptations were accompanied by improvements in systemic insulin sensitivity. According to the NIH Clinial Trials register, PPAR agonists are now being trialled for cardiovascular disease, hypertension, pre-diabetes, and diabetes, and various PPAR agonists (e.g. pioglitazone, rosiglitazone, fibrates) have been FDA-approved for such therapeutic applications. In addition to PPAR ligands, a variety of other common anti-diabetic drugs have pronounced effects on mitochondrial function, with improvements in mitochondrial metabolism likely contributing to the systemic improvements in insulin sensitivity and glycaemic control [79]. While insulin therapy has been shown to improve mitochondrial oxidative phosphorylation [80] and ATP synthesis [81], SGLT2 inhibitors, which primarily act on inhibiting glucose reuptake in the kidney, also improve mitochondrial function in the heart [82–84] and in the brain [85]. However, the positive mitochondrial effects have not been supported by other studies, pointing towards potential inhibitory effects of SGLT2 inhibitors on the mitochondrial respiratory chain [86,87]. Furthermore, conflicting findings have also been reported for one of the most commonly prescribed anti-diabetic agents, the biguanide metformin. While some studies point towards metformin having beneficial effects on mitochondrial oxidative capacity [88] and mitochondrial fission [89], others show the opposite [90–93], with metformin being named 'an energy disruptor' [90]. Lastly, thiazolidinediones (TZDs) such as rosiglitazone have been shown to increase mitochondrial biogenesis [94,95]. For a detailed summary of the effects of anti-diabetic drugs on mitochondrial function, please refer to [79,96].

6. Intercellular Mitochondrial Transfer

In addition to 'boosting' mitochondrial oxidative capacity in the presence of mitochondrial dysfunction through genetic, lifestyle of pharmacological interventions, would it be possible to improve mitochondrial function in a target cell or tissue through mitochondrial transfer? Recent evidence suggests that intact mitochondria, mitochondrial DNA or other mitochondrial components (proteins, lipids or metabolites) can be found in the circulation [97–100] and can be transferred between cells or tissues [101–103]. Mitochondrial transfer between cells was shown in the context of leukaemia [101], acute lung injury [104], asthma [105], and acute respiratory distress syndrome (ARDS) [103], through the use of tunnelling nanotube-like structures between donor and recipient cells. Most importantly, recipient cells showed metabolic impairments which were improved upon transfer of functional mitochondria; e.g., acute myeloid leukaemia (AML) cells were less prone to mitochondrial depolarization after chemotherapy [101]. Other researchers turned to intravenous injections of intact mitochondria as a therapeutic approach for mitochondrial replenishment after cardiac injury [106]. While these studies highlight the protective effects of mitochondrial transfer in a variety of disease conditions, other studies point towards exogenous mitochondria having pro-inflammatory effects [107,108]. In the context of cancer, mitochondrial transfer from benign donor to recipient carcinoma cells elicited a chemo-resistant phenotype [109] and contributed to tumour proliferation [110]. Little is known about mitochondrial transfer in conditions of mitochondrial dysfunction and insulin resistance. Could transfer of intact mitochondria or mitochondrial DNA be a potential therapeutic means to improve mitochondrial dysfunction and subsequently insulin resistance? Could mitochondrial transfer on the other hand further worsen already substantiated metabolic defects? While intercellular transfer using nanotubes-like structures (as described above) is a potential transfer mechanism for cells in close proximity, this pathway is unlikely to 'remodel' whole organs and tissues, as would be required for example for skeletal muscle mitochondrial dysfunction. However, of interest, mitochondrial DNA and mitochondrial proteins have also been shown to be present in extracellular vesicles, particularly exosomes, and the significance of these findings will be discussed below.

7. Exosomes

It has been known for more than 40 years that cells secrete vesicles during apoptosis [111]. More recent studies suggest that also healthy cells have the capacity to release vesicles into the extracellular environment, with exosomes having received substantial attention over the past couple of years, primarily due to early findings such as that dendritic cells secrete antigen-presenting exosomes [112] and that tumour cells can transfer exosomes to dendritic cells to subsequently induce potent antitumor effects [113]. The term exosome is used to distinguish extracellular vesicles with a diameter of 50 to 150 nm, that originate from the late endosomal pathway and are released in the extracellular space upon fusion of multivesicular bodies (MVBs) with the plasma membrane [114] (Figure 1). For detailed info on biogenesis of exosomes, mechanisms of exosome secretion and detailed information on cargo, please refer to a recent review on this topic [115]. Exosomes are lipid-bound vesicles that carry lipids, proteins and nucleic acids. Interestingly, up to 10 percent of exosomal proteins have been described as mitochondrial proteins [116]. However, it should be noted that the relative high number of mitochondrial proteins identified within exosomal preparations could be also due to "contamination" during the preparation procedure. Exosomes are released from a multitude of tissues and cell types, including metabolic tissues, such as skeletal muscle [117], liver [118] and adipose tissue [119,120]. The amount and cargo of released microvesicles differs in obesity and type 2 diabetes [121–124], with adipose-derived exosomes from obese individuals and mouse models being associated with insulin resistance [125,126] and plasma exosomes in obese, T2D individuals showing enrichment in molecules involved in inflammation and immune efficiency [127]. Also, plasma exosomes from obese rats, but not lean rats, induced significant oxidative stress and vascular cell adhesion protein 1 (VCAM-1) expression in endothelial cells, indicative of a pro-inflammatory vesicle phenotype [123].

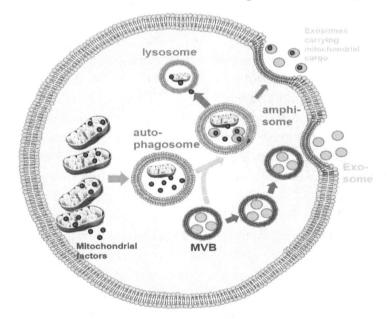

Figure 1. Exosomal secretion of intact mitochondria or mitochondrial factors. Mitochondria or mitochondrial components are packaged into autophagosomes for intracellular degradation. Autophagosomes can fuse with multi-vesicular bodies (MVBs) carrying exosomes, forming amphisomes. Amphisome contents can be either shuttled towards degradation in lysosomes or towards the cell surface where exosomes are released.

Importantly, obesity-associated exosomes released from adipose tissue, macrophages or erythrocytes can transform healthy cells into metabolically defective cells, with robust effects on tissue-specific and systemic insulin sensitivity and overall glucose homeostasis [124,126,128]. Overall, it seems that extracellular vesicles reflect the diverse functional and dysfunctional states of the releasing cells, and it is therefore not surprising that specific vesicle/exosomal signatures are present in distinctive disease states, making exosomes useful biomarkers in the future [129].

8. Exosomes with Mitochondrial Cargo

As mentioned above, up to 10% of exosomal proteins are mitochondria-derived [116]. Initially, vesicles containing mitochondrial cargo were described as being transported within the cytosol towards peroxisomes (i.e., inter-organellar communication) [130], however other vesicle sub-types were also shown fuse with the late endosome or with multi-vesicular bodies for degradation [131], with selective enrichment of oxidized cargo [132]. Of interest, the stress-induced mitochondria-associated proteins Parkin and Pink1 are involved in the generation of these particular multi-vesicular bodies [133], highlighting increased vesicle generation upon autophagy-related stress signals, potentially as a means of mitochondrial quality control. While these studies suggest that these vesicle sub-types and mitochondrial components are destined for degradation, they can also be routed towards the cell surface and fuse with the plasma membrane [134] (Figure 1). It is unclear if increased mitophagy is associated with increased exosomal secretion of mitochondrial components, potentially as a means to get rid of oxidized proteins, in addition to lysosomal degradation.

9. Exosomes with Mitochondrial Cargo—Friend of Foe?

Exosomes containing increased content of mitochondrial lipids, proteins and nucleic acids were found to be released from adipose tissue of obese diabetic and obese non-diabetic rats [135], from pulmonary cells after cigarette smoke injury [136], and are found in plasma upon infection with the human T-lymphotropic retrovirus type 1 (HTLV-1) [99] and in circulating exosomes of breast cancer patients [137], highlighting the broad range of pathological states that are characterized by increased circulating exosomes carrying mitochondrial cargo. Some studies suggest that the cells and tissues releasing these particular exosomes show mitochondrial impairments. For example, it has been shown that mesenchymal stem cells target depolarized mitochondria to the plasma membrane, and that they similarly shed microRNA-containing exosomes, which have the capacity to inhibit macrophage activation, thereby de-sensitizing macrophages to the ingested mitochondria [138]. Cells might use exosomal secretion as a way of quality control, to restore cellular homeostasis and preserve cell viability, to some extent in the presence of mitochondrial dysfunction [139]. This would suggest that mitochondrial cargo within circulating exosomes is largely metabolically defective, and when fusing with recipient cells could either transfer these mitochondrial defects to the recipient cells, or could induce a physiologically adverse response. In support of this hypothesis, it has been shown that leukaemia cells, when challenged with chemotherapeutic drugs that induce oxidative stress, transfer their dysfunctional mitochondria to neighbouring bone marrow mesenchymal stem cells, leading to chemo-resistance [140]. In addition, exosomes can carry mitochondrial electron transport chain (ETC) complexes. Some of these ETC subunits are encoded by mitochondrial DNA. Translation within mitochondria occurs using a formylated initiating methionine (a mechanism still conserved from bacterial origins), and presence of extracellular formylated proteins can lead to an immune response and cytokine release [107].

While mitochondrial proteins are most commonly investigated in the context of exosomal transport, exosomes also carry lipids (a recent paper identified 1,961 lipid species in an exosomal and microvesicle screen [141]), with exosomes from hepatocellular carcinoma cells (Huh7) and human bone marrow-derived mesenchymal stem cells (MSC) specifically enriched in the mitochondrial inner membrane lipid cardiolipin [141]. This enrichment of cardiolipin, but exclusion of other lipid species, such as sphingolipids, within these particular exosomes suggests that cardiolipin might be actively sorted into exosomes of Huh7 cells and MSCs [141]. While the reason for this phenomenon is unknown, the authors suggest that the high concentration of cardiolipin might help in the stability and curvature of the vesicle membrane bilayer. On the other hand, increased secretion of cardiolipin (or other mitochondrial lipids) could impair mitochondrial function of the donor cells, as cardiolipin plays an important role in maintaining optimal mitochondrial function. In this respect, a loss of cardiolipin has been described in the diabetic heart [142–144] and during heart failure [145], while exercise leads to increased cardiolipin content in skeletal muscle [146]. If this is due to differences in synthesis, degradation or exosomal secretion requires further investigation. As mentioned above, exosomal secretion has been considered a way of quality control [139], with the donor cells 'getting rid' of damaged or oxidized cellular components. During conditions of increased mitochondrial ROS production and oxidative stress, as is the case in the presence of insulin resistance and T2D [147], polyunsaturated fatty acids in mitochondrial membranes (such as cardiolipins) are the primary targets of oxidative damage, which may lead to mitochondrial dysfunction [148]. While oxidized cardiolipin can be repaired enzymatically [149], exosomal export is also a likely pathway for clearance of oxidized cellular factors.

Looking at the other side of the coin, a recent study published in the journal *Blood* investigated the metabolic cross-talk between cancer cells and their microenvironment, and found that 'healthy' bone marrow stromal cells (BMSC) were made to transfer their mitochondria to neighbouring acute myeloid leukaemia (AML) cells, supporting the cancer cells' growth [102]. An associated press release in Science Daily termed this phenomenon quite adequately as "Stealing from the body: How cancer recharges its batteries" [150]. A different study identified the complete mitochondrial genome within circulating extracellular vesicles from metastatic breast cancer patients, and showed that these extracellular vesicles can in turn transfer their mtDNA to cells with impaired metabolism, leading to restoration of metabolic activity [151]. The authors suggested that the transfer of mtDNA plays a role in mediating resistance to hormone therapy in these patients.

It seems that, depending on the tissue/cell type and the pathological state examined, mitochondrial cargo can be either transferred from a cell with mitochondrial dysfunction to a cell with 'healthy' metabolic state, leading to metabolic deterioration of the recipient cells; or, on the other hand mitochondrial cargo can be transferred from a 'healthy' cell to a recipient cell with mitochondrial dysfunction, leading to the recipient's metabolic improvement (Figure 2). The impact or physiological importance of exosomal transfer of mitochondrial cargo in the context of mitochondrial dysfunction in insulin resistant and T2D individuals is not known. Does skeletal muscle, heart or liver (or major metabolic tissues in general) have the capacity to shed mitochondria in the presence of mitochondrial dysfunction to rescue the donor's cell energetic state? Could on the other hand mitochondrial cargo be transferred to metabolically deficient cells, to improve mitochondrial dysfunction in the recipient tissue (Figure 2)?

Figure 2. Is mitochondrial transfer in states of insulin resistance and mitochondrial dysfunction a friend or foe? In other pathological conditions, it has been shown that cells with mitochondrial impairments have the capacity to secrete mitochondrial cargo within exosomes that then impairs metabolic state of the recipient cells (i.e., foe). Other studies suggest that 'healthy' cells secrete mitochondrial cargo to improve the recipients cell metabolism (i.e., friend). Future studies will have to show if these phenomena are present states of mitochondrial dysfunction and insulin resistance.

10. Mitochondrial Dysfunction, T2D and Exosomal Transfer of Mitochondrial Cargo

Very little is known about exosomal transfer of mitochondrial cargo in the presence of mitochondrial dysfunction during the development of insulin resistance and T2D. It has been shown that in obese diabetic rats adipose-derived exosomes carry more mitochondrial lipids, proteins and nucleic acids [135]. Furthermore, lower circulating mtDNA content is associated with T2D [152] and severe proliferative diabetic retinopathy [153], with reduced peripheral blood mtDNA content potentially increasing the risk of impaired glucose-stimulated β cell function [152]. In addition, HbA1c, fasting plasma glucose and age of T2D onset are the major factors affecting mtDNA content [154]. While these studies assessed changes in mtDNA content in the circulation, this was not investigated in the context of exosomal transport. In a related matter, point mutations in the mitochondrial genome and decreases in mtDNA copy number have been linked to the pathogenesis of type 2 diabetes [155,156]. Compared with nuclear DNA repair, mtDNA repair mechanisms are significantly less efficient [157] and mtDNA is more susceptible to oxidative stress and mutations [158]. While the secretion of mtDNA within microvesicles has been described previously [159], little is known if mutated mtDNA can be secreted within exosomes and taken up by other cells.

Future studies will have to determine whether metabolic tissues, such as skeletal muscle or liver, have the capacity to shed defective mitochondrial components within exosomes, and if this process is affected in obese T2D individuals. Could on the other hand mitochondrial transfer be used as a means to improve mitochondrial defects (Figure 2)? It would be of interest to assess if targeted transfer of mitochondrial proteins or metabolites, or even fully functioning intact mitochondria, could improve mitochondrial dysfunction and have effects on insulin sensitivity and glucose homeostasis.

11. Conclusions and Future Directions

Mitochondrial impairments have been described in the context of obesity, insulin resistance and T2D, in a variety of metabolic tissues. However, as studies reported opposing findings ranging from decreased mitochondrial function, to unaffected mitochondrial capacity, and even to an increase in mitochondrial oxidative metabolism in individuals and rodent models with insulin resistance or T2D, the requisite for the presence of mitochondrial dysfunction in these pathological states is unclear.

In addition, genetic manipulations of mitochondrial proteins, as well as lifestyle and pharmacological interventions resulted in contradicting findings, and it is still unclear if targeting mitochondrial capacity is a useful therapeutic approach for the treatment of insulin resistance and glycaemic control. In the past years, it has become evident that metabolic tissues secrete microvesicles, such as exosomes, containing mitochondrial cargo, and that these exosomes have the capacity to fuse in a selective targeted manner with recipient cells and tissues, and influence the recipients' cell metabolic status. Future studies will have to show if tissues with mitochondrial impairments in states of obesity and T2D have the capacity to 'shed' their dysfunctional mitochondria to improve their metabolic status, or if dysfunctional tissues have the capacity to 'ingest' exosomes with mitochondrial cargo to improve their oxidative metabolism.

Author Contributions: M.K.M. researched and wrote the manuscript.

References

1. Obesity and Overweight. Available online: http://www.who.int/news-room/fact-sheets/detail/obesity-and-overweight (accessed on 9 September 2018).
2. Type 2 Diabetes. Available online: https://www.niddk.nih.gov/health-information/diabetes/overview/what-is-diabetes/type-2-diabetes (accessed on 8 September 2018).
3. Ye, J. Mechanisms of insulin resistance in obesity. *Front. Med.* **2013**, *7*, 14–24. [CrossRef] [PubMed]
4. Blüher, M. Adipose tissue inflammation: a cause or consequence of obesity-related insulin resistance? *Clin. Sci.* **2016**, *130*, 1603–1614. [CrossRef] [PubMed]
5. Takamura, T.; Misu, H.; Ota, T.; Kaneko, S. Fatty liver as a consequence and cause of insulin resistance: Lessons from type 2 diabetic liver. *Endocr. J.* **2012**, *59*, 745–763. [CrossRef] [PubMed]
6. Keane, K.N.; Cruzat, V.F.; Carlessi, R.; de Bittencourt, P.I.H.; Newsholme, P. Molecular events linking oxidative stress and inflammation to insulin resistance and β-cell dysfunction. *Oxid. Med. Cell Longev.* **2015**, *2015*, 181643. [CrossRef] [PubMed]
7. Daiber, A.; Di Lisa, F.; Oelze, M.; Kröller-Schön, S.; Steven, S.; Schulz, E.; Münzel, T. Crosstalk of mitochondria with NADPH oxidase via reactive oxygen and nitrogen species signalling and its role for vascular function. *Br. J. Pharmacol.* **2017**, *174*, 1670–1689. [CrossRef] [PubMed]
8. Angelova, P.R.; Abramov, A.Y. Functional role of mitochondrial reactive oxygen species in physiology. *Free Radic. Biol. Med.* **2016**, *100*, 81–85. [CrossRef] [PubMed]
9. Owusu-Ansah, E.; Banerjee, U. Reactive oxygen species prime Drosophila haematopoietic progenitors for differentiation. *Nature* **2009**, *461*, 537–541. [CrossRef]
10. Wang, W.; Fang, H.; Groom, L.; Cheng, A.; Zhang, W.; Liu, J.; Wang, X.; Li, K.; Han, P.; Zheng, M.; et al. Superoxide flashes in single mitochondria. *Cell* **2008**, *134*, 279–290. [CrossRef]
11. Redza-Dutordoir, M.; Averill-Bates, D.A. Activation of apoptosis signalling pathways by reactive oxygen species. *Biochim. Biophys. Acta* **2016**, *1863*, 2977–2992. [CrossRef]
12. Estaquier, J.; Vallette, F.; Vayssiere, J.-L.; Mignotte, B. The Mitochondrial Pathways of Apoptosis. In *Advances in Mitochondrial Medicine*; Scatena, R., Bottoni, P., Giardina, B., Eds.; Springer: Dordrecht, The Netherlands; pp. 157–183.
13. Rizzuto, R.; De Stefani, D.; Raffaello, A.; Mammucari, C. Mitochondria as sensors and regulators of calcium signalling. *Nat. Rev. Mol. Cell Biol.* **2012**, *13*, 566. [CrossRef]
14. Chiabrando, D.; Mercurio, S.; Tolosano, E. Heme and erythropoieis: more than a structural role. *Haematologica* **2014**, *99*, 973–983. [CrossRef] [PubMed]
15. Ryu, M.-S.; Zhang, D.; Protchenko, O.; Shakoury-Elizeh, M.; Philpott, C.C. PCBP1 and NCOA4 regulate erythroid iron storage and heme biosynthesis. *J. Clin. Invest.* **2017**, *127*, 1786–1797. [CrossRef] [PubMed]
16. Martin, L.A.; Kennedy, B.E.; Karten, B. Mitochondrial cholesterol: mechanisms of import and effects on mitochondrial function. *J. Bioenerg. Biomembr.* **2016**, *48*, 137–151. [CrossRef] [PubMed]
17. Yamada, T.; Ida, T.; Yamaoka, Y.; Ozawa, K.; Takasan, H.; Honjo, I. Two distinct patterns of glucose intolerance in icteric rats and rabbits. Relationship to impaired liver mitochondria function. *J. Lab. Clin. Med.* **1975**, *86*, 38–45. [PubMed]
18. Heilbronn, L.K.; Gan, S.K.; Turner, N.; Campbell, L.V.; Chisholm, D.J. Markers of mitochondrial biogenesis and metabolism are lower in overweight and obese insulin-resistant subjects. *J. Clin. Endocrinol. Metab.* **2007**, *92*, 1467–1473. [CrossRef] [PubMed]

19. Mootha, V.K.; Lindgren, C.M.; Eriksson, K.F.; Subramanian, A.; Sihag, S.; Lehar, J.; Puigserver, P.; Carlsson, E.; Ridderstrale, M.; Laurila, E.; et al. PGC-1 alpha-responsive genes involved in oxidative phosphorylation are coordinately downregulated in human diabetes. *Nat. Rev. Genet.* **2003**, *34*, 267–273. [CrossRef] [PubMed]

20. Ritov, V.B.; Menshikova, E.V.; He, J.; Ferrell, R.E.; Goodpaster, B.H.; Kelley, D.E. Deficiency of subsarcolemmal mitochondria in obesity and type 2 diabetes. *Diabetes* **2005**, *54*, 8–14. [CrossRef]

21. Kelley, D.E.; He, J.; Menshikova, E.V.; Ritov, V.B. Dysfunction of mitochondria in human skeletal muscle in type 2 diabetes. *Diabetes* **2002**, *51*, 2944–2950. [CrossRef]

22. Kelley, D.E.; Goodpaster, B.; Wing, R.R.; Simoneau, J.A. Skeletal muscle fatty acid metabolism in association with insulin resistance, obesity, and weight loss. *Am. J. Physiol.* **1999**, *277*, E1130–E1141. [CrossRef]

23. Anderson, E.J.; Lustig, M.E.; Boyle, K.E.; Woodlief, T.L.; Kane, D.A.; Lin, C.-T.; Price, J.W., III; Kang, L.; Rabinovitch, P.S.; Szeto, H.H.; et al. Mitochondrial H_2O_2 emission and cellular redox state link excess fat intake to insulin resistance in both rodents and humans. *J. Clin. Invest.* **2009**, *119*, 573–581. [CrossRef]

24. Montgomery, M.K.; Turner, N. Mitochondrial dysfunction and insulin resistance: an update. *Endocr. Connect.* **2015**, *4*, R1–R15. [CrossRef] [PubMed]

25. Boyle, K.E.; Canham, J.P.; Consitt, L.A.; Zheng, D.; Koves, T.R.; Gavin, T.P.; Holbert, D.; Neufer, P.D.; Ilkayeva, O.; Muoio, D.M.; et al. A high-fat diet elicits differential responses in genes coordinating oxidative metabolism in skeletal muscle of lean and obese individuals. *J. Clin. Endocrinol. Metab.* **2011**, *96*, 775–781. [CrossRef] [PubMed]

26. Hwang, H.; Bowen, B.P.; Lefort, N.; Flynn, C.R.; De Filippis, E.A.; Roberts, C.; Smoke, C.C.; Meyer, C.; Højlund, K.; Yi, Z.; et al. Proteomics analysis of human skeletal muscle reveals novel abnormalities in obesity and type 2 diabetes. *Diabetes* **2010**, *59*, 33–42. [CrossRef] [PubMed]

27. Bandyopadhyay, G.K.; Yu, J.G.; Ofrecio, J.; Olefsky, J.M. Increased malonyl-coa levels in muscle from obese and type 2 diabetic subjects lead to decreased fatty acid oxidation and increased lipogenesis; thiazolidinedione treatment reverses these defects. *Diabetes* **2006**, *55*, 2277–2285. [CrossRef] [PubMed]

28. Trenell, M.I.; Hollingsworth, K.G.; Lim, E.L.; Taylor, R. Increased daily walking improves lipid oxidation without changes in mitochondrial function in type 2 diabetes. *Diabetes Care* **2008**, *31*, 1644–1649. [CrossRef] [PubMed]

29. Garcia-Roves, P.; Huss, J.M.; Han, D.-H.; Hancock, C.R.; Iglesias-Gutierrez, E.; Chen, M.; Holloszy, J.O. Raising plasma fatty acid concentration induces increased biogenesis of mitochondria in skeletal muscle. *Proc. Natl. Acad. Sci. USA* **2007**, *104*, 10709–10713. [CrossRef] [PubMed]

30. Hancock, C.R.; Han, D.H.; Chen, M.; Terada, S.; Yasuda, T.; Wright, D.C.; Holloszy, J.O. High-fat diets cause insulin resistance despite an increase in muscle mitochondria. *Proc. Natl. Acad. Sci. USA* **2008**. [CrossRef]

31. Ruegsegger, G.N.; Creo, A.L.; Cortes, T.M.; Dasari, S.; Nair, K.S. Altered mitochondrial function in insulin-deficient and insulin-resistant states. *J. Clin. Invest.* **2018**, *128*, 3671–3681. [CrossRef]

32. Fernández-Vizarra, E.; Enríquez, J.A.; Pérez-Martos, A.; Montoya, J.; Fernández-Silva, P. Tissue-specific differences in mitochondrial activity and biogenesis. *Mitochondrion* **2011**, *11*, 207–213. [CrossRef]

33. Montaigne, D.; Marechal, X.; Coisne, A.; Debry, N.; Modine, T.; Fayad, G.; Potelle, C.; El Arid, J.; Mouton, S.; Sebti, Y.; et al. Myocardial contractile dysfunction is associated with impaired mitochondrial function and dynamics in type 2 diabetic but not in obese patients. *Circulation* **2014**, *130*, 554–564. [CrossRef]

34. Dhalla, N.S.; Takeda, N.; Rodriguez-Leyva, D.; Elimban, V. Mechanisms of subcellular remodeling in heart failure due to diabetes. *Heart Fail. Rev.* **2014**, *19*, 87–99. [CrossRef] [PubMed]

35. Mackenzie, R.M.; Salt, I.P.; Miller, W.H.; Logan, A.; Ibrahim, H.A.; Degasperi, A.; Dymott, J.A.; Hamilton, C.A.; Murphy, M.P.; Delles, C.; et al. Mitochondrial reactive oxygen species enhance AMP-activated protein kinase activation in the endothelium of patients with coronary artery disease and diabetes. *Clin. Sci.* **2013**, *124*, 403–411. [CrossRef] [PubMed]

36. Croston, T.L.; Thapa, D.; Holden, A.A.; Tveter, K.J.; Lewis, S.E.; Shepherd, D.L.; Nichols, C.E.; Long, D.M.; Olfert, I.M.; Jagannathan, R.; et al. Functional deficiencies of subsarcolemmal mitochondria in the type 2 diabetic human heart. *Am. J. Physiol. Heart Circ. Physiol.* **2014**, *307*, H54–H65. [CrossRef] [PubMed]

37. Anderson, E.J.; Rodriguez, E.; Anderson, C.A.; Thayne, K.; Chitwood, W.R.; Kypson, A.P. Increased propensity for cell death in diabetic human heart is mediated by mitochondrial-dependent pathways. *Am. J. Physiol. Heart Circ. Physiol.* **2011**, *300*, H118–H124. [CrossRef] [PubMed]

38. Marciniak, C.; Marechal, X.; Montaigne, D.; Neviere, R.; Lancel, S. Cardiac contractile function and mitochondrial respiration in diabetes-related mouse models. *Cardiovasc. Diabetol.* **2014**, *13*, 118. [CrossRef] [PubMed]

39. Pham, T.; Loiselle, D.; Power, A.; Hickey, A.J.R. Mitochondrial inefficiencies and anoxic ATP hydrolysis capacities in diabetic rat heart. *Am. J. Physiol. Cell Physiol.* **2014**, *307*, C499–C507. [CrossRef]

40. Hicks, S.; Labinskyy, N.; Piteo, B.; Laurent, D.; Mathew, J.E.; Gupte, S.A.; Edwards, J.G. Type II diabetes increases mitochondrial DNA mutations in the left ventricle of the Goto-Kakizaki diabetic rat. *Am. J. Physiol. Heart Circ. Physiol.* **2013**, *304*, H903–H915. [CrossRef] [PubMed]

41. Yan, W.; Zhang, H.; Liu, P.; Wang, H.; Liu, J.; Gao, C.; Liu, Y.; Lian, K.; Yang, L.; Sun, L.; et al. Impaired mitochondrial biogenesis due to dysfunctional adiponectin-AMPK-PGC-1α signaling contributing to increased vulnerability in diabetic heart. *Basic Res. Cardiol.* **2013**, *108*, 329. [CrossRef]

42. Luo, M.; Guan, X.; Luczak, E.D.; Lang, D.; Kutschke, W.; Gao, Z.; Yang, J.; Glynn, P.; Sossalla, S.; Swaminathan, P.D.; et al. Diabetes increases mortality after myocardial infarction by oxidizing CaMKII. *J. Clin. Invest.* **2013**, *123*, 1262–1274. [CrossRef]

43. Vazquez, E.J.; Berthiaume, J.M.; Kamath, V.; Achike, O.; Buchanan, E.; Montano, M.M.; Chandler, M.P.; Miyagi, M.; Rosca, M.G. Mitochondrial complex I defect and increased fatty acid oxidation enhance protein lysine acetylation in the diabetic heart. *Cardiovasc. Res.* **2015**, *107*, 453–465. [CrossRef]

44. Deeds, M.C.; Anderson, J.M.; Armstrong, A.S.; Gastineau, D.A.; Hiddinga, H.J.; Jahangir, A.; Eberhardt, N.L.; Kudva, Y.C. Single dose streptozotocin induced diabetes: considerations for study design in islet transplantation models. *Lab. Anim.* **2011**, *45*, 131–140. [CrossRef] [PubMed]

45. Turkieh, A.; Caubère, C.; Barutaut, M.; Desmoulin, F.; Harmancey, R.; Galinier, M.; Berry, M.; Dambrin, C.; Polidori, C.; Casteilla, L.; et al. Apolipoprotein O is mitochondrial and promotes lipotoxicity in heart. *J. Clin. Invest.* **2014**, *124*, 2277–2286. [CrossRef] [PubMed]

46. Wai, T.; García-Prieto, J.; Baker, M.J.; Merkwirth, C.; Benit, P.; Rustin, P.; Rupérez, F.J.; Barbas, C.; Ibañez, B.; Langer, T. Imbalanced OPA1 processing and mitochondrial fragmentation cause heart failure in mice. *Science* **2015**, *350*. [CrossRef]

47. Liu, W.; Ruiz-Velasco, A.; Wang, S.; Khan, S.; Zi, M.; Jungmann, A.; Dolores Camacho-Muñoz, M.; Guo, J.; Du, G.; Xie, L.; et al. Metabolic stress-induced cardiomyopathy is caused by mitochondrial dysfunction due to attenuated Erk5 signaling. *Nat. Commun.* **2017**, *8*, 494. [CrossRef] [PubMed]

48. Lehmann, L.H.; Jebessa, Z.H.; Kreusser, M.M.; Horsch, A.; He, T.; Kronlage, M.; Dewenter, M.; Sramek, V.; Oehl, U.; Krebs-Haupenthal, J.; et al. A proteolytic fragment of histone deacetylase 4 protects the heart from failure by regulating the hexosamine biosynthetic pathway. *Nat. Med.* **2017**, *24*, 62. [CrossRef] [PubMed]

49. Lopaschuk, G.D.; Ussher, J.R.; Folmes, C.D.L.; Jaswal, J.S.; Stanley, W.C. Myocardial fatty acid metabolism in health and disease. *Physiol. Rev.* **2010**, *90*, 207–258. [CrossRef] [PubMed]

50. Fillmore, N.; Mori, J.; Lopaschuk, G.D. Mitochondrial fatty acid oxidation alterations in heart failure, ischaemic heart disease and diabetic cardiomyopathy. *Br. J. Pharmacol.* **2014**, *171*, 2080–2090. [CrossRef]

51. Szczepaniak, L.S.; Dobbins, R.L.; Metzger, G.J.; Sartoni-D'Ambrosia, G.; Arbique, D.; Vongpatanasin, W.; Unger, R.; Victor, R.G. Myocardial triglycerides and systolic function in humans: In vivo evaluation by localized proton spectroscopy and cardiac imaging. *Magn. Reson. Med.* **2003**, *49*, 417–423. [CrossRef]

52. Peterson, L.; Herrero, P.; Schechtman, K.; Racette, S.; Waggoner, A.; Kisrieva-Ware, Z.; Dence, C.; Klein, S.; Marsala, J.; Meyer, T.; et al. Effect of obesity and insulin resistance on myocardial substrate metabolism and efficiency in young women. *Circulation* **2004**, *109*, 2191–2196. [CrossRef]

53. Mazumder, P.K.; O'Neill, B.T.; Roberts, M.W.; Buchanan, J.; Yun, U.J.; Cooksey, R.C.; Boudina, S.; Abel, E.D. Impaired cardiac efficiency and increased fatty acid oxidation in insulin-resistant ob/ob mouse hearts. *Diabetes* **2004**, *53*, 2366–2374. [CrossRef]

54. Belke, D.D.; Severson, D.L. Diabetes in mice with monogenic obesity: The db/db mouse and its use in the study of cardiac consequences. In *Animal Models in Diabetes Research*. Joost, H.-G.; Al-Hasani, H.; Schürmann, A., Eds.; Humana Press: Totowa, NJ, USA, 2012; pp. 47–57.

55. Ansley, D.M.; Wang, B. Oxidative stress and myocardial injury in the diabetic heart. *J. Pathol.* **2013**, *229*, 232–241. [CrossRef] [PubMed]

56. Zhang, L.; Ussher, J.R.; Oka, T.; Cadete, V.J.J.; Wagg, C.; Lopaschuk, G.D. Cardiac diacylglycerol accumulation in high fat-fed mice is associated with impaired insulin-stimulated glucose oxidation. *Cardiovasc. Res.* **2011**, *89*, 148–156. [CrossRef] [PubMed]

57. Kuramoto, K.; Okamura, T.; Yamaguchi, T.; Nakamura, T.Y.; Wakabayashi, S.; Morinaga, H.; Nomura, M.; Yanase, T.; Otsu, K.; Usuda, N.; et al. Perilipin 5, a lipid droplet-binding protein, protects heart from oxidative burden by sequestering fatty acid from excessive oxidation. *J. Biol. Chem.* **2012**, *287*, 23852–23863. [CrossRef] [PubMed]

58. Chatham, J.C.; Forder, J.R. A 13C-NMR Study of glucose oxidation in the intact functioning rat heart following diabetes-induced cardiomyopathy. *J. Mol. Cell. Cardiol.* **1993**, *25*, 1203–1213. [CrossRef] [PubMed]

59. Chatham, J.C.; Forder, J.R. Relationship between cardiac function and substrate oxidation in hearts of diabetic rats. *Am. J. Physiol. Heart Circ. Physiol.* **1997**, *273*, H52–H58. [CrossRef] [PubMed]

60. Wu, C.-Y.; Satapati, S.; Gui, W.; Wynn, R.M.; Sharma, G.; Lou, M.; Qi, X.; Burgess, S.C.; Malloy, C.; Khemtong, C.; et al. A novel inhibitor of pyruvate dehydrogenase kinase stimulates myocardial carbohydrate oxidation in diet-induced obesity. *J. Biol. Chem.* **2018**, *293*, 9604–9613. [CrossRef]

61. Saeedi, R.; Grist, M.; Wambolt, R.B.; Bescond-Jacquet, A.; Lucien, A.; Allard, M.F. Trimetazidine normalizes postischemic function of hypertrophied rat hearts. *J. Pharmacol. Exp. Ther.* **2005**, *314*, 446–454. [CrossRef]

62. Dyck, J.R.; Cheng, J.F.; Stanley, W.C.; Barr, R.; Chandler, M.P.; Brown, S.; Wallace, D.; Arrhenius, T.; Harmon, C.; Yang, G.; et al. Malonyl coenzyme a decarboxylase inhibition protects the ischemic heart by inhibiting fatty acid oxidation and stimulating glucose oxidation. *Circ. Res.* **2004**, *94*, e78–e84.

63. Keung, W.; Ussher, J.R.; Jaswal, J.S.; Raubenheimer, M.; Lam, V.H.M.; Wagg, C.S.; Lopaschuk, G.D. Inhibition of carnitine palmitoyltransferase-1 activity alleviates insulin resistance in diet-induced obese mice. *Diabetes* **2013**, *62*, 711–720. [CrossRef]

64. Timmers, S.; Nabben, M.; Bosma, M.; van Bree, B.; Lenaers, E.; van Beurden, D.; Schaart, G.; Westerterp-Plantenga, M.S.; Langhans, W.; Hesselink, M.K.C.; et al. Augmenting muscle diacylglycerol and triacylglycerol content by blocking fatty acid oxidation does not impede insulin sensitivity. *Proc. Natl. Acad. Sci. USA* **2012**, *109*, 11711–11716. [CrossRef]

65. Henstridge, D.C.; Bruce, C.R.; Drew, B.G.; Tory, K.; Kolonics, A.; Estevez, E.; Chung, J.; Watson, N.; Gardner, T.; Lee-Young, R.S.; et al. Activating HSP72 in rodent skeletal muscle increases mitochondrial number and oxidative capacity and decreases insulin resistance. *Diabetes* **2014**, *63*, 1881–1894. [CrossRef]

66. Henstridge, D.C.; Estevez, E.; Allen, T.L.; Heywood, S.E.; Gardner, T.; Yang, C.; Mellett, N.A.; Kingwell, B.A.; Meikle, P.J.; Febbraio, M.A. Genetic manipulation of cardiac Hsp72 levels does not alter substrate metabolism but reveals insights into high-fat feeding-induced cardiac insulin resistance. *Cell Stress Chaperones* **2015**, *20*, 461–472. [CrossRef] [PubMed]

67. Holloway, G.P.; Chou, C.J.; Lally, J.; Stellingwerff, T.; Maher, A.C.; Gavrilova, O.; Haluzik, M.; Alkhateeb, H.; Reitman, M.L.; Bonen, A. Increasing skeletal muscle fatty acid transport protein 1 (FATP1) targets fatty acids to oxidation and does not predispose mice to diet-induced insulin resistance. *Diabetologia* **2011**, *54*, 1457. [CrossRef] [PubMed]

68. Snowling, N.J.; Hopkins, W.G. Effects of different modes of exercise training on glucose control and risk factors for complications in type 2 diabetic patients. *A Meta. Analysis* **2006**, *29*, 2518–2527. [CrossRef] [PubMed]

69. Perry, R.J.; Peng, L.; Cline, G.W.; Wang, Y.; Rabin-Court, A.; Song, J.D.; Zhang, D.; Zhang, X.-M.; Nozaki, Y.; Dufour, S.; et al. Mechanisms by which a Very-Low-Calorie Diet Reverses Hyperglycemia in a Rat Model of Type 2 Diabetes. *Cell Metab.* **2018**, *27*, 210–217.e213. [CrossRef] [PubMed]

70. Meex, R.C.R.; Schrauwen-Hinderling, V.B.; Moonen-Kornips, E.; Schaart, G.; Mensink, M.; Phielix, E.; van de Weijer, T.; Sels, J.-P.; Schrauwen, P.; Hesselink, M.K.C. Restoration of muscle mitochondrial function and metabolic flexibility in type 2 diabetes by exercise training is paralleled by increased myocellular fat storage and improved insulin sensitivity. *Diabetes* **2010**, *59*, 572–579. [CrossRef] [PubMed]

71. Finckenberg, P.; Eriksson, O.; Baumann, M.; Merasto, S.; Lalowski, M.M.; Levijoki, J.; Haasio, K.; Kytö, V.; Muller, D.N.; Luft, F.C.; et al. Caloric restriction ameliorates angiotensin II-induced mitochondrial remodeling and cardiac hypertrophy. *Hypertension* **2012**, *59*, 76–84. [CrossRef]

72. Holloszy, J.O. Regulation of mitochondrial biogenesis and GLUT4 expression by exercise. *Compr. Physiol.* **2011**, *1*, 921–940.

73. Johnson, M.L.; Distelmaier, K.; Lanza, I.R.; Irving, B.A.; Robinson, M.M.; Konopka, A.R.; Shulman, G.I.; Nair, K.S. Mechanism by which caloric restriction improves insulin sensitivity in sedentary obese adults. *Diabetes* **2016**, *65*, 74–84. [CrossRef]

74. Rabøl, R.; Svendsen, P.F.; Skovbro, M.; Boushel, R.; Haugaard, S.B.; Schjerling, P.; Schrauwen, P.; Hesselink, M.K.C.; Nilas, L.; Madsbad, S.; Dela, F. Reduced skeletal muscle mitochondrial respiration and improved glucose metabolism in nondiabetic obese women during a very low calorie dietary intervention leading to rapid weight loss. *Metab. Clin. Exp.* **2009**, *58*, 1145–1152. [CrossRef]

75. Veiga, F.M.S.; Graus-Nunes, F.; Rachid, T.L.; Barreto, A.B.; Mandarim-de-Lacerda, C.A.; Souza-Mello, V. Anti-obesogenic effects of WY14643 (PPAR-alpha agonist): Hepatic mitochondrial enhancement and suppressed lipogenic pathway in diet-induced obese mice. *Biochimie* **2017**, *140*, 106–116. [CrossRef] [PubMed]

76. Rasouli, N.; Kern, P.A.; Elbein, S.C.; Sharma, N.K.; Das, S.K. Improved insulin sensitivity after treatment with PPARγ and PPARα ligands is mediated by genetically modulated transcripts. *Pharmacogenet. Genomics* **2012**, *22*, 484–497. [CrossRef] [PubMed]

77. Coletta, D.K.; Fernandez, M.; Cersosimo, E.; Gastaldelli, A.; Musi, N.; DeFronzo, R.A. The effect of muraglitazar on adiponectin signalling, mitochondrial function and fat oxidation genes in human skeletal muscle in vivo. *Diabet. Med.* **2015**, *32*, 657–664. [CrossRef] [PubMed]

78. Tanaka, T.; Yamamoto, J.; Iwasaki, S.; Asaba, H.; Hamura, H.; Ikeda, Y.; Watanabe, M.; Magoori, K.; Ioka, R.X.; Tachibana, K.; et al. Activation of peroxisome proliferator-activated receptor δ induces fatty acid β-oxidation in skeletal muscle and attenuates metabolic syndrome. *Proc. Natl. Acad. Sci. USA* **2003**, *100*, 15924–15929. [CrossRef] [PubMed]

79. Yaribeygi, H.; Atkin, S.L.; Sahebkar, A. Mitochondrial dysfunction in diabetes and the regulatory roles of antidiabetic agents on the mitochondrial function. *J. Cell. Physiol.* **2018**. [CrossRef] [PubMed]

80. Nisr, R.B.; Affourtit, C. Insulin acutely improves mitochondrial function of rat and human skeletal muscle by increasing coupling efficiency of oxidative phosphorylation. *Biochim. Biophys. Acta* **2014**, *1837*, 270–276. [CrossRef]

81. Petersen, K.F.; Dufour, S.; Shulman, G.I. Decreased insulin-stimulated ATP synthesis and phosphate transport in muscle of insulin-resistant offspring of type 2 diabetic parents. *PLoS Med.* **2005**, *2*, e233. [CrossRef] [PubMed]

82. Mizuno, M.; Kuno, A.; Yano, T.; Miki, T.; Oshima, H.; Sato, T.; Nakata, K.; Kimura, Y.; Tanno, M.; Miura, T. Empagliflozin normalizes the size and number of mitochondria and prevents reduction in mitochondrial size after myocardial infarction in diabetic hearts. *Physiol. Rep.* **2018**, *6*, e13741. [CrossRef]

83. Vettor, R.; Inzucchi, S.E.; Fioretto, P. The cardiovascular benefits of empagliflozin: SGLT2-dependent and -independent effects. *Diabetologia* **2017**, *60*, 395–398. [CrossRef]

84. Zhou, H.; Wang, S.; Zhu, P.; Hu, S.; Chen, Y.; Ren, J. Empagliflozin rescues diabetic myocardial microvascular injury via AMPK-mediated inhibition of mitochondrial fission. *Redox Biol.* **2017**, *15*, 335–346. [CrossRef]

85. Sa-nguanmoo, P.; Tanajak, P.; Kerdphoo, S.; Jaiwongkam, T.; Pratchayasakul, W.; Chattipakorn, N.; Chattipakorn, S.C. SGLT2-inhibitor and DPP-4 inhibitor improve brain function via attenuating mitochondrial dysfunction, insulin resistance, inflammation, and apoptosis in HFD-induced obese rats. *Toxicol. Appl. Pharmacol.* **2017**, *333*, 43–50. [CrossRef] [PubMed]

86. Hawley, S.A.; Ford, R.J.; Smith, B.K.; Gowans, G.J.; Mancini, S.J.; Pitt, R.D.; Day, E.A.; Salt, I.P.; Steinberg, G.R.; Hardie, D.G. The Na$^+$/Glucose cotransporter inhibitor canagliflozin activates AMPK by inhibiting mitochondrial function and increasing cellular AMP levels. *Diabetes* **2016**, *65*, 2784–2794. [CrossRef] [PubMed]

87. Secker, P.F.; Beneke, S.; Schlichenmaier, N.; Delp, J.; Gutbier, S.; Leist, M.; Dietrich, D.R. Canagliflozin mediated dual inhibition of mitochondrial glutamate dehydrogenase and complex I: an off-target adverse effect. *Cell Death Dis.* **2018**, *9*, 226. [CrossRef] [PubMed]

88. Sun, D.; Yang, F. Metformin improves cardiac function in mice with heart failure after myocardial infarction by regulating mitochondrial energy metabolism. *Biochemical and Biophysical Research Communications* **2017**, *486*, 329–335. [CrossRef] [PubMed]

89. Wang, Q.; Zhang, M.; Torres, G.; Wu, S.; Ouyang, C.; Xie, Z.; Zou, M.-H. Metformin suppresses diabetes-accelerated atherosclerosis via the inhibition of Drp1-mediated mitochondrial fission. *Diabetes* **2017**, *66*, 193–205. [CrossRef] [PubMed]

90. Loubiere, C.; Clavel, S.; Gilleron, J.; Harisseh, R.; Fauconnier, J.; Ben-Sahra, I.; Kaminski, L.; Laurent, K.; Herkenne, S.; Lacas-Gervais, S.; et al. The energy disruptor metformin targets mitochondrial integrity via modification of calcium flux in cancer cells. *Sci. Rep.* **2017**, *7*, 5040. [CrossRef] [PubMed]

91. Wheaton, W.W.; Weinberg, S.E.; Hamanaka, R.B.; Soberanes, S.; Sullivan, L.B.; Anso, E.; Glasauer, A.; Dufour, E.; Mutlu, G.M.; Budigner, G.S.; et al. Metformin inhibits mitochondrial complex I of cancer cells to reduce tumorigenesis. *eLife* **2014**, *3*, e02242. [CrossRef] [PubMed]

92. Cameron, A.R.; Logie, L.; Patel, K.; Erhardt, S.; Bacon, S.; Middleton, P.; Harthill, J.; Forteath, C.; Coats, J.T.; Kerr, C.; et al. Metformin selectively targets redox control of complex I energy transduction. *Redox Biol.* **2017**, *14*, 187–197. [CrossRef]

93. Gui, D.Y.; Sullivan, L.B.; Luengo, A.; Hosios, A.M.; Bush, L.N.; Gitego, N.; Davidson, S.M.; Freinkman, E.; Thomas, C.J.; Vander Heiden, M.G. Environment dictates dependence on mitochondrial complex i for nad+ and aspartate production and determines cancer cell sensitivity to Metformin. *Cell Metab.* **2016**, *24*, 716–727. [CrossRef]

94. Ghosh, S.; Patel, N.; Rahn, D.; McAllister, J.; Sadeghi, S.; Horwitz, G.; Berry, D.; Wang, K.X.; Swerdlow, R.H. The thiazolidinedione pioglitazone alters mitochondrial function in human neuron-like cells. *Mol. Pharmacol.* **2007**, *71*, 1695–1702. [CrossRef]

95. Bogacka, I.; Xie, H.; Bray, G.A.; Smith, S.R. Pioglitazone induces mitochondrial biogenesis in human subcutaneous adipose tissue in vivo. *Diabetes* **2005**, *54*, 1392–1399. [CrossRef]

96. Wang, W.; Karamanlidis, G.; Tian, R. Novel targets for mitochondrial medicine. *Sci. Transl. Med.* **2016**, *8*, 326rv323. [CrossRef] [PubMed]

97. Nakahira, K.; Kyung, S.-Y.; Rogers, A.J.; Gazourian, L.; Youn, S.; Massaro, A.F.; Quintana, C.; Osorio, J.C.; Wang, Z.; Zhao, Y.; et al. Circulating mitochondrial dna in patients in the icu as a marker of mortality: derivation and validation. *PLoS Med.* **2014**, *10*, e1001577. [CrossRef] [PubMed]

98. Gu, X.; Yao, Y.; Wu, G.; Lv, T.; Luo, L.; Song, Y. The plasma mitochondrial dna is an independent predictor for post-traumatic systemic inflammatory response syndrome. *PLoS ONE* **2013**, *8*, e72834. [CrossRef] [PubMed]

99. Jeannin, P.; Chaze, T.; Giai Gianetto, Q.; Matondo, M.; Gout, O.; Gessain, A.; Afonso, P.V. Proteomic analysis of plasma extracellular vesicles reveals mitochondrial stress upon HTLV-1 infection. *Sci. Rep.* **2018**, *8*, 5170. [CrossRef] [PubMed]

100. Tretter, L.; Patocs, A.; Chinopoulos, C. Succinate, an intermediate in metabolism, signal transduction, ROS, hypoxia, and tumorigenesis. *Biochim. Biophys. Acta* **2016**, *1857*, 1086–1101. [CrossRef] [PubMed]

101. Moschoi, R.; Imbert, V.; Nebout, M.; Chiche, J.; Mary, D.; Prebet, T.; Saland, E.; Castellano, R.; Pouyet, L.; Collette, Y.; et al. Protective mitochondrial transfer from bone marrow stromal cells to acute myeloid leukemic cells during chemotherapy. *Blood* **2016**, *128*, 253–264. [CrossRef] [PubMed]

102. Marlein, C.R.; Zaitseva, L.; Piddock, R.E.; Robinson, S.D.; Edwards, D.R.; Shafat, M.S.; Zhou, Z.; Lawes, M.; Bowles, K.M.; Rushworth, S.A. NADPH oxidase-2 derived superoxide drives mitochondrial transfer from bone marrow stromal cells to leukemic blasts. *Blood* **2017**, *130*, 1649–1660. [CrossRef] [PubMed]

103. Jackson, M.V.; Morrison, T.J.; Doherty, D.F.; McAuley, D.F.; Matthay, M.A.; Kissenpfennig, A.; O'Kane, C.M.; Krasnodembskaya, A.D. Mitochondrial transfer via tunneling nanotubes is an important mechanism by which mesenchymal stem cells enhance macrophage phagocytosis in the in vitro and in vivo models of ARDS. *Stem Cells* **2016**, *34*, 2210–2223. [CrossRef]

104. Islam, M.N.; Das, S.R.; Emin, M.T.; Wei, M.; Sun, L.; Westphalen, K.; Rowlands, D.J.; Quadri, S.K.; Bhattacharya, S.; Bhattacharya, J. Mitochondrial transfer from bone-marrow–derived stromal cells to pulmonary alveoli protects against acute lung injury. *Nat. Med.* **2012**, *18*, 759. [CrossRef]

105. Ahmad, T.; Mukherjee, S.; Pattnaik, B.; Kumar, M.; Singh, S.; Kumar, M.; Rehman, R.; Tiwari, B.K.; Jha, K.A.; Barhanpurkar, A.P.; et al. Miro1 regulates intercellular mitochondrial transport & enhances mesenchymal stem cell rescue efficacy. *EMBO J.* **2014**, *33*, 994–1010. [PubMed]

106. Masuzawa, A.; Black, K.M.; Pacak, C.A.; Ericsson, M.; Barnett, R.J.; Drumm, C.; Seth, P.; Bloch, D.B.; Levitsky, S.; Cowan, D.B.; et al. Transplantation of autologously derived mitochondria protects the heart from ischemia-reperfusion injury. *Am. J. Physiol. Heart Circ. Physiol.* **2013**, *304*, H966–H982. [CrossRef] [PubMed]

107. Zhang, Q.; Raoof, M.; Chen, Y.; Sumi, Y.; Sursal, T.; Junger, W.; Brohi, K.; Itagaki, K.; Hauser, C.J. Circulating mitochondrial DAMPs cause inflammatory responses to injury. *Nature* **2010**, *464*, 104. [CrossRef] [PubMed]

108. Boudreau, L.H.; Duchez, A.-C.; Cloutier, N.; Soulet, D.; Martin, N.; Bollinger, J.; Paré, A.; Rousseau, M.; Naika, G.S.; Lévesque, T.; et al. Platelets release mitochondria serving as substrate for bactericidal group IIA-secreted phospholipase A2 to promote inflammation. *Blood* **2014**, *124*, 2173–2183. [CrossRef] [PubMed]

109. Pasquier, J.; Guerrouahen, B.S.; Al Thawadi, H.; Ghiabi, P.; Maleki, M.; Abu-Kaoud, N.; Jacob, A.; Mirshahi, M.; Galas, L.; Rafii, S.; et al. Preferential transfer of mitochondria from endothelial to cancer cells through tunneling nanotubes modulates chemoresistance. *J. Transl. Med.* **2013**, *11*, 94. [CrossRef] [PubMed]

110. Antanavičiūtė, I.; Rysevaitė, K.; Liutkevičius, V.; Marandykina, A.; Rimkutė, L.; Sveikatienė, R.; Uloza, V.; Skeberdis, V.A. Long-Distance communication between laryngeal carcinoma cells. *PLoS ONE* **2014**, *9*, e99196. [CrossRef]

111. Searle, J.; Lawson, T.A.; Abbott, P.J.; Harmon, B.; Kerr, J.F.R. An electron-microscope study of the mode of cell death induced by cancer-chemotherapeutic agents in populations of proliferating normal and neoplastic cells. *J. Pathol.* **1975**, *116*, 129–138. [CrossRef]

112. Zitvogel, L.; Regnault, A.; Lozier, A.; Wolfers, J.; Flament, C.; Tenza, D.; Ricciardi-Castagnoli, P.; Raposo, G.; Amigorena, S. Eradication of established murine tumors using a novel cell-free vaccine: dendritic cell derived exosomes. *Nat. Med.* **1998**, *4*, 594. [CrossRef]

113. Wolfers, J.; Lozier, A.; Raposo, G.; Regnault, A.; Théry, C.; Masurier, C.; Flament, C.; Pouzieux, S.; Faure, F.; Tursz, T.; et al. Tumor-derived exosomes are a source of shared tumor rejection antigens for CTL cross-priming. *Nat. Med.* **2001**, *7*, 297. [CrossRef]

114. Théry, C.; Ostrowski, M.; Segura, E. Membrane vesicles as conveyors of immune responses. *Nat. Rev. Immunol.* **2009**, *9*, 581. [CrossRef]

115. Hessvik, N.P.; Llorente, A. Current knowledge on exosome biogenesis and release. *Cell. Mol. Life Sci.* **2018**, *75*, 193–208. [CrossRef] [PubMed]

116. Choi, D.-S.; Kim, D.-K.; Kim, Y.-K.; Gho, Y.S. Proteomics, transcriptomics and lipidomics of exosomes and ectosomes. *Proteomics* **2013**, *13*, 1554–1571. [CrossRef] [PubMed]

117. Whitham, M.; Parker, B.L.; Friedrichsen, M.; Hingst, J.R.; Hjorth, M.; Hughes, W.E.; Egan, C.L.; Cron, L.; Watt, K.I.; Kuchel, R.P.; et al. Extracellular vesicles provide a means for tissue crosstalk during exercise. *Cell Metab.* **2018**, *27*, 237–251.e4. [CrossRef] [PubMed]

118. Hirsova, P.; Ibrahim, S.H.; Krishnan, A.; Verma, V.K.; Bronk, S.F.; Werneburg, N.W.; Charlton, M.R.; Shah, V.H.; Malhi, H.; Gores, G.J. Lipid-induced signaling causes release of inflammatory extracellular vesicles from hepatocytes. *Gastroenterology* **2016**, *150*, 956–967. [CrossRef] [PubMed]

119. Crewe, C.; Joffin, N.; Rutkowski, J.M.; Kim, M.; Zhang, F.; Towler, D.A.; Gordillo, R.; Scherer, P.E. An endothelial-to-adipocyte extracellular vesicle axis governed by metabolic state. *Cell* **2018**, *175*, 695–708.e13. [CrossRef] [PubMed]

120. Thomou, T.; Mori, M.A.; Dreyfuss, J.M.; Konishi, M.; Sakaguchi, M.; Wolfrum, C.; Rao, T.N.; Winnay, J.N.; Garcia-Martin, R.; Grinspoon, S.K.; et al. Adipose-derived circulating miRNAs regulate gene expression in other tissues. *Nature* **2017**, *542*, 450. [CrossRef] [PubMed]

121. Murakami, T.; Horigome, H.; Tanaka, K.; Nakata, Y.; Ohkawara, K.; Katayama, Y.; Matsui, A. Impact of weight reduction on production of platelet-derived microparticles and fibrinolytic parameters in obesity. *Thromb. Res.* **2007**, *119*, 45–53. [CrossRef]

122. Eguchi, A.; Lazic, M.; Armando, A.M.; Phillips, S.A.; Katebian, R.; Maraka, S.; Quehenberger, O.; Sears, D.D.; Feldstein, A.E. Circulating adipocyte-derived extracellular vesicles are novel markers of metabolic stress. *J. Cell Mol. Med.* **2016**, *94*, 1241–1253. [CrossRef]

123. Heinrich, L.F.; Andersen, D.K.; Cleasby, M.E.; Lawson, C. Long-term high fat feeding of rats results in increased numbers of circulating microvesicles with pro-inflammatory effects on endothelial cells. *Br. J. Nutr.* **2015**, *113*, 1704–1711. [CrossRef]

124. Freeman, D.W.; Hooten, N.N.; Eitan, E.; Green, J.; Mode, N.A.; Bodogai, M.; Zhang, Y.; Lehrmann, E.; Zonderman, A.B.; Biragyn, A.; et al. Altered extracellular vesicle concentration, cargo and function in diabetes mellitus. *Diabetes* **2018**, *67*, 2377–2388. [CrossRef]

125. Hubal, M.J.; Nadler, E.P.; Ferrante, S.C.; Barberio, M.D.; Suh, J.-H.; Wang, J.; Dohm, G.L.; Pories, W.J.; Mietus-Snyder, M.; Freishtat, R.J. Circulating adipocyte-derived exosomal MicroRNAs associated with decreased insulin resistance after gastric bypass. *Obesity* **2017**, *25*, 102–110. [CrossRef] [PubMed]

126. Ying, W.; Riopel, M.; Bandyopadhyay, G.; Dong, Y.; Birmingham, A.; Seo, J.B.; Ofrecio, J.M.; Wollam, J.; Hernandez-Carretero, A.; Fu, W.; et al. Adipose tissue macrophage-derived exosomal miRNAs can modulate In Vivo and In Vitro insulin sensitivity. *Cell* **2017**, *171*, 372–384.e12. [CrossRef] [PubMed]

127. Pardo, F.; Villalobos-Labra, R.; Sobrevia, B.; Toledo, F.; Sobrevia, L. Extracellular vesicles in obesity and diabetes mellitus. *Mol. Aspects Med.* **2018**, *60*, 81–91. [CrossRef] [PubMed]

128. Deng, Z.-b.; Poliakov, A.; Hardy, R.W.; Clements, R.; Liu, C.; Liu, Y.; Wang, J.; Xiang, X.; Zhang, S.; Zhuang, X.; et al. Adipose tissue exosome-like vesicles mediate activation of macrophage-induced insulin resistance. *Diabetes* **2009**, *58*, 2498–2505. [CrossRef] [PubMed]

129. Müller, G. Microvesicles/exosomes as potential novel biomarkers of metabolic diseases. *Diabetes Metab. Syndr. Obes.* **2012**, *5*, 247–282. [CrossRef] [PubMed]

130. Neuspiel, M.; Schauss, A.C.; Braschi, E.; Zunino, R.; Rippstein, P.; Rachubinski, R.A.; Andrade-Navarro, M.A.; McBride, H.M. Cargo-selected transport from the mitochondria to peroxisomes is mediated by vesicular carriers. *Curr. Biol.* **2008**, *18*, 102–108. [CrossRef] [PubMed]

131. Soubannier, V.; McLelland, G.-L.; Zunino, R.; Braschi, E.; Rippstein, P.; Fon, E.A.; McBride, H.M. A vesicular transport pathway shuttles cargo from mitochondria to lysosomes. *Curr. Biol.* **2012**, *22*, 135–141. [CrossRef]

132. Soubannier, V.; Rippstein, P.; Kaufman, B.A.; Shoubridge, E.A.; McBride, H.M. Reconstitution of mitochondria derived vesicle formation demonstrates selective enrichment of oxidized cargo. *PLoS ONE* **2012**, *7*, e52830. [CrossRef]

133. McLelland, G.-L.; Soubannier, V.; Chen, C.X.; McBride, H.M.; Fon, E.A. Parkin and PINK1 function in a vesicular trafficking pathway regulating mitochondrial quality control. *EMBO J.* **2014**, *33*, 282–295. [CrossRef]

134. Raposo, G.; Stoorvogel, W. Extracellular vesicles: exosomes, microvesicles, and friends. *J. Cell Biol.* **2013**, *200*, 373–383. [CrossRef]

135. Lee, J.; Moon, P.; Lee, I.; Baek, M. Proteomic analysis of extracellular vesicles released by adipocytes of otsuka long-evans tokushima fatty (OLETF) rats. *Protein J.* **2015**, *34*, 220–235. [PubMed]

136. Szczesny, B.; Marcatti, M.; Ahmad, A.; Montalbano, M.; Brunyánszki, A.; Bibli, S.-I.; Papapetropoulos, A.; Szabo, C. Mitochondrial DNA damage and subsequent activation of Z-DNA binding protein 1 links oxidative stress to inflammation in epithelial cells. *Sci. Rep.* **2018**, *8*, 914. [PubMed]

137. Kannan, A.; Wells, R.B.; Sivakumar, S.; Komatsu, S.; Singh, K.P.; Samten, B.; Philley, J.V.; Sauter, E.R.; Ikebe, M.; Idell, S.; et al. Mitochondrial reprogramming regulates breast cancer progression. *Clin. Cancer Res.* **2016**, *22*, 3348–3360. [PubMed]

138. Phinney, D.G.; Di Giuseppe, M.; Njah, J.; Sala, E.; Shiva, S.; St Croix, C.M.; Stolz, D.B.; Watkins, S.C.; Di, Y.P.; Leikauf, G.D.; et al. Mesenchymal stem cells use extracellular vesicles to outsource mitophagy and shuttle microRNAs. *Nat. Commun.* **2015**, *6*, 8472. [PubMed]

139. Baixauli, F.; López-Otín, C.; Mittelbrunn, M. Exosomes and autophagy: coordinated mechanisms for the maintenance of cellular fitness. *Front. Immunol.* **2014**, *5*, 403. [PubMed]

140. Wang, J.; Liu, X.; Qiu, Y.; Shi, Y.; Cai, J.; Wang, B.; Wei, X.; Ke, Q.; Sui, X.; Wang, Y.; et al. Cell adhesion-mediated mitochondria transfer contributes to mesenchymal stem cell-induced chemoresistance on T cell acute lymphoblastic leukemia cells. *J. Hematol. Oncol.* **2018**, *11*, 11. [PubMed]

141. Haraszti, R.A.; Didiot, M.-C.; Sapp, E.; Leszyk, J.; Shaffer, S.A.; Rockwell, H.E.; Gao, F.; Narain, N.R.; DiFiglia, M.; Kiebish, M.A.; et al. High-resolution proteomic and lipidomic analysis of exosomes and microvesicles from different cell sources. *J. Extracell. Vesicles* **2016**, *5*, 32570. [PubMed]

142. Croston, T.L.; Shepherd, D.L.; Thapa, D.; Nichols, C.E.; Lewis, S.E.; Dabkowski, E.R.; Jagannathan, R.; Baseler, W.A.; Hollander, J.M. Evaluation of the cardiolipin biosynthetic pathway and its interactions in the diabetic heart. *Life Sci.* **2013**, *93*, 313–322.

143. Han, X.; Yang, J.; Yang, K.; Zhao, Z.; Abendschein, D.R.; Gross, R.W. Alterations in myocardial cardiolipin content and composition occur at the very earliest stages of diabetes: a shotgun lipidomics study. *Biochemistry* **2007**, *46*, 6417–6428.

144. Han, X.; Yang, J.; Cheng, H.; Yang, K.; Abendschein, D.R.; Gross, R.W. Shotgun lipidomics identifies cardiolipin depletion in diabetic myocardium linking altered substrate utilization with mitochondrial dysfunction. *Biochemistry* **2005**, *44*, 16684–16694.

145. Dolinsky, V.W.; Cole, L.K.; Sparagna, G.C.; Hatch, G.M. Cardiac mitochondrial energy metabolism in heart failure: Role of cardiolipin and sirtuins. *Biochim. Biophys. Acta* **2016**, *1861*, 1544–1554. [CrossRef] [PubMed]

146. Menshikova, E.V.; Ritov, V.B.; Dube, J.J.; Amati, F.; Stefanovic-Racic, M.; Toledo, F.G.S.; Coen, P.M.; Goodpaster, B.H. Calorie restriction-induced weight loss and exercise have differential effects on skeletal muscle mitochondria despite similar effects on insulin sensitivity. *J. Gerontol.* **2018**, *73*, 81–87. [CrossRef] [PubMed]

147. Li, J.; Romestaing, C.; Han, X.L.; Li, Y.A.; Hao, X.B.; Wu, Y.Y.; Sun, C.; Liu, X.L.; Jefferson, L.S.; Xiong, J.W.; et al. Cardiolipin remodeling by alcat1 links oxidative stress and mitochondrial dysfunction to obesity. *Cell Metab.* **2010**, *12*, 154–165. [CrossRef]

148. Xiao, M.; Zhong, H.; Xia, L.; Tao, Y.; Yin, H. Pathophysiology of mitochondrial lipid oxidation: Role of 4-hydroxynonenal (4-HNE) and other bioactive lipids in mitochondria. *Free Radic. Biol. Med.* **2017**, *111*, 316–327. [CrossRef] [PubMed]

149. Zhao, Z.; Zhang, X.; Zhao, C.; Choi, J.; Shi, J.; Song, K.; Turk, J.; Ma, Z.A. Protection of pancreatic beta-cells by group VIA phospholipase A(2)-mediated repair of mitochondrial membrane peroxidation. *Endocrinology* **2010**, *151*, 3038–3048. [CrossRef]

150. Stealing from the Body: How Cancer Recharges Its Batteries. Available online: https://www.uea.ac.uk/about/-/stealing-from-the-body-how-cancer-recharges-its-batteries (accessed on 1 September 2018).

151. Sansone, P.; Savini, C.; Kurelac, I.; Chang, Q.; Amato, L.B.; Strillacci, A.; Stepanova, A.; Iommarini, L.; Mastroleo, C.; Daly, L.; et al. Packaging and transfer of mitochondrial DNA via exosomes regulate escape from dormancy in hormonal therapy-resistant breast cancer. *Proc. Natl. Acad. Sci. USA* **2017**, *114*, E9066–E9075. [CrossRef] [PubMed]

152. Zhou, M.C.; Zhu, L.; Cui, X.; Feng, L.; Zhao, X.; He, S.; Ping, F.; Li, W.; Li, Y. Reduced peripheral blood mtDNA content is associated with impaired glucose-stimulated islet β cell function in a Chinese population with different degrees of glucose tolerance. *Diabetes Metab. Res. Rev.* **2016**, *32*, 768–774. [CrossRef] [PubMed]

153. Malik, A.N.; Parsade, C.K.; Ajaz, S.; Crosby-Nwaobi, R.; Gnudi, L.; Czajka, A.; Sivaprasad, S. Altered circulating mitochondrial DNA and increased inflammation in patients with diabetic retinopathy. *Diabetes Res. Clin. Pract.* **2015**, *110*, 257–265. [CrossRef] [PubMed]

154. Xu, F.X.; Zhou, X.; Shen, F.; Pang, R.; Liu, S.M. Decreased peripheral blood mitochondrial DNA content is related to HbA1c, fasting plasma glucose level and age of onset in Type 2 diabetes mellitus. *Diabet. Med.* **2012**, *29*, e47–e54. [CrossRef]

155. Oexle, K.; Oberle, J.; Finckh, B.; Kohlschütter, A.; Nagy, M.; Seibel, P.; Seissler, J.; Hübner, C. Islet cell antibodies in diabetes mellitus associated with a mitochondrial tRNALeu(UUR) gene mutation. *Exp. Clin. Endocrinol. Diabetes* **1996**, *104*, 212–217. [CrossRef]

156. Li, J.-Y.; Kong, K.-W.; Chang, M.-H.; Cheung, S.-C.; Lee, H.-C.; Pang, C.-Y.; Wei, Y.-H. MELAS syndrome associated with a tandem duplication in the D-loop of mitochondrial DNA. *Acta Neurol. Scand.* **1996**, *93*, 450–455. [CrossRef] [PubMed]

157. Boesch, P.; Weber-Lotfi, F.; Ibrahim, N.; Tarasenko, V.; Cosset, A.; Paulus, F.; Lightowlers, R.N.; Dietrich, A. DNA repair in organelles: Pathways, organization, regulation, relevance in disease and aging. *Biochim. Biophys. Acta* **2011**, *1813*, 186–200. [CrossRef] [PubMed]

158. Gilkerson, R. Commentary: Mitochondrial DNA damage and loss in diabetes. *Diabetes Metab. Res. Rev.* **2016**, *32*, 672–674. [CrossRef] [PubMed]

159. Guescini, M.; Genedani, S.; Stocchi, V.; Agnati, L.F. Astrocytes and Glioblastoma cells release exosomes carrying mtDNA. *J. Neural. Transm.* **2009**, *117*, 1. [CrossRef] [PubMed]

4

Mitochondrial Transport and Turnover in the Pathogenesis of Amyotrophic Lateral Sclerosis

Veronica Granatiero and Giovanni Manfredi *

Feil Family Brain and Mind Research Institute, Weill Cornell Medicine, 407 East 61st Street,
New York, NY 10065, USA; veg2003@med.cornell.edu
* Correspondence: gim2004@med.cornell.edu

Abstract: Neurons are high-energy consuming cells, heavily dependent on mitochondria for ATP generation and calcium buffering. These mitochondrial functions are particularly critical at specific cellular sites, where ionic currents impose a large energetic burden, such as at synapses. The highly polarized nature of neurons, with extremely large axoplasm relative to the cell body, requires mitochondria to be efficiently transported along microtubules to reach distant sites. Furthermore, neurons are post-mitotic cells that need to maintain pools of healthy mitochondria throughout their lifespan. Hence, mitochondrial transport and turnover are essential processes for neuronal survival and function. In neurodegenerative diseases, the maintenance of a healthy mitochondrial network is often compromised. Numerous lines of evidence indicate that mitochondrial impairment contributes to neuronal demise in a variety of neurodegenerative diseases, including amyotrophic lateral sclerosis (ALS), where degeneration of motor neurons causes a fatal muscle paralysis. Dysfunctional mitochondria accumulate in motor neurons affected by genetic or sporadic forms of ALS, strongly suggesting that the inability to maintain a healthy pool of mitochondria plays a pathophysiological role in the disease. This article critically reviews current hypotheses on mitochondrial involvement in the pathogenesis of ALS, focusing on the alterations of mitochondrial axonal transport and turnover in motor neurons.

Keywords: mitochondria; ALS; axonal transport; mitophagy; SOD1; Miro1; PINK1; Parkin

1. Introduction

Amyotrophic lateral sclerosis (ALS) is a devastating neurodegenerative disorder that causes the death of both upper and lower motor neurons. It is the most common among the motor neuron diseases. Loss of motor neurons results in muscle denervation leading to progressive muscle weakness, causing respiratory failure, difficulty in speaking and swallowing, and eventually paralysis and death, typically between one and five years from the time of disease onset [1]. There are currently no effective treatments for ALS, with only two food and drug administration (FDA) approved drugs, which only extend survival by a few months [2]. Approximately, 10% of ALS cases are due to genetic causes, the remaining 90% are sporadic with unknown etiology [3]. The last decade has brought tremendous advances in the understanding of ALS genetics with over 20 different genes identified that account for almost 80% of all familial forms [4].

The nature of the genes involved in ALS indicates that this is an etiologically heterogeneous disease [5] with a multiplicity of initiating factors that trigger diverse pathogenic pathways, ultimately converging in motor neuron toxicity. In the majority of genetic forms of ALS, motor neuron degeneration is accompanied by the involvement of other neural systems, frequently resulting in frontotemporal dementia (FTD). Some of the most prominent alterations observed in ALS/FTD involve protein homeostasis, autophagy, RNA metabolism, axonal transport and mitochondrial abnormalities [5–12].

Mitochondrial abnormalities have often been implicated as secondary mechanisms of disease, because until recently no genetic forms of ALS have been ascribed to mutations in nuclear or mitochondrial DNA encoded proteins. Only in 2014, the first mutation in a mitochondrial gene, coiled–coiled helix containing domain 10 have been identified in pedigrees presenting with ALS, FTD, and myopathy [13]. Despite the scarcity of primary mitochondrial forms of ALS, mitochondrial alterations can be caused by mutant proteins that are not exclusively localized in mitochondria. Notable examples are mutations in Cu, Zn superoxide dismutase (SOD1), the first genetic form of ALS identified [14], and TAR DNA-binding protein (TDP43, [15]).

While motor neurons are the most affected cells in ALS, studies on the pathophysiology of the disease have highlighted the importance of non-cell autonomous mechanisms, which implicate other cell types in the central nervous system. Glial cells, including astrocytes [16–18], oligodendrocytes [19], and microglia [20,21] play toxic roles in mutant SOD1 mouse models of ALS. Particularly in astrocytes, mitochondria can play a significant role in causing toxicity to motor neurons. For example, failure of astrocytes to clear synaptic glutamate as a result of altered mitochondrial glutamate intermediary metabolism, can trigger neuronal excitotoxicity.

Importantly, in ALS neurons mitochondrial alterations are accompanied by defects of organelle dynamics, involving fusion, fission, and transport [12]. These impairments result not only in morphologically and functionally defective mitochondria, but also in mislocalized mitochondrial network [22]. In excitable cells with large axoplasm, such as motor neurons, loss of viable mitochondria at sites of high energy demand, such as the synapses that motor neurons form with muscle (neuromuscular junctions, NMJ), can have catastrophic consequences leading to muscle denervation.

This review article focuses on the alterations of mitochondrial transport in neurons and the role of mitochondrial quality control mechanisms in ALS.

2. Mitochondrial Axonal Transport in ALS

2.1. The Mitochondrial Transport Machinery

In neurons, mitochondria are highly dynamic organelles. They are characterized by fast transport along neuronal axons, in both anterograde and retrograde directions (i.e., from the soma to the periphery and vice versa). Mitochondria from the soma are anterogradely transported to sites where metabolic demand is high, such as the synapse [23,24], while retrograde transport provides essential information regarding the status and environment of distal sites. Thus, mitochondrial transport plays an essential role in maintaining healthy motor neurons, and alterations of rate-limiting components of the mitochondrial transport machinery may cause an imbalance of mitochondrial distribution in neurons. Furthermore, as active lysosomes are mostly localized in the soma, damaged mitochondria in axons are engulfed in autophagosomes and retro-transported to the soma to be degraded upon fusion with lysosomes [25]. Defective retrograde transport of autophagosomes could result in a delay of mitochondrial autophagy (mitophagy) fluxes and accumulation of damaged mitochondria. Thus, axonal transport and mitophagy are intimately interconnected processes.

For long-range axonal transport mitochondria move along microtubules. The kinesin superfamily of proteins and cytoplasmic dynein are the main microtubule-based motor proteins. They drive long distance transport of mitochondria and other membranous organelles through ATP-dependent mechanisms [26]. In axons, cytoplasmic dynein is responsible for the retrograde transport, moving mitochondria towards the soma, whereas kinesin drives anterograde mitochondrial transport from the soma to distal axonal regions and synaptic terminals. In dendritic spines, where microtubules exhibit mixed polarity in proximal regions, kinesin and dynein motors can transport mitochondria in either direction, depending on the microtubule polarity [26,27]. There are two main mechanisms by which molecular motors connect with their cargoes, direct linkage through cargo motor proteins or indirect linkage via linker/adaptor molecules. Several adaptor complexes have been identified, which ensure a precise regulation of mitochondrial motility. Among them, the best studied linkers are Milton and

Miro, first identified in Drosophila. Milton is a kinesin heavy chain-binding protein. In mammals, there are two Milton orthologues, TRAK1 and 2. Milton is linked indirectly with the mitochondrial outer membrane through interaction with an atypical Rho GTPase, Miro. Mammals have 2 orthologues of Miro (Miro1 and 2) [28,29]. Together Miro, Milton and kinesin provide mitochondria-specific axonal transport mechanisms.

The ATP/ADP ratio is part of the signaling involved in regulating mitochondrial transport. In regions with high ATP level, mitochondrial velocity increases, while upon ATP depletion mitochondrial velocity decreases [30]. Another important signal is provided by neuronal Ca^{2+} concentration. Miro contains two Ca^{2+}-sensitive helix-loop-helix structural domain, also called EF hand motifs, facing the cytosolic side, which sense cytosolic Ca^{2+} levels. Two different mechanisms have been proposed to explain how Miro regulates mitochondrial motility in a Ca^{2+}-dependent manner. According to the "motor-Miro binding" model, when Ca^{2+} around mitochondria is low, the C-terminal tail of kinesin is bound to the mitochondrion through its interaction with the Milton–Miro complex, thereby allowing for mitochondrial transport. When Ca^{2+} is high, it binds to Miro EF hands, causing a conformational change that results in the direct interaction of kinesin with Miro, which prevents mitochondrial movement [31]. According to the "motor-releasing model", upon Ca^{2+} increase, Miro remains attached to Milton and the mitochondrion, but dissociates from the kinesin, thereby arresting mitochondrial transport [32].

2.2. Alterations of the Mitochondrial Transport Machinery in ALS

There are two main hypotheses on the process of motor neuron degeneration in ALS, the "dying-forward" and the "dying-back" hypotheses. The former proposes that ALS is mainly a cortical motor neuron disorder, which mediates anterograde degeneration of anterior horn cells via glutamate excitotoxicity [33]. On the other hand, the "dying-back" hypothesis proposes that motor neurons degeneration in ALS starts distally at the nerve terminal or at the NMJ and progresses towards the soma [34]. In support to the latter, it was shown that early degeneration of the NMJ precedes the loss of neurons in the spinal cord of mutant SOD1 mice [35,36]. Mitochondrial transport abnormalities could significantly contribute to dying-back processes, because the distal regions of motor neurons may not be appropriately supplied with healthy, functional mitochondria, while damaged mitochondria may not be correctly turned over. A significant body of evidence points towards a causal relationship between deficits in axonal transport and degeneration of susceptible motor neurons in ALS [37,38]. For example, defects in neuronal mitochondrial morphology and axonal mitochondrial transport have been demonstrated in primary neuronal cultures from ALS mouse models [12,39,40]. Importantly, these abnormalities have also been observed in vivo in mutant SOD1 and TDP-43 ALS mouse models [41,42] and in Drosophila models [43]. Other studies in primary neuronal cultures and in vivo demonstrated that mutant FUS, a RNA-binding protein causative of familial ALS/FTD [44], induces motor neuron degeneration preceded by abnormalities in synaptic transmission [45] and mitochondrial abnormalities at the NMJ [46]. The common denominator of these studies was the finding that mitochondrial abnormalities and the impairment of mitochondrial axonal transport precede motor neuron degeneration. This evidence supports the "dying-back" hypothesis [34,47,48], in which mitochondrial transport abnormalities may play an instrumental role. Indeed, in mutant SOD1 mice deficits in bidirectional transport of mitochondria are described at the pre-symptomatic disease stage [49], suggesting that these alterations play an early causative role in NMJ degeneration.

The causes of mitochondrial transport abnormalities in ALS motor neurons are not fully understood. In some cases, alterations of the axonal transport machinery are directly involved. For example, studies suggest that SOD1 mutations impair dynein functions, as mutant SOD1 directly interacts with the dynein–dynactin complex, forming aggregates in the spinal cord and sciatic nerve of SOD1 transgenic mice [50,51]. Furthermore, a large body of evidence in models of familial ALS with mutations in SOD1 or TDP-43 indicates that mitochondrial damage and dysfunction is the result of the pathological accumulation of aggregated mutant proteins inside or on the surface of mitochondria [42,52–58].

Therefore, another possibility is that ALS mutant proteins damage mitochondria and impair their bioenergetics [59–61], thereby decreasing ATP availability for axonal transport. This is an attractive hypothesis, because it could provide a mechanism whereby unhealthy mitochondria are immobilized to facilitate their removal by autophagy, similar to the Ca^{2+} dependent mitochondrial arrest described above [31,32]. While it was shown that ATP levels affect mitochondrial motility [30], to our knowledge, the question of whether subpopulations of energy defective mitochondria have a selective decrease in transport, has not been addressed experimentally. This could be achieved, for example, by causing a mild impairment in ATP synthesis in a targeted subset of mitochondria in the neuronal soma and tracking their movement to neuronal processes over time, in comparison with healthy mitochondria.

Although long-range mitochondrial transport is microtubule-based, short range movement in presynaptic terminals and dendritic spines, where actin filaments form the cytoskeletal architecture, is mediated by actin-myosin motors. In cultured neurons, axonal mitochondria have been shown to travel along microtubules and actin microfilaments with different velocities and mechanisms [62]. The actin cytoskeleton is especially relevant to motor neuron diseases with altered actin dynamics [63]. Profilin1 (PFN1) is one of four isoforms of profilin, and the first actin-binding protein associated with familial ALS [64]. Initial studies suggested that the main function of profilin was to sequester actin monomers, thereby inhibiting F-actin formation [65,66]. However, later studies revealed that the amount of profilin present in cells is not sufficient to sequester abundant actin monomers, and a different function for profilin was proposed, as a catalytic converter for actin monomer recycling [67,68]. There are several hypotheses on the pathogenic mechanisms of mutant PFN1 in ALS. Both gain and loss of function have been proposed. The former is based on mutant PFN1 forming aggregates in motor neurons [69,70]. The latter on studies showing that mutant PFN1 causes the formation of cavities in its protein core structure, compromising protein stability and leading to misfolding and degradation [71]. Motor neurons of mutant PFN1 transgenic mice show aggregation of the protein and disruption of the actin cytoskeleton, accompanied by elevated ubiquitin and p62/SQSTM levels in motor neurons [72]. Another transgenic mouse model of mutant PFN1 revealed alterations of actin dynamics and reduced filamentous versus globular actin ratio [73]. Although mitochondrial transport and turnover have not yet been investigated in these mouse models, alterations in mitochondrial ultrastructure was reported in motor neuron axons [73], suggesting that cytoskeletal alterations in these mice affect mitochondria, possibly through impairment of their dynamics.

Myosins allow for cargo movement along actin cytoskeleton. Myo19 is the only myosin localized to mitochondria, and plays a physiological role in mitochondrial movement under conditions of glucose-starvation [74]. Recently, a new intersection point between microtubule-dependent and actin-dependent mitochondrial movement was described through Miro [75,76]. It was shown that, upon activation of pathways of mitochondrial degradation, Myo19 was digested together with Miro, thereby regulating mitochondrial movement and distribution. These findings raise the possibility that detachment of mitochondria from the actin cytoskeleton may be an important step in altering mitochondrial transport. Together these findings strongly suggest that microtubule- and actin-dependent mitochondrial transport mechanisms may be connected and that both mechanisms could be dysregulated in ALS.

3. Mitochondrial Turnover in ALS

3.1. Mitochondrial Quality Control Mechanisms

Mitochondrial quality control (MQC) is an important process in cellular homeostasis. Mitochondria with loss of membrane potential or subject to protein oxidation and misfolding become targets of MQC. There are three main known pathways of MQC: Protein degradation, vesicular degradation, and mitophagy. The first involves proteostatic selective elimination of damaged proteins. Mitochondria have internal proteases, such as the AAA-protease complex of the inner membrane [77] and the Lon protease of the matrix [78]. Mitochondria are also endowed with their own unfolded protein response, which is activated when misfolded proteins accumulate in the matrix [79] or in the intermembrane space [80]. Mitochondria rely on the cytosolic ubiquitin-proteasome system to eliminate damaged proteins destined to the outer membrane or in the case of the intermembrane space, before they engage in the mitochondrial import pathway [81,82]. Ubiquitin-ligases, such as Parkin, ubiquitinate oxidized or misfolded outer membrane proteins [83]. Parkin recruitment has been ascribed to the kinase PINK1, following its incomplete processing and import across the outer membrane of depolarized mitochondria [84–86]. Instead, maintenance of Parkin cytosolic localization has been attributed to its interaction with cleaved PINK1 released in the cytosol after processing by healthy mitochondria [87]. If its degradation fails in damaged mitochondria, PINK1 phosphorylates ubiquitin residues and Parkin, thereby activating a cascade of ubiquitination of outer membrane proteins [88]. Ubiquitination of outer membrane proteins is not exclusively performed by Parkin, as it can also be carried out by resident outer membrane ligases, such as MULAN [89] and MITOL/MARCH5, which ubiquitinate outer membrane proteins involved in mitochondrial fusion, Mfn1 and Mfn2, and fission, Drp1 [90,91]. Interestingly, MARCH5 ubiquitinates and increases the turnover of mutant SOD1 on the outer membrane [92].

Ubiquitination of outer membrane proteins is one of the best characterized signals for the activation of mitophagy and the regulation of mitochondrial motility through degradation of proteins involved in mitochondrial fusion/fission and transport (reviewed in [93]). Fragmentation of the network and immobilization facilitate the engulfment of damaged mitochondria in autophagic vesicles. The regulation of PINK1 by phosphorylation of specific amino acid residues [94] could provide an additional link between energetic defects in unhealthy mitochondria and the activation of MQC. What drives the switch from proteostasis to mitophagy is unclear, but the extent of mitochondrial damage is likely a discriminating factor: When proteostasis cannot repair mitochondria, mitophagy ensues. However, in some cases, a Parkin-dependent vesicular degradation of sections of mitochondrial membranes containing oxidized proteins, can be sufficient to repair the damage and prevent full-blown mitophagy [95]. Mitophagy involves ubiquitin-binding adaptors that recruit mitochondria to the autophagosome by binding to LC3 [88].

3.2. Mitochondrial Quality Control in ALS

The best characterized MQC pathway is mediated by the activation of PINK1 and Parkin [96]. Impairment of MQC is most commonly linked to Parkinson's disease, due to the discovery of inactivating mutations of these proteins in recessive forms of the disease [97–99]. However, MQC disturbances have also been associated with ALS, for example through the involvement of the mitophagy adaptor optineurin, which has been found to be mutated in familial forms of the disease [100]. Optineurin plays a role in PINK1-Parkin mediated mitophagy. After Parkin recruitment to the outer membrane, optineurin binds to ubiquitinated mitochondria, inducing autophagosome nucleation through LC3 recruitment [101]. ALS-associated optineurin mutations cause mitochondrial clearance impairment [102]. The link between optineurin and LC3, which finalizes autophagic clearance of damaged mitochondria, is Tank-binding kinase (TBK1). It was reported that TBK1 interacts with optineurin and by phosphorylating it at specific serine residues regulates its ability to bind to ubiquitinated mitochondrial proteins [103]. Therefore, TBK1-mediated phosphorylation of optineurin amplifies and reinforces mitophagy. As a consequence, inhibition or depletion of TBK1 delays mitophagy, resulting in accumulation of damaged mitochondria [104]. TBK1 mutations have been causally linked to familial forms of ALS [105], further reinforcing the relevance of MQC in ALS pathophysiology. Mutations in two additional genes involved in mitophagy were reported in familial ALS, p62 and VCP. p62/SQSTMQ1 is an adaptor for the binding of ubiquitin to LC3, recruiting mitochondria to the autophagosome [106,107]. Valosin-containing protein (VCP) is an ATPase with segregase activity, which can extract ubiquitinated proteins from organelle membranes and target them to proteasomal degradation [108]. Parkin-mediated outer membrane protein ubiquitination recruit VCP to mitochondria [109]. Mutations in VCP are associated with ALS [110]. VCP mutations cause mitochondrial structural changes in transgenic mice, and loss of VCP impairs the clearance of damaged mitochondria [109]. Overall, the genetics of familial ALS strongly emphasizes the relevance of MQC in disease pathogenesis.

Mitochondrial damage with loss of mitochondrial membrane potential may result in Parkin-mediated degradation of Miro [111]. Furthermore, it was reported that PINK1 directly interacts with Miro and Milton [112], and that it phosphorylates Miro in response to mitochondrial damage, thereby promoting its interaction with Parkin and its degradation [113]. Interestingly, Miro is decreased in ALS models [114,115], which may contribute to impairing mitochondrial axonal transport. Moreover, Miro overexpression in mutant SOD1 neurons restores mitochondrial axonal transport deficits [116]. Taken together, these data point to a role for Miro as a converging point between the mechanisms regulating MQC and axonal transport.

The actin cytoskeleton emerges as an additional converging point between mitochondrial turnover and mitochondrial motility. A recent study showed that, after Parkin recruitment to depolarized mitochondria, F-actin encapsulates damaged mitochondria through myosin VI (MYO6) complexing with Parkin [117]. Hence, damaged mitochondria are completely isolated from the rest of the mitochondrial network, and are prevented from fusing with healthy mitochondria. They also showed that lack of MYO6 induces accumulation of damaged mitochondria, because of a severe impairment in the clearance machinery, highlighting the importance of actin-related players in MQC and maintenance of mitochondrial homeostasis.

The therapeutic value of modulating autophagy and mitophagy in ALS is the object of debate. Stimulation of autophagy was attempted mostly in the SOD1 mouse model, using both pharmacological and genetic approaches [118–123]. There were discrepancies in the outcomes, with either beneficial or detrimental effects. This divergence of results could derive from the different approaches used and their effects on different central nervous system (CNS) cell types. A genetic approach to test the cell type specificity of autophagy modulation was implemented by deleting the critical autophagy gene Atg7 specifically in motor neurons of mutant SOD1 mice [124]. Autophagy inhibition accelerated early neuromuscular denervation and the onset of motor symptoms. Surprisingly, removal of Atg7 also extended the lifespan of the animals. The authors proposed that motor neuron autophagy contributes to maintaining neuromuscular innervation early on, but later causes a non-cell-autonomous effect that promotes disease progression. Although mitophagy was not investigated specifically, the findings raise the intriguing possibility of a phase-dependent involvement of MQC in ALS progression.

Mitophagy induction in ALS is supported by the finding of LC3 II increase in neurons of mutant SOD1 mice [125,126], accompanied by the accumulation of p62 and optineurin [115,127]. Furthermore, an increase in mitochondria-containing autophagosomes and autophagolysosomes was described in human ALS spinal cord [128]. Currently, there are no pharmaceutical approaches to selectively modulate MQC in ALS. However, it is possible to target genetically the main components of the machinery, such as Parkin. Interestingly, a progressive decrease in Parkin levels was documented in both cellular and animal models of ALS [115,129,130], suggesting that chronic activation of MQC secondary to mitochondrial damage causes Parkin depletion. In cultured ALS neurons, it was demonstrated that Parkin is responsible for Miro degradation and actively contributes to mitochondrial transport impairment [116]. Overexpression of Miro or ablation of PINK1 rescued the mitochondrial axonal transport deficits. However, genetic constitutive ablation of Parkin in mutant SOD1 mice delayed the decline of Miro and other components of the mitochondrial dynamics machinery, and resulted in a significant delay of neuromuscular degeneration and extension of lifespan [115]. Taken together, these findings support the notion that MQC is involved in ALS pathophysiology. Importantly, they also show that autophagy, and specifically MQC, may be a double-edge sword, with initial protective effects, which can become maladaptive and detrimental in the chronic phase of the disease.

4. Conclusions

Mitochondrial dynamics, axonal transport, and MQC are tightly intertwined processes that play a fundamental role in the homeostasis of neuronal mitochondrial network, in health and disease.

The genetics of familial ALS strongly suggest that these processes are affected during the course of the disease. Figure 1 summarizes the main molecular players of mitochondrial transport and turnover, whose alterations have been proposed to participate in ALS pathogenesis. More work is needed to achieve a detailed mechanistic understanding of the pathogenic pathways linking mitochondria transport and turnover with mitochondrial dysfunction and motor neuron degeneration in ALS. In particular, whether altered MQC in ALS motor neurons is the cause or the consequence of impaired mitochondrial function remains to be elucidated. Nevertheless, a wealth of clues indicate that alterations of these processes can be disease initiators or disease modifiers, with potentially interesting therapeutic implications. Studies focused on these important aspects of ALS pathophysiology will unveil novel disease mechanisms that could be addressed therapeutically by targeted approaches aimed at modulating mitochondrial transport and MQC through pharmacological intervention.

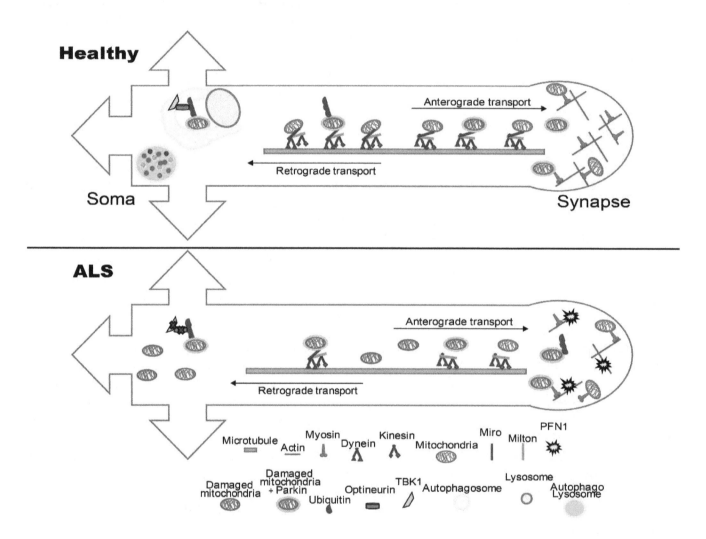

Figure 1. Schematic representation of key players in mitochondrial transport and turnover in healthy and amyotrophic lateral sclerosis (ALS) neurons. Mitochondria are transported in axons along microtubule tracks by dynein and kinesins, which are connected to mitochondria through cargo adaptors Milton and Miro. In ALS axons, the interactions between mitochondria and microtubules are disrupted, resulting in impaired transport. At synapses, mitochondria interact with the actin cytoskeleton, and mutations in proteins involved in actin dynamics, such as PFN1, can alter mitochondrial localization at this neuronal site. Ubiquitination of unhealthy mitochondria by Ub-ligases, such as Parkin, target mitochondria for degradation through the autophagy pathway. TBK1 and optineurin promote PINK1-Parkin ubiquitination of mitochondrial dynamics proteins, such as Miro. In ALS neurons, the quality control mechanisms are affected by dysfunction occurring at various steps of the mitophagy process.

References

1. Hardiman, O.; van den Berg, L.H.; Kiernan, M.C. Clinical diagnosis and management of amyotrophic lateral sclerosis. *Nat. Rev. Neurol.* **2011**, *7*, 639–649. [CrossRef]

2. De Vos, K.J.; Hafezparast, M. Neurobiology of axonal transport defects in motor neuron diseases: Opportunities for translational research? *Neurobiol. Dis.* **2017**, *105*, 283–299. [CrossRef]

3. Emery, A.E.; Holloway, S. Familial motor neuron diseases. *Adv. Neurol.* **1982**, *36*, 139–147. [PubMed]

4. Cirulli, E.T.; Lasseigne, B.N.; Petrovski, S.; Sapp, P.C.; Dion, P.A.; Leblond, C.S.; Couthouis, J.; Lu, Y.F.; Wang, Q.; Krueger, B.J.; et al. Exome sequencing in amyotrophic lateral sclerosis identifies risk genes and pathways. *Science* **2015**, *347*, 1436–1441. [CrossRef]

5. Taylor, J.P.; Brown, R.H., Jr.; Cleveland, D.W. Decoding ALS: From genes to mechanism. *Nature* **2016**, *539*, 197–206. [CrossRef]

6. Andrus, P.K.; Fleck, T.J.; Gurney, M.E.; Hall, E.D. Protein oxidative damage in a transgenic mouse model of familial amyotrophic lateral sclerosis. *J. Neurochem.* **1998**, *71*, 2041–2048. [CrossRef]

7. Wood, J.D.; Beaujeux, T.P.; Shaw, P.J. Protein aggregation in motor neurone disorders. *Neuropathol. Appl. Neurobiol.* **2003**, *29*, 529–545. [CrossRef]

8. Chang, Y.; Kong, Q.; Shan, X.; Tian, G.; Ilieva, H.; Cleveland, D.W.; Rothstein, J.D.; Borchelt, D.R.; Wong, P.C.; Lin, C.L. Messenger RNA oxidation occurs early in disease pathogenesis and promotes motor neuron degeneration in ALS. *PLoS ONE* **2008**, *3*, e2849. [CrossRef] [PubMed]

9. Shaw, P.J.; Ince, P.G.; Falkous, G.; Mantle, D. Oxidative damage to protein in sporadic motor neuron disease spinal cord. *Ann. Neurol.* **1995**, *38*, 691–695. [CrossRef] [PubMed]

10. Wiedemann, F.R.; Manfredi, G.; Mawrin, C.; Beal, M.F.; Schon, E.A. Mitochondrial DNA and respiratory chain function in spinal cords of ALS patients. *J. Neurochem.* **2002**, *80*, 616–625. [CrossRef]

11. Sasaki, S.; Iwata, M. Mitochondrial alterations in the spinal cord of patients with sporadic amyotrophic lateral sclerosis. *J. Neuropathol. Exp. Neurol.* **2007**, *66*, 10–16. [CrossRef] [PubMed]

12. De Vos, K.J.; Chapman, A.L.; Tennant, M.E.; Manser, C.; Tudor, E.L.; Lau, K.F.; Brownlees, J.; Ackerley, S.; Shaw, P.J.; McLoughlin, D.M.; et al. Familial amyotrophic lateral sclerosis-linked SOD1 mutants perturb fast axonal transport to reduce axonal mitochondria content. *Hum. Mol. Genet.* **2007**, *16*, 2720–2728. [CrossRef]

13. Bannwarth, S.; Ait-El-Mkadem, S.; Chaussenot, A.; Genin, E.C.; Lacas-Gervais, S.; Fragaki, K.; Berg-Alonso, L.; Kageyama, Y.; Serre, V.; Moore, D.G.; et al. A mitochondrial origin for frontotemporal dementia and amyotrophic lateral sclerosis through CHCHD10 involvement. *Brain J. Neurol.* **2014**, *137*, 2329–2345. [CrossRef]

14. Rosen, D.R.; Siddique, T.; Patterson, D.; Figlewicz, D.A.; Sapp, P.; Hentati, A.; Donaldson, D.; Goto, J.; O'Regan, J.P.; Deng, H.X.; et al. Mutations in Cu/Zn superoxide dismutase gene are associated with familial amyotrophic lateral sclerosis. *Nature* **1993**, *362*, 59–62. [CrossRef] [PubMed]

15. Sreedharan, J.; Blair, I.P.; Tripathi, V.B.; Hu, X.; Vance, C.; Rogelj, B.; Ackerley, S.; Durnall, J.C.; Williams, K.L.; Buratti, E.; et al. TDP-43 mutations in familial and sporadic amyotrophic lateral sclerosis. *Science* **2008**, *319*, 1668–1672. [CrossRef]

16. Yamanaka, K.; Chun, S.J.; Boillee, S.; Fujimori-Tonou, N.; Yamashita, H.; Gutmann, D.H.; Takahashi, R.; Misawa, H.; Cleveland, D.W. Astrocytes as determinants of disease progression in inherited amyotrophic lateral sclerosis. *Nat. Neurosci.* **2008**, *11*, 251–253. [CrossRef] [PubMed]

17. Nagai, M.; Re, D.B.; Nagata, T.; Chalazonitis, A.; Jessell, T.M.; Wichterle, H.; Przedborski, S. Astrocytes expressing ALS-linked mutated SOD1 release factors selectively toxic to motor neurons. *Nat. Neurosci.* **2007**, *10*, 615–622. [CrossRef] [PubMed]

18. Ferraiuolo, L.; Higginbottom, A.; Heath, P.R.; Barber, S.; Greenald, D.; Kirby, J.; Shaw, P.J. Dysregulation of astrocyte-motoneuron cross-talk in mutant superoxide dismutase 1-related amyotrophic lateral sclerosis. *Brain J. Neurol.* **2011**, *134*, 2627–2641. [CrossRef] [PubMed]

19. Yamanaka, K.; Boillee, S.; Roberts, E.A.; Garcia, M.L.; McAlonis-Downes, M.; Mikse, O.R.; Cleveland, D.W.; Goldstein, L.S. Mutant SOD1 in cell types other than motor neurons and oligodendrocytes accelerates onset of disease in ALS mice. *Proc. Natl. Acad. Sci. USA* **2008**, *105*, 7594–7599. [CrossRef] [PubMed]

20. Di Giorgio, F.P.; Carrasco, M.A.; Siao, M.C.; Maniatis, T.; Eggan, K. Non-cell autonomous effect of glia on motor neurons in an embryonic stem cell-based ALS model. *Nat. Neurosci.* **2007**, *10*, 608–614. [CrossRef]

21. Sargsyan, S.A.; Monk, P.N.; Shaw, P.J. Microglia as potential contributors to motor neuron injury in amyotrophic lateral sclerosis. *Glia* **2005**, *51*, 241–253. [CrossRef] [PubMed]

22. Vande Velde, C.; McDonald, K.K.; Boukhedimi, Y.; McAlonis-Downes, M.; Lobsiger, C.S.; Bel Hadj, S.; Zandona, A.; Julien, J.P.; Shah, S.B.; Cleveland, D.W. Misfolded SOD1 associated with motor neuron mitochondria alters mitochondrial shape and distribution prior to clinical onset. *PLoS ONE* **2011**, *6*, e22031. [CrossRef] [PubMed]

23. Hollenbeck, P.J.; Saxton, W.M. The axonal transport of mitochondria. *J. Cell Sci.* **2005**, *118*, 5411–5419. [CrossRef] [PubMed]

24. Kang, J.S.; Tian, J.H.; Pan, P.Y.; Zald, P.; Li, C.; Deng, C.; Sheng, Z.H. Docking of axonal mitochondria by syntaphilin controls their mobility and affects short-term facilitation. *Cell* **2008**, *132*, 137–148. [CrossRef] [PubMed]

25. Maday, S.; Holzbaur, E.L. Autophagosome assembly and cargo capture in the distal axon. *Autophagy* **2012**, *8*, 858–860. [CrossRef]

26. Hirokawa, N.; Niwa, S.; Tanaka, Y. Molecular motors in neurons: Transport mechanisms and roles in brain function, development, and disease. *Neuron* **2010**, *68*, 610–638. [CrossRef] [PubMed]

27. Sheng, Z.H.; Cai, Q. Mitochondrial transport in neurons: Impact on synaptic homeostasis and neurodegeneration. *Nat. Rev. Neurosci.* **2012**, *13*, 77–93. [CrossRef]

28. Fransson, A.; Ruusala, A.; Aspenstrom, P. Atypical Rho GTPases have roles in mitochondrial homeostasis and apoptosis. *J. Biol. Chem.* **2003**, *278*, 6495–6502. [CrossRef]

29. Fransson, S.; Ruusala, A.; Aspenstrom, P. The atypical Rho GTPases Miro-1 and Miro-2 have essential roles in mitochondrial trafficking. *Biochem. Biophys. Res. Commun.* **2006**, *344*, 500–510. [CrossRef]

30. Mironov, S.L. ADP regulates movements of mitochondria in neurons. *Biophys. J.* **2007**, *92*, 2944–2952. [CrossRef]

31. Wang, X.; Schwarz, T.L. The mechanism of Ca^{2+}-dependent regulation of kinesin-mediated mitochondrial motility. *Cell* **2009**, *136*, 163–174. [CrossRef]

32. Macaskill, A.F.; Rinholm, J.E.; Twelvetrees, A.E.; Arancibia-Carcamo, I.L.; Muir, J.; Fransson, A.; Aspenstrom, P.; Attwell, D.; Kittler, J.T. Miro1 is a calcium sensor for glutamate receptor-dependent localization of mitochondria at synapses. *Neuron* **2009**, *61*, 541–555. [CrossRef]

33. Eisen, A.; Weber, M. The motor cortex and amyotrophic lateral sclerosis. *Muscle Nerve* **2001**, *24*, 564–573. [CrossRef]

34. Kiernan, M.C.; Vucic, S.; Cheah, B.C.; Turner, M.R.; Eisen, A.; Hardiman, O.; Burrell, J.R.; Zoing, M.C. Amyotrophic lateral sclerosis. *Lancet* **2011**, *377*, 942–955. [CrossRef]

35. Fischer, L.R.; Culver, D.G.; Tennant, P.; Davis, A.A.; Wang, M.; Castellano-Sanchez, A.; Khan, J.; Polak, M.A.; Glass, J.D. Amyotrophic lateral sclerosis is a distal axonopathy: Evidence in mice and man. *Exp. Neurol.* **2004**, *185*, 232–240. [CrossRef]

36. Martineau, E.; Di Polo, A.; Vande Velde, C.; Robitaille, R. Dynamic neuromuscular remodeling precedes motor-unit loss in a mouse model of ALS. *eLife* **2018**, *7*. [CrossRef]

37. De Vos, K.J.; Grierson, A.J.; Ackerley, S.; Miller, C.C. Role of axonal transport in neurodegenerative diseases. *Annu. Rev. Neurosci.* **2008**, *31*, 151–173. [CrossRef]

38. Morfini, G.A.; Burns, M.; Binder, L.I.; Kanaan, N.M.; LaPointe, N.; Bosco, D.A.; Brown, R.H., Jr.; Brown, H.; Tiwari, A.; Hayward, L.; et al. Axonal transport defects in neurodegenerative diseases. *J. Neurosci. Off. J. Soc. Neurosci.* **2009**, *29*, 12776–12786. [CrossRef]

39. Wang, W.; Li, L.; Lin, W.L.; Dickson, D.W.; Petrucelli, L.; Zhang, T.; Wang, X. The ALS disease-associated mutant TDP-43 impairs mitochondrial dynamics and function in motor neurons. *Hum. Mol. Genet.* **2013**, *22*, 4706–4719. [CrossRef]

40. Magrane, J.; Sahawneh, M.A.; Przedborski, S.; Estevez, A.G.; Manfredi, G. Mitochondrial dynamics and bioenergetic dysfunction is associated with synaptic alterations in mutant SOD1 motor neurons. *J. Neurosci. Off. J. Soc. Neurosci.* **2012**, *32*, 229–242. [CrossRef]

41. Marinkovic, P.; Reuter, M.S.; Brill, M.S.; Godinho, L.; Kerschensteiner, M.; Misgeld, T. Axonal transport deficits and degeneration can evolve independently in mouse models of amyotrophic lateral sclerosis. *Proc. Natl. Acad. Sci. USA* **2012**, *109*, 4296–4301. [CrossRef] [PubMed]

42. Magrane, J.; Cortez, C.; Gan, W.B.; Manfredi, G. Abnormal mitochondrial transport and morphology are common pathological denominators in SOD1 and TDP43 ALS mouse models. *Hum. Mol. Genet.* **2014**, *23*, 1413–1424. [CrossRef] [PubMed]

43. Shahidullah, M.; Le Marchand, S.J.; Fei, H.; Zhang, J.; Pandey, U.B.; Dalva, M.B.; Pasinelli, P.; Levitan, I.B. Defects in synapse structure and function precede motor neuron degeneration in Drosophila models of FUS-related ALS. *J. Neurosci. Off. J. Soc. Neurosci.* **2013**, *33*, 19590–19598. [CrossRef] [PubMed]

44. Kwiatkowski, T.J., Jr.; Bosco, D.A.; Leclerc, A.L.; Tamrazian, E.; Vanderburg, C.R.; Russ, C.; Davis, A.; Gilchrist, J.; Kasarskis, E.J.; Munsat, T.; et al. Mutations in the FUS/TLS gene on chromosome 16 cause familial amyotrophic lateral sclerosis. *Science* **2009**, *323*, 1205–1208. [CrossRef] [PubMed]

45. Sharma, A.; Lyashchenko, A.K.; Lu, L.; Nasrabady, S.E.; Elmaleh, M.; Mendelsohn, M.; Nemes, A.; Tapia, J.C.; Mentis, G.Z.; Shneider, N.A. ALS-associated mutant FUS induces selective motor neuron degeneration through toxic gain of function. *Nat. Commun.* **2016**, *7*, 10465. [CrossRef] [PubMed]

46. So, E.; Mitchell, J.C.; Memmi, C.; Chennell, G.; Vizcay-Barrena, G.; Allison, L.; Shaw, C.E.; Vance, C. Mitochondrial abnormalities and disruption of the neuromuscular junction precede the clinical phenotype and motor neuron loss in hFUSWT transgenic mice. *Hum. Mol. Genet.* **2018**, *27*, 463–474. [CrossRef]

47. Dadon-Nachum, M.; Melamed, E.; Offen, D. The "dying-back" phenomenon of motor neurons in ALS. *J. Mol. Neurosci.* **2011**, *43*, 470–477. [CrossRef]

48. Krakora, D.; Macrander, C.; Suzuki, M. Neuromuscular junction protection for the potential treatment of amyotrophic lateral sclerosis. *Neurol. Res. Int.* **2012**, *2012*, 379657. [CrossRef]

49. Bilsland, L.G.; Sahai, E.; Kelly, G.; Golding, M.; Greensmith, L.; Schiavo, G. Deficits in axonal transport precede ALS symptoms in vivo. *Proc. Natl. Acad. Sci. USA* **2010**, *107*, 20523–20528. [CrossRef]

50. Ligon, L.A.; LaMonte, B.H.; Wallace, K.E.; Weber, N.; Kalb, R.G.; Holzbaur, E.L. Mutant superoxide dismutase disrupts cytoplasmic dynein in motor neurons. *Neuroreport* **2005**, *16*, 533–536. [CrossRef]

51. Zhang, F.; Strom, A.L.; Fukada, K.; Lee, S.; Hayward, L.J.; Zhu, H. Interaction between familial amyotrophic lateral sclerosis (ALS)-linked SOD1 mutants and the dynein complex. *J. Biol. Chem.* **2007**, *282*, 16691–16699. [CrossRef] [PubMed]

52. Igoudjil, A.; Magrane, J.; Fischer, L.R.; Kim, H.J.; Hervias, I.; Dumont, M.; Cortez, C.; Glass, J.D.; Starkov, A.A.; Manfredi, G. In vivo pathogenic role of mutant SOD1 localized in the mitochondrial intermembrane space. *J. Neurosci. Off. J. Soc. Neurosci.* **2011**, *31*, 15826–15837. [CrossRef]

53. Pickles, S.; Destroismaisons, L.; Peyrard, S.L.; Cadot, S.; Rouleau, G.A.; Brown, R.H., Jr.; Julien, J.P.; Arbour, N.; Vande Velde, C. Mitochondrial damage revealed by immunoselection for ALS-linked misfolded SOD1. *Hum. Mol. Genet.* **2013**, *22*, 3947–3959. [CrossRef] [PubMed]

54. Pickles, S.; Semmler, S.; Broom, H.R.; Destroismaisons, L.; Legroux, L.; Arbour, N.; Meiering, E.; Cashman, N.R.; Vande Velde, C. ALS-linked misfolded SOD1 species have divergent impacts on mitochondria. *Acta Neuropathol. Commun.* **2016**, *4*, 43. [CrossRef] [PubMed]

55. Li, Q.; Vande Velde, C.; Israelson, A.; Xie, J.; Bailey, A.O.; Dong, M.Q.; Chun, S.J.; Roy, T.; Winer, L.; Yates, J.R.; et al. ALS-linked mutant superoxide dismutase 1 (SOD1) alters mitochondrial protein composition and decreases protein import. *Proc. Natl. Acad. Sci. USA* **2010**, *107*, 21146–21151. [CrossRef]

56. Liu, J.; Lillo, C.; Jonsson, P.A.; Vande Velde, C.; Ward, C.M.; Miller, T.M.; Subramaniam, J.R.; Rothstein, J.D.; Marklund, S.; Andersen, P.M.; et al. Toxicity of familial ALS-linked SOD1 mutants from selective recruitment to spinal mitochondria. *Neuron* **2004**, *43*, 5–17. [CrossRef]

57. Magrane, J.; Hervias, I.; Henning, M.S.; Damiano, M.; Kawamata, H.; Manfredi, G. Mutant SOD1 in neuronal mitochondria causes toxicity and mitochondrial dynamics abnormalities. *Hum. Mol. Genet.* **2009**, *18*, 4552–4564. [CrossRef]

58. Cozzolino, M.; Pesaresi, M.G.; Amori, I.; Crosio, C.; Ferri, A.; Nencini, M.; Carri, M.T. Oligomerization of mutant SOD1 in mitochondria of motoneuronal cells drives mitochondrial damage and cell toxicity. *Antioxid. Redox Signal.* **2009**, *11*, 1547–1558. [CrossRef]

59. Mattiazzi, M.; D'Aurelio, M.; Gajewski, C.D.; Martushova, K.; Kiaei, M.; Beal, M.F.; Manfredi, G. Mutated human SOD1 causes dysfunction of oxidative phosphorylation in mitochondria of transgenic mice. *J. Biol. Chem.* **2002**, *277*, 29626–29633. [CrossRef]

60. Kawamata, H.; Manfredi, G. Different regulation of wild-type and mutant Cu,Zn superoxide dismutase localization in mammalian mitochondria. *Hum. Mol. Genet.* **2008**, *17*, 3303–3317. [CrossRef]

61. Ferri, A.; Cozzolino, M.; Crosio, C.; Nencini, M.; Casciati, A.; Gralla, E.B.; Rotilio, G.; Valentine, J.S.; Carri, M.T. Familial ALS-superoxide dismutases associate with mitochondria and shift their redox potentials. *Proc. Natl. Acad. Sci. USA* **2006**, *103*, 13860–13865. [CrossRef] [PubMed]

62. Morris, R.L.; Hollenbeck, P.J. Axonal transport of mitochondria along microtubules and F-actin in living vertebrate neurons. *J. Cell Biol.* **1995**, *131*, 1315–1326. [CrossRef] [PubMed]

63. Hensel, N.; Claus, P. The Actin Cytoskeleton in SMA and ALS: How Does It Contribute to Motoneuron Degeneration? *Neurosci. Rev. J. Bringing Neurobiol. Neurol. Psychiatry* **2018**, *24*, 54–72. [CrossRef]

64. Wu, C.H.; Fallini, C.; Ticozzi, N.; Keagle, P.J.; Sapp, P.C.; Piotrowska, K.; Lowe, P.; Koppers, M.; McKenna-Yasek, D.; Baron, D.M.; et al. Mutations in the profilin 1 gene cause familial amyotrophic lateral sclerosis. *Nature* **2012**, *488*, 499–503. [CrossRef] [PubMed]

65. Carlsson, L.; Nystrom, L.E.; Sundkvist, I.; Markey, F.; Lindberg, U. Actin polymerizability is influenced by profilin, a low molecular weight protein in non-muscle cells. *J. Mol. Biol.* **1977**, *115*, 465–483. [CrossRef]

66. Birbach, A. Profilin, a multi-modal regulator of neuronal plasticity. *Bioessays News Rev. Mol. Cell. Dev. Biol.* **2008**, *30*, 994–1002. [CrossRef]

67. Kang, F.; Purich, D.L.; Southwick, F.S. Profilin promotes barbed-end actin filament assembly without lowering the critical concentration. *J. Biol. Chem.* **1999**, *274*, 36963–36972. [CrossRef]

68. Yarmola, E.G.; Bubb, M.R. How depolymerization can promote polymerization: The case of actin and profilin. *Bioessays News Rev. Mol. Cell. Dev. Biol.* **2009**, *31*, 1150–1160. [CrossRef]

69. Smith, B.N.; Vance, C.; Scotter, E.L.; Troakes, C.; Wong, C.H.; Topp, S.; Maekawa, S.; King, A.; Mitchell, J.C.; Lund, K.; et al. Novel mutations support a role for Profilin 1 in the pathogenesis of ALS. *Neurobiol. Aging* **2015**, *36*, 1602.e17-27. [CrossRef]

70. Tanaka, Y.; Nonaka, T.; Suzuki, G.; Kametani, F.; Hasegawa, M. Gain-of-function profilin 1 mutations linked to familial amyotrophic lateral sclerosis cause seed-dependent intracellular TDP-43 aggregation. *Hum. Mol. Genet.* **2016**, *25*, 1420–1433. [CrossRef]

71. Boopathy, S.; Silvas, T.V.; Tischbein, M.; Jansen, S.; Shandilya, S.M.; Zitzewitz, J.A.; Landers, J.E.; Goode, B.L.; Schiffer, C.A.; Bosco, D.A. Structural basis for mutation-induced destabilization of profilin 1 in ALS. *Proc. Natl. Acad. Sci. USA* **2015**, *112*, 7984–7989. [CrossRef]

72. Yang, C.; Danielson, E.W.; Qiao, T.; Metterville, J.; Brown, R.H., Jr.; Landers, J.E.; Xu, Z. Mutant PFN1 causes ALS phenotypes and progressive motor neuron degeneration in mice by a gain of toxicity. *Proc. Natl. Acad. Sci. USA* **2016**, *113*, E6209–E6218. [CrossRef]

73. Fil, D.; DeLoach, A.; Yadav, S.; Alkam, D.; MacNicol, M.; Singh, A.; Compadre, C.M.; Goellner, J.J.; O'Brien, C.A.; Fahmi, T.; et al. Mutant Profilin1 transgenic mice recapitulate cardinal features of motor neuron disease. *Hum. Mol. Genet.* **2017**, *26*, 686–701. [CrossRef]

74. Shneyer, B.I.; Usaj, M.; Henn, A. Myo19 is an outer mitochondrial membrane motor and effector of starvation-induced filopodia. *J. Cell Sci.* **2016**, *129*, 543–556. [CrossRef]

75. Lopez-Domenech, G.; Covill-Cooke, C.; Ivankovic, D.; Halff, E.F.; Sheehan, D.F.; Norkett, R.; Birsa, N.; Kittler, J.T. Miro proteins coordinate microtubule- and actin-dependent mitochondrial transport and distribution. *Embo J.* **2018**, *37*, 321–336. [CrossRef]

76. Oeding, S.J.; Majstrowicz, K.; Hu, X.P.; Schwarz, V.; Freitag, A.; Honnert, U.; Nikolaus, P.; Bahler, M. Identification of Miro1 and Miro2 as mitochondrial receptors for myosin XIX. *J. Cell Sci.* **2018**, *131*, jcs219469. [CrossRef]

77. Gerdes, F.; Tatsuta, T.; Langer, T. Mitochondrial AAA proteases—Towards a molecular understanding of membrane-bound proteolytic machines. *Biochim. Biophys. Acta* **2012**, *1823*, 49–55. [CrossRef]

78. Matsushima, Y.; Kaguni, L.S. Matrix proteases in mitochondrial DNA function. *Biochim. Biophys. Acta* **2012**, *1819*, 1080–1087. [CrossRef]

79. Pellegrino, M.W.; Nargund, A.M.; Haynes, C.M. Signaling the mitochondrial unfolded protein response. *Biochim. Biophys. Acta* **2013**, *1833*, 410–416. [CrossRef]

80. Papa, L.; Germain, D. Estrogen receptor mediates a distinct mitochondrial unfolded protein response. *J. Cell Sci.* **2011**, *124*, 1396–1402. [CrossRef]

81. Radke, S.; Chander, H.; Schafer, P.; Meiss, G.; Kruger, R.; Schulz, J.B.; Germain, D. Mitochondrial protein quality control by the proteasome involves ubiquitination and the protease Omi. *J. Biol. Chem.* **2008**, *283*, 12681–12685. [CrossRef] [PubMed]

82. Karbowski, M.; Youle, R.J. Regulating mitochondrial outer membrane proteins by ubiquitination and proteasomal degradation. *Curr. Opin. Cell Biol.* **2011**, *23*, 476–482. [CrossRef]

83. Heo, J.M.; Rutter, J. Ubiquitin-dependent mitochondrial protein degradation. *Int. J. Biochem. Cell Biol.* **2011**, *43*, 1422–1426. [CrossRef]

84. Narendra, D.; Tanaka, A.; Suen, D.F.; Youle, R.J. Parkin is recruited selectively to impaired mitochondria and promotes their autophagy. *J. Cell Biol.* **2008**, *183*, 795–803. [CrossRef]

85. Narendra, D.P.; Jin, S.M.; Tanaka, A.; Suen, D.F.; Gautier, C.A.; Shen, J.; Cookson, M.R.; Youle, R.J. PINK1 is selectively stabilized on impaired mitochondria to activate Parkin. *PLoS Biol.* **2010**, *8*, e1000298. [CrossRef] [PubMed]

86. Deas, E.; Plun-Favreau, H.; Gandhi, S.; Desmond, H.; Kjaer, S.; Loh, S.H.; Renton, A.E.; Harvey, R.J.; Whitworth, A.J.; Martins, L.M.; et al. PINK1 cleavage at position A103 by the mitochondrial protease PARL. *Hum. Mol. Genet.* **2011**, *20*, 867–879. [CrossRef]

87. Vives-Bauza, C.; de Vries, R.L.; Tocilescu, M.; Przedborski, S. PINK1/Parkin direct mitochondria to autophagy. *Autophagy* **2010**, *6*, 315–316. [CrossRef]

88. Lazarou, M.; Sliter, D.A.; Kane, L.A.; Sarraf, S.A.; Wang, C.; Burman, J.L.; Sideris, D.P.; Fogel, A.I.; Youle, R.J. The ubiquitin kinase PINK1 recruits autophagy receptors to induce mitophagy. *Nature* **2015**, *524*, 309–314. [CrossRef]

89. Li, W.; Bengtson, M.H.; Ulbrich, A.; Matsuda, A.; Reddy, V.A.; Orth, A.; Chanda, S.K.; Batalov, S.; Joazeiro, C.A. Genome-wide and functional annotation of human E3 ubiquitin ligases identifies MULAN, a mitochondrial E3 that regulates the organelle's dynamics and signaling. *PLoS ONE* **2008**, *3*, e1487. [CrossRef] [PubMed]

90. Yonashiro, R.; Ishido, S.; Kyo, S.; Fukuda, T.; Goto, E.; Matsuki, Y.; Ohmura-Hoshino, M.; Sada, K.; Hotta, H.; Yamamura, H.; et al. A novel mitochondrial ubiquitin ligase plays a critical role in mitochondrial dynamics. *Embo J.* **2006**, *25*, 3618–3626. [CrossRef]

91. Karbowski, M.; Neutzner, A.; Youle, R.J. The mitochondrial E3 ubiquitin ligase MARCH5 is required for Drp1 dependent mitochondrial division. *J. Cell Biol.* **2007**, *178*, 71–84. [CrossRef] [PubMed]

92. Yonashiro, R.; Sugiura, A.; Miyachi, M.; Fukuda, T.; Matsushita, N.; Inatome, R.; Ogata, Y.; Suzuki, T.; Dohmae, N.; Yanagi, S. Mitochondrial ubiquitin ligase MITOL ubiquitinates mutant SOD1 and attenuates mutant SOD1-induced reactive oxygen species generation. *Mol. Biol. Cell* **2009**, *20*, 4524–4530. [CrossRef] [PubMed]

93. Ashrafi, G.; Schwarz, T.L. The pathways of mitophagy for quality control and clearance of mitochondria. *Cell Death Differ.* **2013**, *20*, 31–42. [CrossRef] [PubMed]

94. Aerts, L.; Craessaerts, K.; De Strooper, B.; Morais, V.A. PINK1 kinase catalytic activity is regulated by phosphorylation on serines 228 and 402. *J. Biol. Chem.* **2015**, *290*, 2798–2811. [CrossRef]

95. Soubannier, V.; McLelland, G.L.; Zunino, R.; Braschi, E.; Rippstein, P.; Fon, E.A.; McBride, H.M. A vesicular transport pathway shuttles cargo from mitochondria to lysosomes. *Curr. Biol.* **2012**, *22*, 135–141. [CrossRef]

96. Ravikumar, B.; Sarkar, S.; Davies, J.E.; Futter, M.; Garcia-Arencibia, M.; Green-Thompson, Z.W.; Jimenez-Sanchez, M.; Korolchuk, V.I.; Lichtenberg, M.; Luo, S.; et al. Regulation of mammalian autophagy in physiology and pathophysiology. *Physiol. Rev.* **2010**, *90*, 1383–1435. [CrossRef]

97. Kitada, T.; Asakawa, S.; Hattori, N.; Matsumine, H.; Yamamura, Y.; Minoshima, S.; Yokochi, M.; Mizuno, Y.; Shimizu, N. Mutations in the parkin gene cause autosomal recessive juvenile parkinsonism. *Nature* **1998**, *392*, 605–608. [CrossRef]

98. Valente, E.M.; Abou-Sleiman, P.M.; Caputo, V.; Muqit, M.M.; Harvey, K.; Gispert, S.; Ali, Z.; Del Turco, D.; Bentivoglio, A.R.; Healy, D.G.; et al. Hereditary early-onset Parkinson's disease caused by mutations in PINK1. *Science* **2004**, *304*, 1158–1160. [CrossRef]

99. Youle, R.J.; Narendra, D.P. Mechanisms of mitophagy. *Nat. Rev. Mol. Cell Biol.* **2011**, *12*, 9–14. [CrossRef]

100. Maruyama, H.; Morino, H.; Ito, H.; Izumi, Y.; Kato, H.; Watanabe, Y.; Kinoshita, Y.; Kamada, M.; Nodera, H.; Suzuki, H.; et al. Mutations of optineurin in amyotrophic lateral sclerosis. *Nature* **2010**, *465*, 223–226. [CrossRef]

101. Poole, A.C.; Thomas, R.E.; Yu, S.; Vincow, E.S.; Pallanck, L. The mitochondrial fusion-promoting factor mitofusin is a substrate of the PINK1/parkin pathway. *PLoS ONE* **2010**, *5*, e10054. [CrossRef]

102. Wong, Y.C.; Holzbaur, E.L. Optineurin is an autophagy receptor for damaged mitochondria in parkin-mediated mitophagy that is disrupted by an ALS-linked mutation. *Proc. Natl. Acad. Sci. USA* **2014**, *111*, E4439–E4448. [CrossRef]

103. Richter, B.; Sliter, D.A.; Herhaus, L.; Stolz, A.; Wang, C.; Beli, P.; Zaffagnini, G.; Wild, P.; Martens, S.; Wagner, S.A.; et al. Phosphorylation of OPTN by TBK1 enhances its binding to Ub chains and promotes selective autophagy of damaged mitochondria. *Proc. Natl. Acad. Sci. USA* **2016**, *113*, 4039–4044. [CrossRef]

104. Moore, A.S.; Holzbaur, E.L. Dynamic recruitment and activation of ALS-associated TBK1 with its target optineurin are required for efficient mitophagy. *Proc. Natl. Acad. Sci. USA* **2016**, *113*, E3349–E3358. [CrossRef]

105. Freischmidt, A.; Wieland, T.; Richter, B.; Ruf, W.; Schaeffer, V.; Muller, K.; Marroquin, N.; Nordin, F.; Hubers, A.; Weydt, P.; et al. Haploinsufficiency of TBK1 causes familial ALS and fronto-temporal dementia. *Nat. Neurosci.* **2015**, *18*, 631–636. [CrossRef]

106. Rubino, E.; Rainero, I.; Chio, A.; Rogaeva, E.; Galimberti, D.; Fenoglio, P.; Grinberg, Y.; Isaia, G.; Calvo, A.; Gentile, S.; et al. SQSTM1 mutations in frontotemporal lobar degeneration and amyotrophic lateral sclerosis. *Neurology* **2012**, *79*, 1556–1562. [CrossRef]

107. Goode, A.; Butler, K.; Long, J.; Cavey, J.; Scott, D.; Shaw, B.; Sollenberger, J.; Gell, C.; Johansen, T.; Oldham, N.J.; et al. Defective recognition of LC3B by mutant SQSTM1/p62 implicates impairment of autophagy as a pathogenic mechanism in ALS-FTLD. *Autophagy* **2016**, *12*, 1094–1104. [CrossRef]

108. Ye, Y.; Shibata, Y.; Kikkert, M.; van Voorden, S.; Wiertz, E.; Rapoport, T.A. Recruitment of the p97 ATPase and ubiquitin ligases to the site of retrotranslocation at the endoplasmic reticulum membrane. *Proc. Natl. Acad. Sci. USA* **2005**, *102*, 14132–14138. [CrossRef]

109. Kim, N.C.; Tresse, E.; Kolaitis, R.M.; Molliex, A.; Thomas, R.E.; Alami, N.H.; Wang, B.; Joshi, A.; Smith, R.B.; Ritson, G.P.; et al. VCP is essential for mitochondrial quality control by PINK1/Parkin and this function is impaired by VCP mutations. *Neuron* **2013**, *78*, 65–80. [CrossRef]

110. Johnson, J.O.; Mandrioli, J.; Benatar, M.; Abramzon, Y.; Van Deerlin, V.M.; Trojanowski, J.Q.; Gibbs, J.R.; Brunetti, M.; Gronka, S.; Wuu, J.; et al. Exome sequencing reveals VCP mutations as a cause of familial ALS. *Neuron* **2010**, *68*, 857–864. [CrossRef]

111. Wang, X.; Winter, D.; Ashrafi, G.; Schlehe, J.; Wong, Y.L.; Selkoe, D.; Rice, S.; Steen, J.; LaVoie, M.J.; Schwarz, T.L. PINK1 and Parkin target Miro for phosphorylation and degradation to arrest mitochondrial motility. *Cell* **2011**, *147*, 893–906. [CrossRef]

112. Weihofen, A.; Thomas, K.J.; Ostaszewski, B.L.; Cookson, M.R.; Selkoe, D.J. Pink1 forms a multiprotein complex with Miro and Milton, linking Pink1 function to mitochondrial trafficking. *Biochemistry* **2009**, *48*, 2045–2052. [CrossRef]

113. Shlevkov, E.; Kramer, T.; Schapansky, J.; LaVoie, M.J.; Schwarz, T.L. Miro phosphorylation sites regulate Parkin recruitment and mitochondrial motility. *Proc. Natl. Acad. Sci. USA* **2016**, *113*, E6097–E6106. [CrossRef]

114. Zhang, F.; Wang, W.; Siedlak, S.L.; Liu, Y.; Liu, J.; Jiang, K.; Perry, G.; Zhu, X.; Wang, X. Miro1 deficiency in amyotrophic lateral sclerosis. *Front. Aging Neurosci.* **2015**, *7*, 100. [CrossRef]

115. Palomo, G.M.; Granatiero, V.; Kawamata, H.; Konrad, C.; Kim, M.; Arreguin, A.J.; Zhao, D.; Milner, T.A.; Manfredi, G. Parkin is a disease modifier in the mutant SOD1 mouse model of ALS. *Embo Mol. Med.* **2018**, *10*. [CrossRef]

116. Moller, A.; Bauer, C.S.; Cohen, R.N.; Webster, C.P.; De Vos, K.J. Amyotrophic lateral sclerosis-associated mutant SOD1 inhibits anterograde axonal transport of mitochondria by reducing Miro1 levels. *Hum. Mol. Genet.* **2017**, *26*, 4668–4679. [CrossRef]

117. Kruppa, A.J.; Kishi-Itakura, C.; Masters, T.A.; Rorbach, J.E.; Grice, G.L.; Kendrick-Jones, J.; Nathan, J.A.; Minczuk, M.; Buss, F. Myosin VI-Dependent Actin Cages Encapsulate Parkin-Positive Damaged Mitochondria. *Dev. Cell* **2018**, *44*, 484–499 e486. [CrossRef]

118. Fornai, F.; Longone, P.; Cafaro, L.; Kastsiuchenka, O.; Ferrucci, M.; Manca, M.L.; Lazzeri, G.; Spalloni, A.; Bellio, N.; Lenzi, P.; et al. Lithium delays progression of amyotrophic lateral sclerosis. *Proc. Natl. Acad. Sci. USA* **2008**, *105*, 2052–2057. [CrossRef]

119. Pizzasegola, C.; Caron, I.; Daleno, C.; Ronchi, A.; Minoia, C.; Carri, M.T.; Bendotti, C. Treatment with lithium carbonate does not improve disease progression in two different strains of SOD1 mutant mice. *Amyotroph. Lateral Scler. Off. Publ. World Fed. Neurol. Res. Group Mot. Neuron Dis.* **2009**, *10*, 221–228. [CrossRef]

120. Zhang, X.; Li, L.; Chen, S.; Yang, D.; Wang, Y.; Zhang, X.; Wang, Z.; Le, W. Rapamycin treatment augments motor neuron degeneration in SOD1(G93A) mouse model of amyotrophic lateral sclerosis. *Autophagy* **2011**, *7*, 412–425. [CrossRef]

121. Zhang, K.; Shi, P.; An, T.; Wang, Q.; Wang, J.; Li, Z.; Duan, W.; Li, C.; Guo, Y. Food restriction-induced autophagy modulates degradation of mutant SOD1 in an amyotrophic lateral sclerosis mouse model. *Brain Res.* **2013**, *1519*, 112–119. [CrossRef]

122. Zhang, X.; Chen, S.; Song, L.; Tang, Y.; Shen, Y.; Jia, L.; Le, W. MTOR-independent, autophagic enhancer trehalose prolongs motor neuron survival and ameliorates the autophagic flux defect in a mouse model of amyotrophic lateral sclerosis. *Autophagy* **2014**, *10*, 588–602. [CrossRef]

123. Kim, J.; Kim, T.Y.; Cho, K.S.; Kim, H.N.; Koh, J.Y. Autophagy activation and neuroprotection by progesterone in the G93A-SOD1 transgenic mouse model of amyotrophic lateral sclerosis. *Neurobiol. Dis.* **2013**, *59*, 80–85. [CrossRef]

124. Rudnick, N.D.; Griffey, C.J.; Guarnieri, P.; Gerbino, V.; Wang, X.; Piersaint, J.A.; Tapia, J.C.; Rich, M.M.; Maniatis, T. Distinct roles for motor neuron autophagy early and late in the SOD1(G93A) mouse model of ALS. *Proc. Natl. Acad. Sci. USA* **2017**, *114*, E8294–E8303. [CrossRef]

125. Li, L.; Zhang, X.; Le, W. Altered macroautophagy in the spinal cord of SOD1 mutant mice. *Autophagy* **2008**, *4*, 290–293. [CrossRef]

126. Morimoto, N.; Nagai, M.; Ohta, Y.; Miyazaki, K.; Kurata, T.; Morimoto, M.; Murakami, T.; Takehisa, Y.; Ikeda, Y.; Kamiya, T.; et al. Increased autophagy in transgenic mice with a G93A mutant SOD1 gene. *Brain Res.* **2007**, *1167*, 112–117. [CrossRef]

127. Xie, Y.; Zhou, B.; Lin, M.Y.; Wang, S.; Foust, K.D.; Sheng, Z.H. Endolysosomal Deficits Augment Mitochondria Pathology in Spinal Motor Neurons of Asymptomatic fALS Mice. *Neuron* **2015**, *87*, 355–370. [CrossRef]

128. Sasaki, S. Autophagy in spinal cord motor neurons in sporadic amyotrophic lateral sclerosis. *J. Neuropathol. Exp. Neurol.* **2011**, *70*, 349–359. [CrossRef]

129. Lagier-Tourenne, C.; Polymenidou, M.; Hutt, K.R.; Vu, A.Q.; Baughn, M.; Huelga, S.C.; Clutario, K.M.; Ling, S.C.; Liang, T.Y.; Mazur, C.; et al. Divergent roles of ALS-linked proteins FUS/TLS and TDP-43 intersect in processing long pre-mRNAs. *Nat. Neurosci.* **2012**, *15*, 1488–1497. [CrossRef]

130. Polymenidou, M.; Lagier-Tourenne, C.; Hutt, K.R.; Huelga, S.C.; Moran, J.; Liang, T.Y.; Ling, S.C.; Sun, E.; Wancewicz, E.; Mazur, C.; et al. Long pre-mRNA depletion and RNA missplicing contribute to neuronal vulnerability from loss of TDP-43. *Nat. Neurosci.* **2011**, *14*, 459–468. [CrossRef]

5

Mitochondrial Dysfunction in the Aging Retina

Janis T. Eells

Department of Biomedical Sciences, University of Wisconsin-Milwaukee, Milwaukee, WI 53211, USA;
jeells@uwm.edu

Abstract: Mitochondria are central in retinal cell function and survival and they perform functions that are critical to cell function. Retinal neurons have high energy requirements, since large amounts of ATP are needed to generate membrane potentials and power membrane pumps. Mitochondria over the course of aging undergo a number of changes. Aged mitochondria exhibit decreased rates of oxidative phosphorylation, increased reactive oxygen species (ROS) generation and increased numbers of mtDNA mutations. Mitochondria in the neural retina and the retinal pigment epithelium are particularly susceptible to oxidative damage with aging. Many age-related retinal diseases, including glaucoma and age-related macular degeneration, have been associated with mitochondrial dysfunction. Therefore, mitochondria are a promising therapeutic target for the treatment of retinal disease.

Keywords: aging; mitochondria; retina; optic nerve; diabetic retinopathy; age-related macular degeneration; glaucoma

1. Retinal Anatomy and Physiology

The fundamental organization of the retina is conserved across vertebrates. The retina contains five major neuronal cell classes (photoreceptors, bipolar cells, amacrine cells, horizontal cells, and retinal ganglion cells) with Müller glial cells and retinal pigment epithelial cells providing metabolic and homeostatic support [1] (Figure 1). The interaction of light with light-sensitive pigments in the outer segments of rod and cone photoreceptors initiates signaling mechanisms that convert light energy to neural activity. Photoreceptors synapse with bipolar cells. Bipolar cells synapse with the retinal ganglion cells that transmit the visual signal along their axons (optic nerve) and, ultimately, to the brain. The retinal pigment epithelium envelopes the photoreceptors, which facilitates the diffusion of nutrients, key metabolites, and oxygen from the choroidal vessels. Horizontal cells, amacrine cells, and Muller cells mediate and support the synapses between the retinal neurons. Unique to the Muller cell, its processes span the inner retina and most of the outer retina, assisting in the maintenance of multiple synapses throughout the retina. Pericytes surround the vascular endothelial cells in all retinal layers, forming the blood-retinal barrier.

The retina is the highest oxygen-consuming organ in the human body [2–6]. The inner retinal neurons have the highest metabolic rate of all central nervous tissue, and the oxygen consumption rate of the photoreceptors is several times higher again. The inner segments of the photoreceptor cells are rich in mitochondria providing the ATP that are required by the ionic pumps that drive the 'dark current'. In addition, photoreceptors also metabolize glucose through aerobic glycolysis [2–6].

The key role of aerobic glycolysis in the vertebrate retina has been long recognized and well established [2,5,6]. The majority of aerobic glycolysis occurs in the photoreceptors. Although aerobic glycolysis dominates energy production in the photoreceptors, the retina requires both glycolysis and oxidative phosphorylation to initiate vision [4]. This has been demonstrated in studies showing that the responses of neurons downstream of photoreceptors are abolished by inhibiting glycolysis or by removing O_2 [2]. Recent studies have proposed a model in which glucose from the choroidal blood passes through the retinal pigment epithelium to the retina, where photoreceptors convert it to lactate [6]. Photoreceptors then export the lactate as fuel for the retinal pigment epithelium and for neighboring Müller glial cells. Aerobic glycolysis not only enables enhanced anabolic metabolism in photoreceptors, but also maximizes their function and adaptability to nutrient stress conditions.

Photoreceptors consume more oxygen per gram of tissue weight than any cell in the body [2,5]. This intense degree of oxidative phosphorylation in their inner segments, coupled with high concentrations of polyunsaturated fatty acids in their outer segments, renders the retina susceptible to oxidative stress and lipid peroxidation [2–4]. The retina is exposed to visible light and it contains abundant photosensitizers [1]. Normally, endogenous antioxidants and repair systems minimize oxidative damage. However, with aging and retinal disease, there is an increase in mitochondrial dysfunction and oxidative damage and corresponding decrements in antioxidants and repair systems, resulting in retinal dysfunction and retinal cell loss, which leads to visual impairment [7–13].

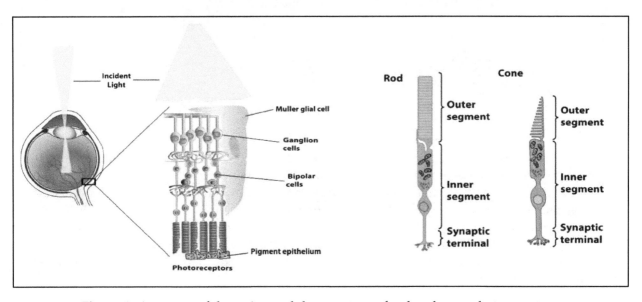

Figure 1. Anatomy of the retina and the structure of rod and cone photoreceptors.

2. Mitochondrial Dysfunction with Aging and Disease

2.1. Age-Related Mitochondrial Changes

Mitochondria are central to retinal cell function and survival and they perform a variety of functions critical to cell metabolism, including oxidative phosphorylation, beta-oxidation of fatty acids, calcium homeostasis, and the regulation of neuronal excitability [7–13]. Retinal neurons have high energy requirements and large amounts of ATP are needed to generate membrane potentials and power membrane pumps. It has been estimated that 90% of mitochondria-generated ATP is used to maintain transmembrane ion gradients [10].

Mitochondria in the aging retina show a decline in the function of the electron transport chain and a significant increase in the generation of reactive oxygen species (ROS) (Figure 2). This increased ROS production leads to increased oxidative damage to mitochondrial DNA, lipids, and proteins [5,6,14–16]. With aging, there is an accumulation of mtDNA mutations and a disruption of mitochondrial structure. Mitochondrial genomic instability has been postulated to play an important role in age-related retinal pathophysiology [16]. However, murine studies have shown that the majority of mtDNA mutations in aged cells appear to be caused by replication errors early in life, rather than by oxidative damage [15]. Mitochondrial DNA repair pathways are limited and they begin to fail with aging, leading to additional mtDNA damage and contributing to the development of retinal degenerative diseases [8,9].

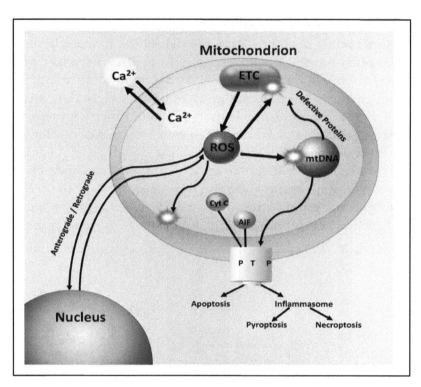

Figure 2. Mitochondria in the aging retina. Mitochondria are essential for many cellular functions including: (1) the synthesis of ATP by oxidative phosphorylation, (2) the regulation of intracellular calcium homeostasis, (3) anterograde and retrograde signaling between the nucleus and mitochondria, (4) the generation of reactive oxygen species (ROS) from the electron transport chain (ETC). ROS act as signaling molecules in low concentrations or as toxic molecules in higher concentrations. ROS oxidize mitochondrial lipids, proteins and DNA and (5) the regulation of apoptosis. Excess ROS or intramitochondrial calcium can lead to the activation of cell death pathways by opening the mitochondrial permeability transition pore (PTP).

2.2. Age-Related Macular Degeneration

Age-related macular degeneration (AMD) is the leading cause of blindness in individuals over 65 in developed countries [17]. As the name implies, AMD primarily affects the central retina or macula. It is characterized by the development of drusen, extracellular lipoprotein deposits under the retinal pigment epithelium (RPE), in the early stages of the disease, followed by the loss of photoreceptors and RPE. Choroidal neovascularization (CNV) develops during later stages of the disease (wet AMD) [17]. Choroidal neovascularization (CNV) is the growth of new blood vessels that originate from the choroid through a break in Bruch's membrane into the subretinal space or sub-retinal pigment epithelium. Dry or atrophic AMD is the most common form of AMD and there are no treatments for this form of AMD.

Aging is a recognized factor that is associated with mitochondrial dysfunction in the outer retina. Other important risk factors for the development of AMD are genetics and environmental stressors, including smoking and exposure to ultraviolet and blue light [18–24]. All of these factors are likely to result in mtDNA damage in the RPE.

Genetic risk factors also contribute to the development of AMD. Genetic polymorphisms of complement factor H (CFH) contribute to AMD pathology. An important relationship between mitochondrial dysfunction and CFH has been recently established [24,25]. These studies have demonstrated mitochondrial abnormalities in Complement factor H null (Cfh$^{-/-}$) mice that are characterized by disrupted mitochondrial morphology and decreased ATP production [24,25]. These findings suggest that CFH plays an important role in retinal oxidative metabolism. Genome wide associated studies have implicated several genes in the cholesterol pathway, including apolipoprotein

E (APOE), in the development of AMD [17]. Recent studies by Lee et al. (2016) have shown that mutations in the transmembrane 135 (Tmem 135) gene that codes for a mitochondrial protein located in RPE and photoreceptors results in accelerated retinal aging in a mouse model of AMD [26].

Although in vitro studies have unequivocally demonstrated that either UV or blue light damage RPE cells [22], epidemiological evidence of the association between exposure to sunlight and AMD is mixed [23]. The ability of the ocular media (cornea, lens, and vitreous humor) to block UV and blue light and the protection of the retina by antioxidant systems, including superoxide dismutase and glutathione peroxidase and macular pigments, including melanin and flavoproteins likely explain these differences [17].

Recent studies suggest that a bioenergetic crisis in the RPE contributes to the pathology of AMD, as illustrated in Figure 3 [20]. Analysis of retinal tissue from human donors with AMD have documented a reduction in the mitochondrial number, a disruption in mitochondrial structure and an increase in mtDNA damage in the RPE that correlates with the severity of disease [15–18]. Recent studies in the primary cultures of RPE derived from human donors with and without AMD have shown decreased rates of ATP synthesis from oxidative phosphorylation and glycolysis in AMD donors consistent with a bioenergetic crisis. Fisher and Ferrington (2018) have suggested that mitochondrial damage is limited to the RPE, because these cells rely nearly exclusively on mitochondrial oxidative phosphorylation, whereas photoreceptors utilize aerobic glycolysis [4–7]. In addition to disruptions in mitochondrial bioenergetics, mitochondrial dysfunction has been shown to disrupt calcium homeostasis and mitochondrial nuclear signaling. Several studies have suggested that therapeutic approaches that target RPE mitochondria may provide an effective early treatment strategy for AMD [18–22].

Figure 3. Mitochondrial involvement in dry age-related macular degeneration (AMD).

2.3. Diabetic Retinopathy

Diabetic Retinopathy (DR) is the most common complication of diabetes mellitus. DR is a leading cause of blindness in many developed countries [27]. Chronic hyperglycemia coupled with other risk factors, including hypertension and dyslipidemia, are postulated to trigger a cascade of biochemical and pathophysiological changes that lead to microvascular damage and retinal dysfunction. Mitochondrial dysfunction is a key component of this cascade.

The pathogenesis of diabetic retinopathy is complex, involving the disruption of multiple intracellular pathways [27]. Early pathologic changes that were observed in diabetic retinopathy include mitochondrial dysfunction, oxidative stress, and inflammation [27–30]. Oxidative stress results from the increased production of reactive oxygen species (ROS), including superoxide and hydrogen peroxide. ROS oxidize intracellular proteins, lipids, and nucleic acids, disrupting normal signaling and culminating in disease. Under physiological conditions, small amounts of superoxide leak from the electron transport chain and they are converted to hydrogen peroxide by mitochondrial superoxide dismutase. Hydrogen peroxide diffuses out of the mitochondria into the cytosol and it serves an important signaling molecule. Intracellular ROS concentrations are regulated by a complex array of antioxidant systems to maintain low intracellular ROS concentrations [29]. Under hyperglycemic conditions, the excess production of ROS overwhelms the antioxidant systems, resulting in oxidative damage [11,28,29].

Hyperglycemia is known to disrupt several metabolic pathways that are involved in the pathogenesis of diabetic retinopathy. These pathways include protein kinase C (PKC) activation, accumulation of advanced glycation products (AGEs), the polyol pathway, and activation of the hexosamine pathway [27,28]. Experimental models have shown that, in the etiology of this progressive disease, the activation of NADPH oxidase (*Nox*) increases cytosolic ROS and this sustained accumulation of ROS damages mitochondria, which further increases oxidative stress [30]. Superoxide radicals (O_2^-) that are produced by the mitochondrial electron transport chain activate these major pathways, and activation, in turn, can damage the mitochondria propagating the vicious cycle of ROS.

A major source of the excess ROS production under hyperglycemic conditions is the mitochondrial electron transport chain (ETC) [28–30]. Under normal physiological conditions, the electrons are donated to complex I or complex II of the ETC and are then passed on to coenzyme Q, complex III, cytochrome C, complex IV, and ultimately to molecular oxygen, the final electron acceptor. The transfer of electrons generates a proton gradient across the mitochondrial intermembrane, which drives the synthesis of ATP by ATP synthase. During this process, small amounts of superoxide are produced, but the cell via antioxidant defense mechanisms easily clears them [20–30].

Complex I of the ETC is generally regarded as the primary source of superoxide production. However, the 2-oxoglutarate dehydrogenase (OGDH), branched-chain 2-oxoacid dehydrogenase (BCKDH), and pyruvate dehydrogenase (PDH) complexes are also capable of considerable superoxide/H_2O_2 production. Moreover, mitochondria can generate ROS, superoxide, or hydrogen peroxide, from at least ten distinct sites on the ETC or associated pathways [31–34].

The precise cause of mitochondrial dysfunction in a diabetic state is unclear. Some studies suggest that the increased glucose concentration overwhelms the electron transport chain by increasing the rate of oxidative phosphorylation [16–19], thus generating ROS. Other studies suggest that mitochondrial DNA is damaged, which results in dysfunctional proteins that are required for ETC complexes, also causing excess ROS and mitochondrial dysfunction [27,28].

Mitochondrial function, structure, and mtDNA are damaged in the retina in diabetic retinopathy [29]. Mitochondrial biogenesis and mtDNA repair mechanisms are compromised [35,36]. The ETC becomes dysfunctional and the import of nuclear DNA encoded proteins is disrupted. These diabetes-induced abnormalities in mitochondria persist after the removal of the hyperglycemic insult and they are implicated in the metabolic memory phenomenon associated with the continued progression of diabetic retinopathy [36,37]. Hyperglycemic insult also results in epigenetic modifications [38]. These epigenetic changes in histones and DNA methylation can be passed to the next generation. Epigenetic modifications also contribute to mitochondrial damage and disrupt mitochondrial homeostasis [38]. Therapeutic strategies directed at mitochondrial homeostasis and epigenetic modifications have the potential to halt or slow the progression of diabetic retinopathy.

2.4. Glaucoma

Glaucoma is a leading cause of blindness, which is characterized by the accelerated death of retinal ganglion cells (RGC), leading to vision loss [39–42]. Age and elevated intraocular pressure (IOP) are two major risk factors in developing glaucoma. Therapies reducing IOP have been shown to slow the progression of glaucoma in many but not all patients. Aging may increase the vulnerability of the optic nerve to various stressors, ultimately resulting in RGC death and optic nerve degeneration [39–41].

A growing body of evidence supports a key role for mitochondrial dysfunction in the pathogenesis of glaucoma [39–51]. Mitochondrial dysfunction has been demonstrated in RGC loss in animal and cultured cell experimental models of glaucoma [47,51]. Mutations in mitochondrial and nuclear genes encoding mitochondrial proteins are known to cause primary optic neuropathies, including Leber's Hereditary Optic Neuropathy (LHON) and Autosomal Dominant Optic Atrophy (AODA) [51]. Recent studies indicate that the bioenergetic consequences of mtDNA and nuclear DNA mutations contribute to the development of Primary Open Angle Glaucoma (POAG) and Normal Tension Glaucoma (NTG) [40–43].

In addition to genetic factors, retinal ganglion cells are profoundly susceptible to mitochondrial dysfunction [42,51]. A combination of the acute energy demand of RGCs and their unique morphology appears to underlie the susceptibility of these neurons to mitochondrial dysfunction. The RGC cell body is located in the ganglion cell layer of the retina. RGCs possess elaborate dendritic arbors that project into the inner plexiform layer to synapse with other retinal neurons. These dendritic arbors are packed with mitochondria that are needed to supply the ATP required to maintain these connections. The long axons of the RGCs form the optic nerve and extend into the brain. The RGC axons make a 90-degree turn at the optic nerve head and pass through the lamina cribrosa, a series of perforated collagen plates, before forming the optic nerve. After passing through the lamina cribrosa, the optic nerve becomes laminated and continues to the visual cortex. The optic nerve has one of the highest oxygen consumption rates and energy demands of any tissue in the body [51]. The mitochondrial density is greater in the unmyelinated region of the optic nerve than in the myelinated region. The unmyelinated prelaminar and laminar regions of the optic nerve require more energy than the myelinated segment of the optic nerve due to the absence of saltatory conduction. This region of the optic nerve has a high density of voltage gated sodium channels and it requires more energy to restore ion gradients.

The combination of genetic susceptibility due to inherited or acquired mutations, energy demand, and unique morphology of retinal ganglion cells in an aging population all contribute to the pathogenesis and incidence of glaucoma (Figure 4).

Figure 4. Mitochondrial dysfunction in glaucoma.

3. Conclusions

Experimental evidence has shown a link between mitochondrial dysfunction and the loss of vision. Most mitochondrial diseases exhibit some form of visual impairment. Many retinal and optic nerve diseases, including AMD, diabetic retinopathy, and glaucoma are also characterized by mitochondrial dysfunction. The development of therapeutic approaches that target retinal mitochondrial dysfunction has the potential to profoundly impact the treatment of retinal and optic nerve disease.

References

1. Sung, C.H.; Chuang, J.Z. The cell biology of vision. *J. Cell Biol.* **2010**, *190*, 953–963. [CrossRef] [PubMed]
2. Winkler, B.S. Glycolytic and oxidative metabolism in relation to retinal function. *J. Gen. Physiol.* **1981**, *77*, 667–692. [CrossRef]
3. Warbug, O. Uber die klassifizierung tierischer gewebe nach ihrem stoffwechsel. *Biochem. Z.* **1927**, *184*, 484–488.
4. Ames, A., 3rd; Li, Y.Y.; Heher, E.C.; Kimble, C.R. Energy metabolism of rabbit retina as related to function: High cost of sodium transport. *J. Neurosci.* **1992**, *12*, 840–853. [CrossRef]
5. Medrano, C.J.; Fox, D.A. Oxygen consumption in the rat outer and inner retina: Light- and pharmacologically-induced inhibition. *Exp. Eye Res.* **1995**, *61*, 273–284. [CrossRef]
6. Hurley, J.B.; Lindsay, K.J.; Du, J. Glucose, lactate and shuttling of metabolites in vertebrate retinas. *J. Neurosci. Res.* **2015**, *93*, 1079–1092. [CrossRef] [PubMed]
7. Yu, D.Y.; Cringle, S.J. Retinal degeneration and local oxygen metabolism. *Exp. Eye Res.* **2005**, *80*, 745–751. [CrossRef]
8. Barot, M.; Gokulgandhi, M.R.; Mitra, A.K. Mitochondrial dysfunction in retinal diseases. *Curr. Eye Res.* **2011**, *36*, 1069–1077. [CrossRef]
9. Wang, A.L.; Lukas, T.J.; Yuan, M.; Neufeld, A.H. Age-related increase in mitochondrial DNA damage and loss of DNA repair capacity in the neural retina. *Neurobiol. Aging* **2010**, *31*, 2002–2010. [CrossRef]
10. Barron, M.J.; Johnson, M.A.; Andrews, R.M.; Clarke, M.P.; Griffiths, P.G.; Bristow, E.; He, L.-P.; Durham, S.; Turnbull, D.M. Mitochondrial abnormalities in aging macular photoreceptors. *Investig. Ophthalmol. Vis. Sci.* **2001**, *42*, 3016–3022.
11. Country, M.W. Retinal metabolism: A comparative look as energetics in the retina. *Brain Res.* **2017**, *1672*, 50–57. [CrossRef] [PubMed]
12. Lefevere, E.; Toft-Kehler, A.K.; Vohra, R.; Kolko, M.; Moons, L.; van Hovea, I. Mitochondrial dysfunction underlying outer retinal diseases. *Mitochondrion* **2017**, *36*, 66–76. [CrossRef]
13. Jarrett, S.G.; Lin, H.; Godley, B.F.; Boultonc, M.E. Mitochondrial DNA damage and its potential role in retinal degeneration. *Prog. Retin. Eye Res.* **2008**, *27*, 596–607. [CrossRef]
14. Kennedy, S.R.; Salk, J.J.; Schmitt, M.W.; Loeb, L.A. Ultra-sensitive sequencing reveals an age-related increase in somatic mitochondrial mutations that are inconsistent with oxidative damage. *PLoS Genet.* **2013**, *9*, e1003794. [CrossRef]
15. Ameur, A.; Stewart, J.B.; Freyer, C.; Hagström, E.; Ingman, M.; Larsson, N.-G.; Gyllensten, U. Ultra-deep sequencing of mouse mitochondrial DNA: Mutational patterns and their origins. *PLoS Genet.* **2011**, *7*, e1002028. [CrossRef] [PubMed]
16. Lopez-Otin, C.; Blasco, M.A.; Partridge, L.; Serrano, M.; Kroemer, G. The hallmarks of aging. *Cell* **2013**, *153*, 1194–1217. [CrossRef]
17. Lim, L.S.; Mitchell, P.; Seddon, J.M.; Holz, F.G.; Wong, T.Y. Age-related macular degeneration. *Lancet* **2012**, *379*, 1728–1738. [CrossRef]
18. Feher, J.; Kovacs, I.; Artico, M.; Cavallotti, C.; Papale, A.; Gabrieli, C.B. Mitochondrial alterations of retinal pigment epithelium in age-related macular degeneration. *Neurobiol. Aging* **2006**, *27*, 983–993. [CrossRef] [PubMed]
19. Ferrington, D.A.; Ebeling, M.C.; Kapphahn, R.J.; Terluk, M.R.; Fisher, C.R.; Polanco, J.R.; Roehrich, H.; Leary, M.M.; Geng, Z.; Dutton, J.R.; et al. Altered bioenergetics and enhanced resistance to oxidative stress in human retinal pigment epithelial cells from donors with age-related macular degeneration. *Redox Biol.* **2017**, *13*, 255–265. [CrossRef]
20. Fisher, C.R.; Ferrington, D.A. Perspective on AMD pathobiology: A bioenergetic crisis in the RPE. *Investig. Ophthalmol. Vis. Sci.* **2018**, *59*, 41–55. [CrossRef]
21. Turluk, M.R.; Kapphahn, R.J.; Soukup, L.M.; Gong, H.; Gallardo, C.; Montezuma, S.R.; Ferrington, D.A. Investigating mitochondria as a target for treating age-related macular degeneration. *J. Neurosci.* **2015**, *35*, 7304–7311. [CrossRef]
22. King, A.; Gottlieb, E.; Brooks, D.G.; Murphy, M.P.; Dunaief, J.L. Mitochondria-derived reactive oxygen species mediate blue light-induced death of retinal pigment epithelial cells. *Photochem. Photobiol.* **2004**, *79*, 470475. [CrossRef]

23. Zhou, H.; Zhang, H.; Yu, A.; Xie, J. Association between sunlight exposure and risk of age-related macular degeneration: A meta-analysis. *BMC Ophthalmol.* **2018**, *18*, 331–338. [CrossRef]

24. Sivapathasuntharam, C.; Hayes, M.J.; Shinhmar, H.; Kam, J.H.; Sivaprasad, S.; Jeffery, G. Complement factor H regulates retinal development and its absence may establish a footprint for age related macular degeneration. *Sci. Rep.* **2019**, *9*, 1082–1092. [CrossRef]

25. Calaza, K.C.; Kam, J.H.; Hogg, C.; Jeffery, G. Mitochondrial decline precedes phenotype development in the complement factor H mouse model of retinal degeneration but can be corrected by near infrared light. *Neurobiol. Aging* **2015**, *36*, 2869–2876. [CrossRef]

26. Lee, W.-H.; Higuchi, H.; Ikeda, S.; Macke, E.L.; Takimoto, T.; Pattnaik, B.R.; Liu, C.; Chu, L.-F.; Siepka, S.M.; Krentz, K.J.; et al. Mouse Tmem135 mutation reveals a mechanism involving mitochondrial dynamics that leads to age-dependent retinal pathologies. *eLife* **2016**, *5*, e19264. [CrossRef] [PubMed]

27. Antonetti, D.A.; Klein, R.; Gardner, T.W. Mechanisms of disease diabetic retinopathy. *N. Engl. J. Med.* **2012**, *366*, 1227–1239. [CrossRef]

28. Brownlee, M. The pathobiology of diabetic complications; a unifying mechanism. *Diabetes* **2005**, *54*, 1615–1625. [CrossRef]

29. Kowluru, R.A.; Mirsha, M. Oxidative stress, mitochondrial damage and diabetic retinopathy. *Biochim. Biophys. Acta* **2015**, *1852*, 2474–2483. [CrossRef]

30. Roy, S.; Kern, T.S.; Song, B.; Stuebe, C. Mechanistic insights into pathological changes in the diabetic retina: Implications for targeting diabetic retinopathy. *Am. J. Pathol.* **2017**, *187*, 9–19. [CrossRef]

31. St-Pierre, J.; Buckingham, J.A.; Roebuck, S.J.; Brand, M.D. Topology of superoxide production from different sites in the mitochondrial electron transport chain. *J. Biol. Chem.* **2002**, *277*, 44784–44790. [CrossRef]

32. Brand, M.D. The sites and topology of mitochondrial superoxide production. *Exp. Gerontol.* **2010**, *45*, 466–472. [CrossRef]

33. Murphy, M.P. How mitochondria produce reactive oxygen species. *Biochem. J.* **2009**, *417*, 1–13. [CrossRef] [PubMed]

34. Quinlan, C.L.; Goncalves, R.L.S.; Hey-Mogensen, M.; Yadava, N.; Bunik, V.I.; Brand, M.D. The 2-oxoacid dehydrogenase complexes in mitochondria can produce superoxide/hydrogen peroxide at much higher rates than complex I. *J. Biol. Chem.* **2014**, *289*, 8312–8325. [CrossRef]

35. Kowluru, R.A. Diabetic retinopathy, metabolic memory and epigenetic modifications. *Vis. Res.* **2017**, *139*, 30–38. [CrossRef]

36. Kowluru, R.A. Mitochondria damage in the pathogenesis of diabetic retinopathy and in the metabolic memory associated with its continued progression. *Curr. Med. Chem.* **2013**, *20*, 3226–3233. [CrossRef]

37. Kowluru, R.A.; Abbas, S.N. Diabetes-induced mitochondrial dysfunction in the retina. *Investig. Ophthalmol. Vis. Sci.* **2003**, *12*, 5327–5334. [CrossRef]

38. Kowluru, R.A.; Kowluru, A.; Mishra, M.; Kumar, B. Oxidative stress and epigenetic modifications in the pathogenesis of diabetic retinopathy. *Prog. Retin. Eye Res.* **2015**, *48*, 40–61. [CrossRef] [PubMed]

39. Ju, W.K.; Liu, Q.; Kim, K.-Y.; Crowston, J.G.; Lindsey, J.D.; Agarwal, N.; Ellisman, M.H.; Perkins, G.A.; Weinreb, R.N. Elevated hydrostatic pressure triggers mitochondrial fission and decreases cellular ATP in differentiated RGC-5 cells. *Investig. Ophthalmol. Vis. Sci.* **2007**, *48*, 2145–2151. [CrossRef]

40. Abu-Amero, K.K.; Morales, J.; Bosley, T.M. Mitochondrial abnormalities in patients with primary open-angle glaucoma. *Investig. Ophthalmol. Vis. Sci.* **2006**, *47*, 2533–2541. [CrossRef]

41. Moreno, M.C.; Campanelli, J.; Sande, P.; Sáenz, D.A.; Sarmiento, M.I.K.; Rosenstein, R.E. Retinal oxidative stress induced by high intraocular pressure. *Free Radic. Biol. Med.* **2004**, *37*, 803–812. [CrossRef] [PubMed]

42. Kong, G.Y.; Van Bergen, N.J.; Trounce, I.A.; Crowston, J.G. Mitochondrial dysfunction and glaucoma. *J. Glaucoma* **2009**, *18*, 93–100. [CrossRef]

43. Harun-or-Rashid, M.; Pappenhagen, N.; Palmer, P.G.; Smith, M.A.; Gevorgyan, V.; Wilson, G.N.; Crish, S.D.; Inman, D.M. Structural and functional rescue of chronic metabolically stressed optic nerves through respiration. *J. Neurosci.* **2018**, *38*, 5122–5139. [CrossRef] [PubMed]

44. Libby, R.T.; Anderson, M.G.; Pang, I.-H.; Robinson, Z.H.; Savinova, O.V.; Cosma, I.M.; Snow, A.; Wilson, L.A.; Smith, R.S.; Clark, A.F.; et al. Inherited glaucoma in DBA/2J mice: Pertinent disease features for studying the neurodegeneration. *Vis. Neurosci.* **2005**, *22*, 637–648. [CrossRef] [PubMed]

45.   Baltan, S.; Inman, D.M.; Danilov, C.A.; Morrison, R.S.; Calkins, D.J.; Horner, P.J. Metabolic vulnerability
      disposes retinal ganglion cell axons to dysfunction in a model of glaucomatous degeneration. *J. Neurosci.*
      2010, *30*, 5644–5652. [CrossRef]

46.   Kleesattel, D.; Crish, S.D.; Inman, D.M. Decreased energy capacity and increased autophagic activity in
      optic nerve axons with defective anterograde transport. *Investig. Ophthalmol. Vis. Sci.* **2015**, *56*, 8215–8227.
      [CrossRef] [PubMed]

47.   Ju, W.-K.; Kim, K.-Y.; Lindsey, J.D.; Angert, M.; Duong-Polk, K.X.; Scott, R.T.; Kim, J.J.; Kukhmazov, I.;
      Ellisman, M.H.; Perkins, G.A.; et al. Intraocular pressure elevation induces mitochondrial fission and triggers
      OPA1 release in glaucomatous optic nerve. *Investig. Ophthalmol. Vis. Sci.* **2008**, *49*, 4903–4911. [CrossRef]

48.   Coughlin, L.; Morrison, R.S.; Horner, P.J.; Inman, D.M. Mitochondrial morphology differences and mitophagy
      deficit in murine glaucomatous optic nerve. *Investig. Ophthalmol. Vis. Sci.* **2015**, *56*, 1437–1446. [CrossRef]

49.   Williams, P.A.; Harder, J.M.; Foxworth, N.E.; Cochran, K.E.; Philip, V.M.; Porciatti, V.; Smithies, O.; John, S.W.M.
      Vitamin B3 modulates mitochondrial vulnerability and prevents glaucoma in aged mice. *Science* **2017**, *760*,
      756–760. [CrossRef]

50.   Ju, W.K.; Kim, K.Y.; Noh, Y.H.; Hoshijima, M.; Lukas, T.J.; Ellisman, M.H.; Weinreb, R.N.; Perkins, G.A.
      Increased mitochondrial fission and volume density by blocking glutamate excitotoxicity protect
      glaucomatous optic nerve head astrocytes. *Glia* **2015**, *63*, 736–753. [CrossRef]

51.   Lee, S. Mitochondrial dysfunction in glaucoma and emerging bioenergetic therapies. *Exp. Eye Res.* **2011**, *93*,
      204–212. [CrossRef]

6

Mitochondrial Dysfunction and the Aging Immune System

Peter J. McGuire

Metabolism, Infection and Immunity Section, National Human Genome Research Institute, National Institutes of Health, Bethesda, MD 20892, USA; peter.mcguire@nih.gov

Abstract: Mitochondria are ancient organelles that have co-evolved with their cellular hosts, developing a mutually beneficial arrangement. In addition to making energy, mitochondria are multifaceted, being involved in heat production, calcium storage, apoptosis, cell signaling, biosynthesis, and aging. Many of these mitochondrial functions decline with age, and are the basis for many diseases of aging. Despite the vast amount of research dedicated to this subject, the relationship between aging mitochondria and immune function is largely absent from the literature. In this review, three main issues facing the aging immune system are discussed: (1) inflamm-aging; (2) susceptibility to infection and (3) declining T-cell function. These issues are re-evaluated using the lens of mitochondrial dysfunction with aging. With the recent expansion of numerous profiling technologies, there has been a resurgence of interest in the role of metabolism in immunity, with mitochondria taking center stage. Building upon this recent accumulation of knowledge in immunometabolism, this review will advance the hypothesis that the decline in immunity and associated pathologies are partially related to the natural progression of mitochondrial dysfunction with aging.

Keywords: aging; mitochondria; inflammation; innate immunity; adaptive immunity; immunosenescence

1. Introduction

The ancestry of the mitochondrion originated ~2.5 billion years ago within the bacterial phylum α-Proteobacteria, during the rise of eukaryotes [1]. The endosymbiotic theory, advanced with microbial evidence by Dr. Lynn Margulis in the 1960s, proposed that one prokaryote engulfed another resulting in a quid pro quo arrangement and survival advantage [2]. The ability of mitochondria to convert organic molecules from the environment to energy led to the persistence of this pact.

Since most cells contain mitochondria, the clinical effects of mitochondrial dysfunction are potentially multisystemic, and involve organs with large energy requirements [3]. In addition to making energy, the basis of life, mitochondria are also involved in heat production, calcium storage, apoptosis, cell signaling, biosynthesis, and aging—all important for cell survival and function [4–7]. A decline in mitochondrial function and oxidant production has been connected to normal aging and with the development of a variety of diseases of aging. These topics are explored more thoroughly in other articles in this special edition. While the human immune system undergoes dramatic changes during aging, eventually progressing to immunosenescence [8], the role of mitochondrial dysfunction in this process remains largely absent in the literature. Consequently, the purpose of this review is to highlight three important issues in the aging immune system: (1) inflammation with aging; (2) susceptibility to viral infections; (3) impaired T-cell immunity. These clinical phenotypes will be related to our current knowledge on the role of the mitochondria in immune function. As the associations discussed are largely speculative, it is hoped that this review will serve as a stimulus for further investigation into these issues.

2. Is There a Mitochondrial Etiology for "Inflamm-Aging"?

The term "inflamm-aging" (IA) refers to a low-grade, chronic inflammatory state that can be found in the elderly [9]. IA increases morbidity and mortality in older adults, and nearly all diseases of aging share an inflammatory pathogenesis including Alzheimer's disease, atherosclerosis, heart disease, type II diabetes, and cancer [9]. Nevertheless, the precise etiology of IA and its causal role in contributing to adverse health outcomes remain largely unknown.

The ability of the innate system to respond to a wide variety of pathogens lies in germline-encoded receptors, whose recognition is based on repetitive molecular signatures. These pattern recognition receptors (PRRs) are present on the cell surface and intracellular compartments. Toll-like receptors (TLRs), retinoic acid-inducible gene I-like receptors (RLRs), nucleotide oligomerization domain-like receptors (NLRs) and cytosolic DNA sensors (cGAS and STING) are prime examples [10]. Ligands for these receptor systems comprise pathogen associated molecular patterns (PAMPs) and damage associated molecular patterns (DAMPs) [11]. PAMPs are derived from components of microorganisms and are recognized by innate immune cells bearing PRRs. In contrast to PAMPs, DAMPs are endogenous "danger signals" that are released by cells during stress, apoptosis or necrosis. DAMPs can arise from a variety of components normally sequestered to the mitochondria, when upon release, induce inflammation via recognition by the same PRRs that recognize PAMPs [12,13]. Events downstream of PRR engagement include caspase-1 activation with the release of pro-inflammatory cytokines [14]. Examples of mitochondrial DAMPs (mtDAMPs) include cardiolipin, n-formyl peptides (e.g., fMet), mitochondrial transcription factor A (TFAM), adenosine triphosphate (ATP), reactive oxygen species (mtROS), and mitochondrial DNA (mtDNA) (Figure 1). From an evolutionary standpoint, select mitochondrial products produce inflammation due to their prokaryotic origins: e.g., cardiolipin (TLR), fMet (formyl peptide receptor 1, FPR1), and mtDNA (TLR, NLR, cGAS) [15–22]. However, mtDAMPs are not just limited to bacterial mimics. TFAM, a nuclear gene and key regulator of mtDNA transcription and replication, activates immune cells via receptors for advanced glycation end products (RAGE) and TLR9 [23,24]. Products of oxidative phosphorylation (OXPHOS) can also stimulate innate immune cells. Released from apoptotic or necrotic cells, ATP binds to purigenic receptors initiating inflammation [25], while mtROS modifies core immune signaling pathways involving hypoxia inducible factor 1 alpha (HIF1α) and nuclear factor kappa light chain enhancer of activated B-cells (NFkB) [26,27].

mtDAMPs contribute to a host of inflammatory diseases, including sepsis, systemic inflammatory response syndrome (SIRS), ischemic reperfusion injury, and aging [28]. One of the consequences of failing mitochondria due to aging, beyond mtROS, is the release of mtDNA. Plasma levels of mtDNA increase gradually after the fifth decade of life, correlating with elevated levels of pro-inflammatory cytokines (i.e., TNF-α, IL-6, RANTES, and IL-1ra) [29]. These data indicate that mtDNA may promote the production of pro-inflammatory cytokines in aging. Because cell stress, senescence and death are a part of the pathophysiology of aging [30], designing new therapeutic strategies against circulating mtDNA, or other mtDAMPs, or their cognate receptors (e.g., TLRs or FPR1) may be a viable strategy to approaching IA and its associated conditions.

Figure 1. Mitochondrial damage associated molecular patterns (DAMPs). DAMPs derived from mitochondrial components may be released during cellular injury, apoptosis or necrosis. Once these mitochondrial components are released into the extracellular space, they can lead to the activation of innate and adaptive immune cells. The recognition of mitochondrial DAMPs involves toll-like receptors (TLR), formyl peptide receptors (FPR) and purigenic receptors (P2RX7). By binding their cognate ligands or by direct interaction (i.e., reactive oxygen species, ROS), intracellular signaling pathways such as NFkB and the NLRP3 inflammasome become activated resulting in a proinflammatory response. TLR4 = toll-like receptor 4, TLR9 = toll-like receptor 9, P2RX7 = purigenic receptor, FPR1 = formyl peptide receptor 1, NLRP3 = NLR Family Pyrin Domain Containing 3, fMet = N-formylmethionine, mtROS = mitochondrial reactive oxygen species, mtDNA = mitochondrial DNA, Tfam = transcription factor A, mitochondrial, RAGE = receptors for advanced glycation end-products, NFkB = nuclear factor kappa-light-chain-enhancer of activated B cells.

3. Is Increased Susceptibility to Viral Infections Related to Depressed Mitochondrial Anti-Viral Signaling Pathways?

In general, older adults are more susceptible to a variety of viral infections, especially respiratory viral infections, resulting in high morbidity and mortality. For example, adults over the age of 65 exhibit a vulnerability to influenza A virus (IAV), and account for ≥90% of IAV-related deaths annually [31,32]. Type I interferons (e.g., IFN-α and IFN-β) are essential cytokines involved in the host antiviral response. Secreted by numerous cell types such as lymphocytes, monocytes, macrophages, dendritic cells, fibroblasts, endothelial cells, osteoblasts and others, type I interferons: (1) limit viral spread by inducing antiviral states in infected and neighboring cells; (2) stimulate antigen presentation and natural killer cell function; and (3) promote antigen-specific T and B cell responses and immunological memory. Interestingly, mitochondria play a major part in innate immune signaling against viruses and the production of type I interferons and will be discussed further.

RLRs (e.g., RIG-I and MDA5) are cytosolic receptors that recognize viral RNA. Consequent to binding viral RNA, RIG-I and MDA5 mobilize the mitochondrial antiviral signaling protein (MAVS) [33,34]. MAVS is a 56 kDa protein which contains an N-terminal caspase recruitment domain (CARD), a proline-rich region and a C-terminal transmembrane domain. Anchored on the outer membrane of the mitochondria, peroxisomes and mitochondrial associated membranes (e.g., endoplasmic reticulum), MAVS assembles into prion-like aggregates following RIG-I or MDA5 binding (Figure 2). MAVS aggregates serve as a scaffold to recruit various TNF receptor associated factors (TRAFs), resulting in phosphorylation and nuclear translocation of interferon regulatory factors

(IRFs) [35]. Downstream of MAVS, IRF3, IRF5 and IRF7 bind to their cognate promoters, leading to the production of type I interferons [36]. The localization of MAVS to the outer mitochondrial membrane is not coincidental. MAVS activity has been found to be dependent upon intact mitochondrial membrane potential, and by extension OXPHOS function [37].

Figure 2. Mitochondrial antiviral response. The recognition of viral nucleic acids involves mitochondria and intact membrane potential (ψ_m). RIG-I and MDA5 recognize cytoplasmic viral nucleic acids, leading to the oligomerization of MAVS. MAVS then sets in motion a signaling pathway that eventually leads to the phosphorylation (*P) of IRF3/7 with subsequent induction of IFNα to offer antiviral cellular protection. RIG-I = retinoic acid inducible gene I, MDA5 = melanoma differentiation-associated protein 5, MAVS = mitochondrial antiviral-signaling protein, TRAFs = TNF receptor associated factors, TBK1 = TANK binding kinase 1, IKKϵ = inhibitor of nuclear factor kappa-B kinase subunit epsilon, IRF 3 = interferon response factor 3, IRF 7 = interferon response factor 7, INFα = interferon alpha.

To date, studies addressing MAVS function during aging and its relationship to waning antiviral immunity are lacking. Decreased mitochondrial membrane potential, mitochondrial dysfunction and declining mitophagy occur in a variety of aging cell types [38,39], raising the question of whether MAVS dysfunction can occur due to mitochondrial failure with aging. Mitochondrial respiratory capacity is impaired in aging monocytes [40] as is phosphorylation of IRF3 and IRF7, suggesting a link with MAVS [41]. As a result, type I IFN synthesis is significantly lower in dendritic cells and monocytes from aging individuals [42,43]. In addition to a decline in mitochondrial respiration, oxidative stress, another consequence of aging, may also be involved in this process [43].

4. Is Impaired T-Cell Immunity in Aging Related to a Decline in Mitochondrial Function?

Aging-related decline in immune function (i.e., immunosenescence) renders older individuals more vulnerable to infectious diseases and cancer, resulting in increased morbidity and mortality. Besides increased susceptibility to infection, vaccine efficacy is significantly reduced in the elderly, limiting the utility of prophylaxis [44,45]. Undeniably, profound changes in T-cell function are evident in older individuals, and these changes may be related to a decline in mitochondrial function.

T-cells play a central role in the coordination of adaptive immune responses and cell-mediated immunity. The ability of T-cells to fulfill this role is dependent upon rapid cellular proliferation and differentiation. In response to infection, T-cells proliferate every 4–6 h, generating >10^{12} cells in one week [46,47]. This is accompanied by an increase in size, DNA remodeling, up-regulation of transcription factors and effector molecules, and increased expression of surface proteins [48,49], thus necessitating a large metabolic demand. To accomplish this task, metabolic fuels including fats, sugars and amino acids are actively transported across the cell membrane to feed the increase in energetic demands [50,51]. Along with this increased transport, T-cells undergo metabolic reprogramming during their transition from a naïve state to activated and differentiated cell types (e.g., effector, regulatory and memory cells).

The diverse roles played by mitochondria in T-cell activation emphasizes the potential mechanisms by which aging-related mitochondrial decline may contribute to immune dysfunction. Following stimulation of the T-cell receptor, T-cells undergo substantial changes in intermediary metabolism including an increase in glycolysis and OXPHOS [52–57]. In the presence of oxygen, pyruvate produced via glycolysis is fully oxidized in the mitochondria for energy in many cell types [58,59]. In T-cells, a significant proportion of glucose is not oxidized, but rather fermented to lactate from pyruvate via lactate dehydrogenase. This is done despite the presence of oxygen, and is termed aerobic glycolysis or Warburg metabolism [50,56,60]. Although Warburg metabolism is viewed as energetically inefficient, the rate of glycolysis is 10–100 times faster than glucose oxidation by the mitochondria, yielding equivalent amounts of ATP [61]. The additional payoff of Warburg metabolism lies in pathways that are branch points off of glycolysis (e.g., pentose phosphate pathway) which yield reducing equivalents for biosynthesis and nucleotides. Despite this adoption of the Warburg phenotype, OXPHOS is still required for T-cell activation [57]. ATP derived from the mitochondrial respiration promotes enhanced glycolysis as well as the initiation of proliferation in activated T-cells [62]. While pyruvate is mostly diverted to lactate rather than acetyl-CoA via pyruvate dehydrogenase, TCA function and the generation of reducing equivalents in highly proliferating cells is still maintained through anapleurosis: glutamine is converted to α-ketoglutarate via glutaminolysis [63,64]. Bioenergetic studies of aging tissues are consistent with a progressive decline in mitochondrial respiratory function due to a decrease in respiratory complex activity, mitochondrial membrane potential, and impaired mitophagy [39,65]. As a result, impaired OXPHOS results in reduced ATP production, thus potentially limiting glycolysis, biosynthesis and the attainment of biomass during T-cell activation and proliferation.

Besides engaging in bioenergetics, mitochondria also function in T-cell activation by modulating secondary messengers including calcium (Ca^{2+}) and reactive oxygen species (ROS). In activated T-cells, mitochondria localize to the immune synapse, and where they regulate Ca^{2+} flux [5,6]. In response to this calcium flux, ROS production via complex III of the respiratory chain is amplified, leading to nuclear factor of activated T-cells (NFAT) activation and subsequent interleukin-2 (IL-2) production [66]. Aged T-cells show reduced Ca^{2+} signaling, which could be partly due to deficits in Ca^{2+} regulation found in mitochondria of aged cells [67,68], theoretically yielding perturbations at the immune synapse causing diminished T-cell signaling and activation.

Depending on the cytokine milieu, helper T-cells (Th), marked by the surface expression of CD4, differentiate into various effector subsets comprising T-helper 1 (Th1), T-helper 2 (Th2), T-helper 17 (Th17), regulatory T-cells (Treg). Each of these T-cell subsets are unique in their responsibilities and are identified by their cytokine signatures. Accompanying these functional distinctions are differences in metabolic reprogramming (Figure 3). For example, for T-cells subsets involved in inflammation (e.g., Th1 and Th17), the Warburg metabolism instituted at T-cell activation persists [69]. Despite this primary use of glycolysis, intact OXPHOS is still necessary for their function [57]. The effects of mitochondrial dysfunction may be more readily seen in regulatory (Treg) and memory (Tmem) T-cells. Tregs, which serve to modulate the immune system and maintain tolerance, revert back to OXPHOS as their main pathway for generating energy upon differentiation [69]. Tmem follow a similar metabolic path. Tmem are critical for adaptive immune responses characterized by robust responses to secondary immune challenges. Unlike effector T-cells, Tmem do not undergo extensive proliferation and produce little or no cytokines. As such, the metabolic profile of Tmem are essentially catabolic, relying on OXPHOS and fatty acid oxidation [70,71]. Therefore, it is not surprising to find that CD8[+] cytotoxic memory T-cells have high respiratory capacity and increased mitochondrial mass, which allows them to rapidly reactivate upon re-exposure to their cognate antigens [62,72]. Given the age-related decline in mitochondrial function as described above, T-cell subsets which are critical for immunosurveillance and the clearance of invading pathogens could be functionally impaired and may partially explain the vulnerability to infection and cancer with aging [57]. Emerging data also suggest that aging significantly affects Treg frequencies, subsets and function [73], potentially leading to the increased incidence of autoimmunity, oftentimes seen with aging [74]. As noted above, Tmem also rely heavily on OXPHOS. Therefore, aging-related deficiencies in Tmem may also be traced to declining OXPHOS, manifesting as impaired immune memory to novel antigens and suboptimal boosts to existing memory [75].

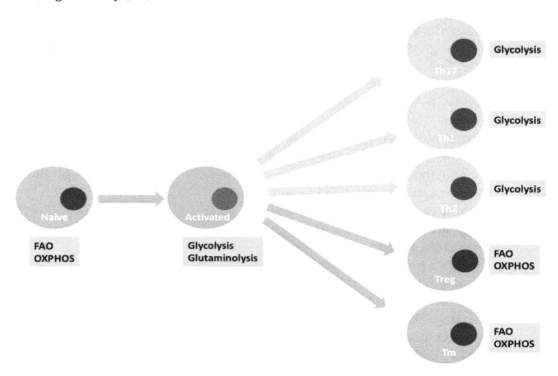

Figure 3. T-cell activation and differentiation involved metabolic reprogramming. At rest, naïve T-cells primarily use OXPHOS to derive their energy. Following activation, T-cells switch to Warburg metabolism and glutaminolysis to support their proliferative needs. Differentiation into T-helper subsets can involve either the maintenance of the Warburg phenotype (i.e., Th17, Th1, Th2), or the reversion to OXPHOS with FAO (i.e., Treg, Tm) as an important fuel. FAO = mitochondrial fatty acid oxidation, OXPHOS = oxidative phosphorylation, Th17 = T-helper cell 17, Th1 = T-helper cell 1, Th2 = T-helper cell 2, Treg = regulatory T-cells, Tm = memory T-cells.

5. Conclusions

Virtually every country in the world is experiencing the challenges associated with accelerated growth in the aging population. With this graying of the population comes an increased incidence in diseases of aging, many of which have an immune component. As a result, understanding the pathophysiology of diseases of aging is now more important than ever. In this review, three main immune issues prevalent in the aging population were addressed: (1) inflamm-aging; (2) increased vulnerability to infection; and (3) declining T-cell immunity. The role of the mitochondria in inflammation and immunity, combined with the knowledge of a decline in mitochondrial function with aging, has been synthesized in this review in an effort to partially explain the immune phenotype associated with aging. However, further examination of this relationship is needed. As the methods of inquiry into mitochondrial biology continue to expand, so will investigations into the relationship between this ancient organelle and immunity in the aging population.

References

1. Martin, W.F.; Garg, S.; Zimorski, V. Endosymbiotic theories for eukaryote origin. *Philos. Trans. R. Soc. Lond. B Biol. Sci.* **2015**, *370*, 20140330. [CrossRef]
2. Gray, M.W. Mitochondrial evolution. *Cold Spring Harb. Perspect. Biol.* **2012**, *4*, a011403. [CrossRef] [PubMed]
3. Vafai, S.B.; Mootha, V.K. Mitochondrial disorders as windows into an ancient organelle. *Nature* **2012**, *491*, 374–383. [CrossRef]
4. Antico Arciuch, V.G.; Elguero, M.E.; Poderoso, J.J.; Carreras, M.C. Mitochondrial regulation of cell cycle and proliferation. *Antioxid. Redox Signal.* **2012**, *16*, 1150–1180. [CrossRef] [PubMed]
5. Quintana, A.; Schwindling, C.; Wenning, A.S.; Becherer, U.; Rettig, J.; Schwarz, E.C.; Hoth, M. T cell activation requires mitochondrial translocation to the immunological synapse. *Proc. Natl. Acad. Sci. USA* **2007**, *104*, 14418–14423. [CrossRef]
6. Schwindling, C.; Quintana, A.; Krause, E.; Hoth, M. Mitochondria positioning controls local calcium influx in T cells. *J. Immunol.* **2010**, *184*, 184–190. [CrossRef]
7. Sena, L.A.; Chandel, N.S. Physiological roles of mitochondrial reactive oxygen species. *Mol. Cell* **2012**, *48*, 158–167. [CrossRef] [PubMed]
8. Weyand, C.M.; Goronzy, J.J. Aging of the Immune System. Mechanisms and Therapeutic Targets. *Ann. Am. Thorac. Soc.* **2016**, *13* (Suppl. 5), S422–S428. [CrossRef]
9. Xia, S.; Zhang, X.; Zheng, S.; Khanabdali, R.; Kalionis, B.; Wu, J.; Wan, W.; Tai, X. An Update on Inflamm-Aging: Mechanisms, Prevention, and Treatment. *J. Immunol. Res.* **2016**, *2016*, 8426874. [CrossRef]
10. Thompson, M.R.; Kaminski, J.J.; Kurt-Jones, E.A.; Fitzgerald, K.A. Pattern recognition receptors and the innate immune response to viral infection. *Viruses* **2011**, *3*, 920–940. [CrossRef]
11. Tang, D.; Kang, R.; Coyne, C.B.; Zeh, H.J.; Lotze, M.T. PAMPs and DAMPs: Signal 0s that spur autophagy and immunity. *Immunol. Rev.* **2012**, *249*, 158–175. [CrossRef]
12. Janeway, C.A., Jr.; Medzhitov, R. Innate immune recognition. *Annu. Rev. Immunol.* **2002**, *20*, 197–216. [CrossRef]
13. Medzhitov, R. Innate immunity: Quo vadis? *Nat. Immunol.* **2010**, *11*, 551–553. [CrossRef]
14. Martinon, F.; Burns, K.; Tschopp, J. The inflammasome: A molecular platform triggering activation of inflammatory caspases and processing of proIL-beta. *Mol. Cell* **2002**, *10*, 417–426. [CrossRef]
15. Wenceslau, C.F.; McCarthy, C.G.; Goulopoulou, S.; Szasz, T.; NeSmith, E.G.; Webb, R.C. Mitochondrial-derived N-formyl peptides: Novel links between trauma, vascular collapse and sepsis. *Med. Hypotheses* **2013**, *81*, 532–535. [CrossRef]
16. Collins, L.V.; Hajizadeh, S.; Holme, E.; Jonsson, I.M.; Tarkowski, A. Endogenously oxidized mitochondrial DNA induces in vivo and in vitro inflammatory responses. *J. Leukoc. Biol.* **2004**, *75*, 995–1000. [CrossRef]
17. Hauser, C.J.; Sursal, T.; Rodriguez, E.K.; Appleton, P.T.; Zhang, Q.; Itagaki, K. Mitochondrial damage associated molecular patterns from femoral reamings activate neutrophils through formyl peptide receptors and P44/42 MAP kinase. *J. Orthop. Trauma* **2010**, *24*, 534–538. [CrossRef]
18. Zhang, Q.; Raoof, M.; Chen, Y.; Sumi, Y.; Sursal, T.; Junger, W.; Brohi, K.; Itagaki, K.; Hauser, C.J. Circulating mitochondrial DAMPs cause inflammatory responses to injury. *Nature* **2010**, *464*, 104–107. [CrossRef]
19. Zhang, Q.; Itagaki, K.; Hauser, C.J. Mitochondrial DNA Is Released by Shock and Activates Neutrophils Via P38 Map Kinase. *Shock* **2010**, *34*, 55–59. [CrossRef]
20. Iyer, S.S.; He, Q.; Janczy, J.R.; Elliott, E.I.; Zhong, Z.; Olivier, A.K.; Sadler, J.J.; Knepper-Adrian, V.; Han, R.; Qiao, L.; et al. Mitochondrial cardiolipin is required for Nlrp3 inflammasome activation. *Immunity* **2013**, *39*, 311–323. [CrossRef]
21. Toksoy, A.; Sennefelder, H.; Adam, C.; Hofmann, S.; Trautmann, A.; Goebeler, M.; Schmidt, M. Potent NLRP3 Inflammasome Activation by the HIV Reverse Transcriptase Inhibitor Abacavir. *J. Biol. Chem.* **2017**, *292*, 2805–2814. [CrossRef]
22. Rossen, R.D.; Michael, L.H.; Hawkins, H.K.; Youker, K.; Dreyer, W.J.; Baughn, R.E.; Entman, M.L. Cardiolipin-Protein Complexes and Initiation of Complement Activation after Coronary-Artery Occlusion. *Circ. Res.* **1994**, *75*, 546–555. [CrossRef]
23. Chaung, W.W.; Wu, R.; Ji, Y.; Dong, W.; Wang, P. Mitochondrial transcription factor A is a proinflammatory mediator in hemorrhagic shock. *Int. J. Mol. Med.* **2012**, *30*, 199–203.
24. Julian, M.W.; Shao, G.; Vangundy, Z.C.; Papenfuss, T.L.; Crouser, E.D. Mitochondrial transcription factor A,

an endogenous danger signal, promotes TNFalpha release via RAGE- and TLR9-responsive plasmacytoid dendritic cells. *PLoS ONE* **2013**, *8*, e72354. [CrossRef]

25. Iyer, S.S.; Pulskens, W.P.; Sadler, J.J.; Butter, L.M.; Teske, G.J.; Ulland, T.K.; Eisenbarth, S.C.; Florquin, S.; Flavell, R.A.; Leemans, J.C.; et al. Necrotic cells trigger a sterile inflammatory response through the Nlrp3 inflammasome. *Proc. Natl. Acad. Sci. USA* **2009**, *106*, 20388–20393. [CrossRef]

26. Brunelle, J.K.; Bell, E.L.; Quesada, N.M.; Vercauteren, K.; Tiranti, V.; Zeviani, M.; Scarpulla, R.C.; Chandel, N.S. Oxygen sensing requires mitochondrial ROS but not oxidative phosphorylation. *Cell Metab.* **2005**, *1*, 409–414. [CrossRef]

27. Chandel, N.S.; Trzyna, W.C.; McClintock, D.S.; Schumacker, P.T. Role of oxidants in NF-kappa B activation and TNF-alpha gene transcription induced by hypoxia and endotoxin. *J. Immunol.* **2000**, *165*, 1013–1021. [CrossRef]

28. Nakahira, K.; Hisata, S.; Choi, A.M. The Roles of Mitochondrial Damage-Associated Molecular Patterns in Diseases. *Antioxid. Redox Signal.* **2015**, *23*, 1329–1350. [CrossRef]

29. Pinti, M.; Cevenini, E.; Nasi, M.; De Biasi, S.; Salvioli, S.; Monti, D.; Benatti, S.; Gibellini, L.; Cotichini, R.; Stazi, M.A.; et al. Circulating mitochondrial DNA increases with age and is a familiar trait: Implications for "inflamm-aging". *Eur. J. Immunol.* **2014**, *44*, 1552–1562. [CrossRef]

30. Childs, B.G.; Durik, M.; Baker, D.J.; van Deursen, J.M. Cellular senescence in aging and age-related disease: From mechanisms to therapy. *Nat. Med.* **2015**, *21*, 1424–1435. [CrossRef]

31. Thompson, W.W.; Shay, D.K.; Weintraub, E.; Brammer, L.; Cox, N.; Anderson, L.J.; Fukuda, K. Mortality associated with influenza and respiratory syncytial virus in the United States. *JAMA* **2003**, *289*, 179–186. [CrossRef]

32. Simonsen, L.; Clarke, M.J.; Schonberger, L.B.; Arden, N.H.; Cox, N.J.; Fukuda, K. Pandemic versus epidemic influenza mortality: A pattern of changing age distribution. *J. Infect. Dis.* **1998**, *178*, 53–60. [CrossRef]

33. Kumar, H.; Kawai, T.; Kato, H.; Sato, S.; Takahashi, K.; Coban, C.; Yamamoto, M.; Uematsu, S.; Ishii, K.J.; Takeuchi, O.; et al. Essential role of IPS-1 in innate immune responses against RNA viruses. *J. Exp. Med.* **2006**, *203*, 1795–1803. [CrossRef]

34. Lin, R.T.; Lacoste, J.; Nakhaei, P.; Sun, Q.; Yang, L.; Paz, S.; Wilkinson, P.; Julkunen, I.; Vitour, D.; Meurs, E.; et al. Dissociation of a MAVS/IPS-1/VISA/Cardif-1KK epsilon molecular complex from the mitochondrial outer membrane by hepatitis C virus NS3-4A proteolytic cleavage. *J. Virol.* **2006**, *80*, 6072–6083. [CrossRef]

35. Liu, B.Y.; Gao, C.J. Regulation of MAVS activation through post-translational modifications. *Curr. Opin. Immunol.* **2018**, *50*, 75–81. [CrossRef]

36. Lazear, H.M.; Lancaster, A.; Wilkins, C.; Suthar, M.S.; Huang, A.; Vick, S.C.; Clepper, L.; Thackray, L.; Brassil, M.M.; Virgin, H.W.; et al. IRF-3, IRF-5, and IRF-7 coordinately regulate the type I IFN response in myeloid dendritic cells downstream of MAVS signaling. *PLoS Pathog.* **2013**, *9*, e1003118. [CrossRef]

37. Koshiba, T.; Yasukawa, K.; Yanagi, Y.; Kawabata, S. Mitochondrial Membrane Potential Is Required for MAVS-Mediated Antiviral Signaling. *Sci. Signal.* **2011**, *4*, ra7. [CrossRef]

38. Sugrue, M.M.; Tatton, W.G. Mitochondrial membrane potential in aging cells. *Neurosignals* **2001**, *10*, 176–188. [CrossRef]

39. Diot, A.; Morten, K.; Poulton, J. Mitophagy plays a central role in mitochondrial ageing. *Mamm. Genome* **2016**, *27*, 381–395. [CrossRef]

40. Pence, B.D.; Yarbro, J.R. Aging impairs mitochondrial respiratory capacity in classical monocytes. *Exp. Gerontol.* **2018**, *108*, 112–117. [CrossRef]

41. Molony, R.D.; Nguyen, J.T.; Kong, Y.; Montgomery, R.R.; Shaw, A.C.; Iwasaki, A. Aging impairs both primary and secondary RIG-I signaling for interferon induction in human monocytes. *Sci. Signal.* **2017**, *10*, eaan2392. [CrossRef]

42. Qian, F.; Wang, X.; Zhang, L.; Lin, A.; Zhao, H.; Fikrig, E.; Montgomery, R.R. Impaired interferon signaling in dendritic cells from older donors infected in vitro with West Nile virus. *J. Infect. Dis.* **2011**, *203*, 1415–1424. [CrossRef]

43. Stout-Delgado, H.W.; Yang, X.; Walker, W.E.; Tesar, B.M.; Goldstein, D.R. Aging impairs IFN regulatory factor 7 up-regulation in plasmacytoid dendritic cells during TLR9 activation. *J. Immunol.* **2008**, *181*, 6747–6756. [CrossRef]

44. Burns, E.A.; Lum, L.G.; L'Hommedieu, G.; Goodwin, J.S. Specific humoral immunity in the elderly: In vivo and in vitro response to vaccination. *J. Gerontol.* **1993**, *48*, B231–B236. [CrossRef]

45. Musher, D.M.; Chapman, A.J.; Goree, A.; Jonsson, S.; Briles, D.; Baughn, R.E. Natural and vaccine-related immunity to Streptococcus pneumoniae. *J. Infect. Dis.* **1986**, *154*, 245–256. [CrossRef]

46. Badovinac, V.P.; Haring, J.S.; Harty, J.T. Initial T cell receptor transgenic cell precursor frequency dictates critical aspects of the CD8(+) T cell response to infection. *Immunity* **2007**, *26*, 827–841. [CrossRef]

47. Yoon, H.; Kim, T.S.; Braciale, T.J. The Cell Cycle Time of CD8(+) T Cells Responding In Vivo Is Controlled by the Type of Antigenic Stimulus. *PLoS ONE* **2010**, *5*, e15423. [CrossRef]

48. Gray, S.M.; Kaech, S.M.; Staron, M.M. The interface between transcriptional and epigenetic control of effector and memory CD8(+) T-cell differentiation. *Immunol. Rev.* **2014**, *261*, 157–168. [CrossRef]

49. Zhang, N.; Bevan, M.J. CD8(+) T cells: Foot soldiers of the immune system. *Immunity* **2011**, *35*, 161–168. [CrossRef]

50. Macintyre, A.N.; Gerriets, V.A.; Nichols, A.G.; Michalek, R.D.; Rudolph, M.C.; Deoliveira, D.; Anderson, S.M.; Abel, E.D.; Chen, B.J.; Hale, L.P.; et al. The Glucose Transporter Glut1 Is Selectively Essential for CD4 T Cell Activation and Effector Function. *Cell Metab.* **2014**, *20*, 61–72. [CrossRef]

51. Sinclair, L.V.; Rolf, J.; Emslie, E.; Shi, Y.B.; Taylor, P.M.; Cantrell, D.A. Control of amino-acid transport by antigen receptors coordinates the metabolic reprogramming essential for T cell differentiation. *Nat. Immunol.* **2013**, *14*, 500–508. [CrossRef]

52. Frauwirth, K.A.; Riley, J.L.; Harris, M.H.; Parry, R.V.; Rathmell, J.C.; Plas, D.R.; Elstrom, R.L.; June, C.H.; Thompson, C.B. The CD28 signaling pathway regulates glucose metabolism. *Immunity* **2002**, *16*, 769–777. [CrossRef]

53. Marjanovic, S.; Eriksson, I.; Nelson, B.D. Expression of a new set of glycolytic isozymes in activated human peripheral lymphocytes. *Biochim. Biophys. Acta* **1990**, *1087*, 1–6. [CrossRef]

54. Marjanovic, S.; Wielburski, A.; Nelson, B.D. Effect of phorbol myristate acetate and concanavalin A on the glycolytic enzymes of human peripheral lymphocytes. *Biochim. Biophys. Acta* **1988**, *970*, 1–6. [CrossRef]

55. O'Rourke, A.M.; Rider, C.C. Glucose, glutamine and ketone body utilisation by resting and concanavalin A activated rat splenic lymphocytes. *Biochim. Biophys. Acta* **1989**, *1010*, 342–345. [CrossRef]

56. Wang, R.N.; Dillon, C.P.; Shi, L.Z.; Milasta, S.; Carter, R.; Finkelstein, D.; McCormick, L.L.; Fitzgerald, P.; Chi, H.B.; Munger, J.; et al. The Transcription Factor Myc Controls Metabolic Reprogramming upon T Lymphocyte Activation. *Immunity* **2011**, *35*, 871–882. [CrossRef]

57. Tarasenko, T.N.; Pacheco, S.E.; Koenig, M.K.; Gomez-Rodriguez, J.; Kapnick, S.M.; Diaz, F.; Zerfas, P.M.; Barca, E.; Sudderth, J.; DeBerardinis, R.J.; et al. Cytochrome c Oxidase Activity Is a Metabolic Checkpoint that Regulates Cell Fate Decisions During T Cell Activation and Differentiation. *Cell Metab.* **2017**, *25*, 1268 e1257. [CrossRef]

58. Jones, R.G.; Thompson, C.B. Revving the engine: Signal transduction fuels T cell activation. *Immunity* **2007**, *27*, 173–178. [CrossRef]

59. Krebs, H.A. The tricarboxylic acid cycle. *Harvey Lect.* **1948**, *Series 44*, 165–199.

60. Macintyre, A.N.; Rathmell, J.C. Activated lymphocytes as a metabolic model for carcinogenesis. *Cancer Metab.* **2013**, *1*, 5. [CrossRef]

61. Shestov, A.A.; Liu, X.J.; Ser, Z.; Cluntun, A.A.; Hung, Y.P.; Huang, L.; Kim, D.; Le, A.; Yellen, G.; Albeck, J.G.; et al. Quantitative determinants of aerobic glycolysis identify flux through the enzyme GAPDH as a limiting step. *eLife* **2014**, *3*, e03342. [CrossRef]

62. Van der Windt, G.J.; O'Sullivan, D.; Everts, B.; Huang, S.C.; Buck, M.D.; Curtis, J.D.; Chang, C.H.; Smith, A.M.; Ai, T.; Faubert, B.; et al. CD8 memory T cells have a bioenergetic advantage that underlies their rapid recall ability. *Proc. Natl. Acad. Sci. USA* **2013**, *110*, 14336–14341. [CrossRef]

63. DeBerardinis, R.J.; Mancuso, A.; Daikhin, E.; Nissim, I.; Yudkoff, M.; Wehrli, S.; Thompson, C.B. Beyond aerobic glycolysis: Transformed cells can engage in glutamine metabolism that exceeds the requirement for protein and nucleotide synthesis. *Proc. Natl. Acad. Sci. USA* **2007**, *104*, 19345–19350. [CrossRef]

64. Csibi, A.; Fendt, S.M.; Li, C.; Poulogiannis, G.; Choo, A.Y.; Chapski, D.J.; Jeong, S.M.; Dempsey, J.M.; Parkhitko, A.; Morrison, T.; et al. The mTORC1 pathway stimulates glutamine metabolism and cell proliferation by repressing SIRT4. *Cell* **2013**, *153*, 840–854. [CrossRef]

65. Lee, H.C.; Wei, Y.H. Mitochondria and aging. *Adv. Exp. Med. Biol.* **2012**, *942*, 311–327.

66. Sena, L.A.; Li, S.; Jairaman, A.; Prakriya, M.; Ezponda, T.; Hildeman, D.A.; Wang, C.R.; Schumacker, P.T.; Licht, J.D.; Perlman, H.; et al. Mitochondria are required for antigen-specific T cell activation through reactive oxygen species signaling. *Immunity* **2013**, *38*, 225–236. [CrossRef]

67. Mather, M.W.; Rottenberg, H. The inhibition of calcium signaling in T lymphocytes from old mice results from enhanced activation of the mitochondrial permeability transition pore. *Mech. Ageing Dev.* **2002**, *123*, 707–724. [CrossRef]

68. Murchison, D.; Zawieja, D.C.; Griffith, W.H. Reduced mitochondrial buffering of voltage-gated calcium influx in aged rat basal forebrain neurons. *Cell Calcium* **2004**, *36*, 61–75. [CrossRef]

69. Buck, M.D.; O'Sullivan, D.; Klein Geltink, R.I.; Curtis, J.D.; Chang, C.H.; Sanin, D.E.; Qiu, J.; Kretz, O.; Braas, D.; van der Windt, G.J.; et al. Mitochondrial Dynamics Controls T Cell Fate through Metabolic Programming. *Cell* **2016**, *166*, 63–76. [CrossRef]

70. Fox, C.J.; Hammerman, P.S.; Thompson, C.B. Fuel feeds function: Energy metabolism and the T-cell response. *Nat. Rev. Immunol.* **2005**, *5*, 844–852. [CrossRef]

71. Yusuf, I.; Fruman, D.A. Regulation of quiescence in lymphocytes. *Trends Immunol.* **2003**, *24*, 380–386. [CrossRef]

72. Van der Windt, G.J.; Everts, B.; Chang, C.H.; Curtis, J.D.; Freitas, T.C.; Amiel, E.; Pearce, E.J.; Pearce, E.L. Mitochondrial respiratory capacity is a critical regulator of CD8+ T cell memory development. *Immunity* **2012**, *36*, 68–78. [CrossRef]

73. Jagger, A.; Shimojima, Y.; Goronzy, J.J.; Weyand, C.M. Regulatory T cells and the immune aging process: A mini-review. *Gerontology* **2014**, *60*, 130–137. [CrossRef]

74. Vadasz, Z.; Haj, T.; Kessel, A.; Toubi, E. Age-related autoimmunity. *BMC Med.* **2013**, *11*, 94. [CrossRef]

75. Goronzy, J.J.; Weyand, C.M. Successful and Maladaptive T Cell Aging. *Immunity* **2017**, *46*, 364–378. [CrossRef]

7

From Powerhouse to Perpetrator—Mitochondria in Health and Disease

**Nima B. Fakouri [1], Thomas Lau Hansen [2], Claus Desler [2], Sharath Anugula [2]
and Lene Juel Rasmussen [2,*]**

[1]   Laboratory of Molecular Gerontology, National Institute on Aging, National Institutes of Health, Baltimore,
    MD 21224, USA; nima.borhanfakouri@nih.gov
[2]   Center for Healthy Aging, Department of Cellular and Molecular Medicine, University of Copenhagen,
    2200 Copenhagen, Denmark; tlhansen@sund.ku.dk (T.L.H.); cdesler@sund.ku.dk (C.D.);
    sharath@sund.ku.dk (S.A.)
*   Correspondence: lenera@sund.ku.dk

Abstract: In this review we discuss the interaction between metabolic stress, mitochondrial dysfunction, and genomic instability. Unrepaired DNA damage in the nucleus resulting from excess accumulation of DNA damages and stalled replication can initiate cellular signaling responses that negatively affect metabolism and mitochondrial function. On the other hand, mitochondrial pathologies can also lead to stress in the nucleus, and cause sensitivity to DNA-damaging agents. These are examples of how hallmarks of cancer and aging are connected and influenced by each other to protect humans from disease.

Keywords: mitochondria; cancer; nucleotide metabolism; DNA damage; NAD$^+$

1. Introduction

It has been almost two decades since Hanahan and Weinberg for the first time classified the hallmarks of cancer [1]. Ten years later, they updated that list and introduced genomic instability and dysregulation of cellular energetics and mitochondrial function as emerging hallmarks [2]. Recently, both genomic instability and mitochondrial dysfunction are considered as two of the key hallmarks of aging [3]. Both of these have been implicated in several pathologies, as reviewed in References [4–6]. There are other hallmarks that are common between cancer and aging, such as epigenetic changes and altered cellular communication. Moreover, other hallmarks are in opposition to each other in cancer and aging. These include the dysregulation of apoptosis and senescence, which are stimulated in aging cells and suppressed in cancer cells [2,3]. Whether we can consider cancer as the disease of aging is a topic that is beyond the scope of this review, but age is the largest risk factor in the development of cancer [7].

One of the key questions that remain to be answered is, how are these hallmarks are connected and influenced by each other [3]? As these pathologic cellular changes occur gradually, understanding the connection between them would help to develop more effective therapeutic strategies to treat cancer or rather prevent it.

It has long been known that byproducts of cellular metabolism such as reactive oxygen and nitrogen species (ROS and RNS) can damage cellular components and macromolecules including DNA [8,9]. Damage to DNA can have severe effects on cells by blocking replication, transcription, generation of DNA double and single strand breaks, as well as chromosome rearrangements [10,11]. Activation of the DNA damage response (DDR) following DNA damage is an energy-demanding process [12], and can deplete cells of substrates such as NAD$^+$ and ATP, which can in turn lead to additional metabolic stress and mitochondrial dysfunction (Figure 1) [13–15].

Figure 1. Illustration of the mitochondrial-nuclear interactions in aging or cancer. Abnormal metabolism and/or metabolic defects lead to metabolic stress and mitochondrial dysfunction. This is followed by the increased generation of reactive oxygen and nitrogen species (ROS and RNS) as well as reactive aldehydes. These reactive species can react and damage macromolecules such as proteins and DNA. Damage to DNA causes genomic instability via stalled replication and transcription, and the generation of double- and single-strand breaks (DSBs and SSBs, respectively) within the genome. Increased activities of the DNA damage response (DDR) deplete cells of key cellular substrates and cofactors, mainly ATP and NAD$^+$. This generates a positive feedback that enhances metabolic stress and mitochondrial dysfunction.

In this review, we aim to discuss the interaction between metabolic stress and mitochondrial dysfunction with genomic instability. Stress in the nucleus, such as the accumulation of DNA damage and stalled replication, negatively affects metabolism and mitochondrial function [13–17], while mitochondrial pathologies lead to stress in the nucleus [18] and cause sensitivity to DNA-damaging agents [19], as reviewed by Desler et al. in 2012 [20].

First, we explain how the accumulation of DNA damages and the activation of the DDR leads to mitochondrial dysfunction. Next, we explain how the dysregulation of mitochondrial function and metabolism contributes to the epigenetic changes, imbalanced dNTP pools, and genomic instability.

2. From DNA Damage to Mitochondrial Dysfunction

Activation of the main components of the DDR, including poly (ADP-ribose) polymerase (PARP) enzymes (mainly PARP1 and PARP2) as well as ataxia telangiectasia mutated (ATM) [21], DNA-dependent protein kinase (DNA-PK) [22,23] and P53 [24–27], is able to influence mitochondrial function and cellular metabolism. Chronic activation of PARP1 negatively affects cellular physiology and mitochondrial function [28]. Activation of ATM, DNA-PK, and P53 can influence mitochondrial and cellular metabolism to promote either cell survival or death (Figure 2). Here, we briefly describe how each of these enzymes are able to influence mitochondrial function.

Figure 2. Core DNA damage response proteins are able to influence mitochondrial activity and quality control via multiple pathways. Abnormal DNA structure and certain genomic lesions, such as strand breaks, activate poly (ADP-ribose) polymerase (PARP) enzymes, mainly PARP1. Chronic activation of PARP1 can deplete the cell of NAD^+, which is a rate-limiting substrate for SIRT1. SIRT1 together with AMP-activated kinase (AMPK) can enhance metabolism and mitochondrial function by enhancing mitochondrial biogenesis and mitophagy. Activation of ataxia telangiectasia mutated (ATM), Rad3-related (ATR) and DNA-dependent protein kinase (DNA-PK) following DNA damage can promote the activation AKT and P53. Activation of AKT rewires cellular metabolism by inhibiting Forkhead box (FOXO) enzymes. Deacetylation of P53 by SIRT1 targets P53 for degradation. Decrease in SIRT1 activity stabilizes P53. P53 decreases mitophagy via inhibition of PTEN-induced kinase 1 (PINK1) and PARKIN transcription. SIRT1 promotes AMPK activity indirectly. Decrease in SIRT1 activity is followed by the decrease in activated AMPK.

3. PARP Modulates Mitochondrial Function and Cellular Metabolism

PARPs are a group of enzymes (16 in mice and 17 in humans) that are the main constituent of the cellular stress response [29]. PARPs cleave NAD^+ to nicotinamide (NAM) and ADP-ribose (ADPR), and the ADPR is subsequently transferred to certain amino acids within the target protein. The attachment of poly ADP-ribose (PAR) to the target proteins is referred to as PARylation, and it can affect protein–protein and protein–DNA interaction as well as protein localization [30]. PAR has a short half-life and is degraded almost directly after its formation by the activity of the PAR-degrading enzyme, poly(ADP-ribose) glycohydrolase (PARG) [31]. PARylation modulates several key cellular processes such as chromatin structure, transcription, translation, cell cycle, DNA repair, mitochondrial homeostasis, apoptosis, and metabolism [29,32]. PARP1 is activated by several mechanisms, including mono(ADP-ribosyl)ation, phosphorylation, and acetylation [29]. PARP1 possesses a DNA-binding domain that recognizes abnormal DNA structures such as gapped DNA, single- and double strand breaks, cruciform structures, and nucleosome linker DNA [33,34]. In the initial steps of the repair, PARP1 PARylates histones and facilitates the chromatin relaxation that provides more space for the recruitment of DNA repair proteins. Subsequent PAR generation recruits the DNA repair proteins via their PAR-binding domains [35,36]. Under mild genotoxic stress, PARP activation results in repair and survival. However, in response to DNA damage, PARP hyper-activation results in decrease in NAD^+ and ATP levels, mitochondrial dysfunction, and eventually cell death [32,35,37].

4. DNA Damage can Activate Both Pro-Survival and Pro-Death Pathways That Involve the Mitochondria

DNA damage and DDR can activate pathways that promote cell survival or death depending on the extent and type of DNA damages [38]. In addition to PARP1, other immediate sensors of DDR are enzymes belonging to the superfamily of phosphatidylinositol 3-kinase-related kinases (PIKKs), including ATM, ataxia telangiectasia and Rad3-related (ATR), and DNA-PK. Activated ATR and ATM, in turn, activate P53 through CHK1 and CHK2, respectively. Apart from preventing cell cycle progression and the recruitment of DNA repair proteins, these enzymes can modulate mitochondrial function and survival [23,39]. ATM, ATR, and DNA-PK are able to promote survival via the direct phosphorylation of AKT (also known as protein kinase B, PKB) independently of growth factor signaling [22,40–43]. However, the mechanism of this interaction is not fully understood [44]. This is particularly interesting, as in many cancer cells, the AKT is activated independently of growth factors [45]. Activated AKT stimulates glucose uptake and ATP production through glycolysis, one of the main hallmarks of cancer, also known as the Warburg effect [46]. In addition, activated AKT inhibits Forkhead box (FOXO) transcription factors [47,48]. FOXO proteins regulate the expression of key genes that are involved in mitochondrial biogenesis and homeostasis, such as peroxisome proliferator-activated receptor gamma co-activator 1alpha (PGC1a) and PTEN-induced kinase 1 (PINK1). Decrease in FOXO activity results in the decrease of mitochondrial biogenesis, mitophagy, autophagy, and lipolysis [49].

5. Mito-Nuclear Signaling in Aging and Cancer

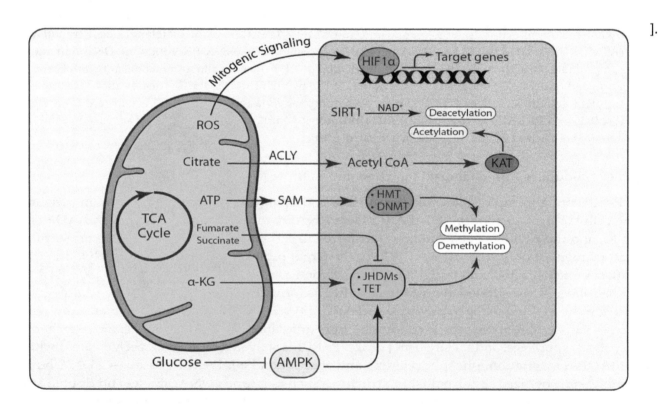

Figure 3. Mitochondrial function and metabolites influence nuclear processes. Mitochondrial ROS and secondary metabolites act as signaling molecules and cofactors that regulate fundamental nuclear processes. Mitochondrial ROS that are released into the cytosol stabilize hypoxia-inducible factor 1- α

(HIF1α) and activate the transcription of genes that are involved in proliferation. Citrate generated through the TCA cycle is released into the cytosol and in the nucleus. It is further converted into acetyl-coenzyme A (acetyl CoA) that is used for the acetylation of target proteins. Through a reverse reaction, SIRT1 uses NAD$^+$ to deacetylate the target proteins. S-adenosylmethionine (SAM) is a methyl donor that is generated from methionine and ATP in the cytosol. Demethylases such as Jumonji C (JMJC) family members and the ten-eleven translocation (TET) methylcytosine hydroxylases use α-ketoglutarate (α-KG) as cofactor to remove methyl groups from proteins and DNA. AMPK stimulates the activity of TET enzymes, and thus the inhibition of AMPK by glucose impairs the function TET enzymes. The accumulation of fumarate and succinate due to impaired fumarate hydratase (FH) and succinate dehydrogenase (SDH) can inhibit α-KG-dependent demethylases and even cause defects in homologous recombination (HR) DNA repair.

For a long time, it was believed that mitochondria are regulated from the nucleus by the nuclear genome, and changes in mitochondria follow changes in the nucleus [50,51]. However, during recent years, accumulative evidence suggest that mitochondria and mitochondrial metabolites can influence nuclear processes and gene expression in response to various stimuli and environmental cues [52–54].

Mitochondrially generated ROS and intermediate metabolites are essential for several processes, including proliferation, epigenetic modifications, and post-translational modifications [54,55]. In addition, mitochondria contribute to genomic stability by replenishing dNTP pools for replication and repair of the genome (Figure 3) [56,57]. In this section we will discuss nuclear processes that are dependent on mitochondrial function and intermediate metabolites.

6. Mitochondrial ROS Are Involved in Signaling and Determine Cell Fate

The mitochondrial electron transport chain (ETC) generates reactive oxygen species (ROS) as the byproduct of oxidative phosphorylation (OXPHOS) from different complexes, though mainly complexes I, II, and III. While complexes I and II exclusively create $O_2\cdot$ in the mitochondrial matrix, complex III produces $O_2\cdot$ in both the matrix and intermembrane space [58]. However, the ROS that are released outside of the matrix are converted into H_2O_2 by cytosolic superoxide dismutase 1 (SOD1) and participate in mitochondrial signaling through reversible cysteine oxidation [59]. Mitochondrially produced ROS can serve as second-messenger molecules. Mitochondrial ROS (mtROS) are required for the stabilization of HIFα (hypoxia-inducible factor 1-α) and the activation of downstream pathways that promote proliferation [60].

It is possible that the type of cell and energy demand determine the effect of ROS and mtDNA mutation over the cell. Cells that mostly rely on glycolysis will probably not be affected by mutation in mtDNA under physiological conditions. During the exposure to stress and stimuli, however, these cells might not be able to trigger an adaptive response to an increase in demand for ATP and NAD$^+$ [61]. During stress and increased energy demand, cells respond by boosting cellular respiration and mitochondrial activity to provide the cells with ATP and NAD$^+$ [12,62]. This is accompanied by increased mitochondrial membrane potential and ROS above the physiological level [61,63]. Increased ROS cause damage to macromolecules such as DNA, proteins, and lipids, which can cause cell death or malignancy, as reviewed by Sies et al. in 2017 [64]. The inability to enhance ATP production in response to stress and increased energy demand probably contributes to cellular deterioration during aging [65].

In contrast to increased ROS generation, a decrease in ROS in metabolically active or proliferative tissues interferes with cellular metabolism or proliferation that can promote senescence, as reviewed by Diebold and Chandel in 2016 [66].

Hematopoietic stem cells (HSCs) represent an excellent example for both situations [67]. HSCs are mainly quiescent, and they rely on glycolysis for ATP production [68]. While low levels of ROS prevent the proliferation of HSCs and maintain their quiescent state, stress and increased energy demand promote a shift toward ATP production by mitochondria and OXPHOS. This is accompanied by increased ROS and proliferation [67]. Chronic stress followed by enhanced mitochondrial activity and ROS generation leads to the depletion of HSCs, which is one of the hallmarks of aging [69–71].

7. Mitochondria Influence Post-Translational Modifications (PTMs) and Epigenetic Marks

Reversible acetylation and methylation are two frequently employed post-translational modifications that regulate a variety of protein functions, protein stability, gene expression [72], as well as DNA repair [73]. Epigenetic changes are also one of the main hallmarks of both aging and cancer [2,3]. The modifications include alterations in DNA methylation, modifications of histones, and chromatin remodeling. While DNA methylations show similar patterns in aging and cancer, the histone modifications show distinct patterns, as reviewed by Zane et al. in 2014 [74].

The multiple enzymatic systems assuring the generation and maintenance of epigenetic patterns include DNA methyltransferases, histone acetylases, deacetylases, methylases, and demethylases, as well as protein complexes implicated in chromatin remodeling. Most PTMs, such as phosphorylation, acetylation, methylation, and O-linked N-acetylglucosamine modification (O-GlcNAcylation), require metabolites as substrates [75]. If not all, the majority of substrates required for PTMs are intermediate metabolites generated by mitochondria [54]. Chromatin modifiers use metabolic intermediates as cofactors or substrates, but are also regulated by their availability. These metabolites include NAD^+ for deacetylation, acetyl-CoA for histone acetylation, S-adenosylmethionine (SAM) for histone as well as DNA methylation, and α-ketoglutarate (α-KG) for demethylation [54].

Lysine acetyltransferases (KATs) add acetyl groups to proteins while lysine deacetylases (KDACs) remove acetyl groups from proteins [76,77]. KATs such as GCN5, CBP/p300, and MYST use acetyl-coenzyme A (acetyl CoA) as an acetyl group donor for protein acetylation [78]. KDACs are classified into two groups with different catalytic mechanisms: Zn^{2+}-dependent histone deacetylases (HDAC1-11) and NAD^+-dependent deacetylases (SIRT1-7) [76,77]. Acetyl CoA is generated in mitochondria and converted to citrate through the TCA cycle. Citrate can then be exported from mitochondria. In the cytoplasm and nucleus, citrate is converted back into acetyl CoA via the function of ATP-citrate lyase (ACLY). Citrate is the major source of acetyl CoA in the cytoplasm and the nucleus. Depletion of mtDNA and the subsequent decrease in NAD negatively affect the TCA cycle and lead to a decrease in histone acetylation. This can be rescued by the restoration of electron flow and TCA cycle [60,79]. The degree of acetylation directly correlates with the availability of cofactors such as acetyl CoA and NAD^+. While increased nuclear acetyl CoA promotes increased acetylation and the formation of euchromatin, an increase in NAD^+ promotes deacetylation and the formation of heterochromatin, resulting in a decrease of gene expression [79]. MYC and AKT stimulate nutrient uptake and promote acetyl CoA production via ACLY. AKT can directly phosphorylate and activate ACLY to maintain the acetyl CoA levels, regardless of glucose concentrations [80].

Another key chromatin modification that is strongly interconnected with metabolism is methylation [54,81]. Methylation is regulated by S-adenosylmethionine (SAM) abundance, whereby SAM serves as a universal methyl donor, synthesized from methionine and ATP by methionine adenosyltransferases (MATs) [54,81]. Histone and DNA methylation is removed by demethylases such as Jumonji C (JMJC) family members and the ten-eleven translocation (TET) methylcytosine hydroxylases, which use a dioxygenation reaction that requires Fe^{2+}, O_2, and α-ketoglutarate (α-KG) as cofactors [82]. α-KG is generated in the TCA cycle via the catabolism of glucose and glutamine. The function of lysine-specific histone demethylase 1A (LSD1; KDM1A) and LSD2 (KDM1B), which catalyze an amine oxidation reaction, is dependent on flavin adenine dinucleotide (FAD) [83,84].

The dysregulation of the TCA cycle and cellular metabolism affect PTMs, epigenetic changes, and choice of DNA repair pathway. Accumulation of succinate or fumarate, which occurs respectively in tumors deficient for succinate dehydrogenase (SDH) or fumarate hydratase (FH), similarly inhibits α-KG-dependent enzymes, leading to defects in homologous recombination (HR) DNA repair [53]. Changes in nutrient availability can directly affect chromatin modifications. The tumor suppressor ten-eleven translocation (TET) protein family of dioxygenases (TET1, TET2, and TET3) converts a 5mC DNA methylation to a hydroxymethylation, 5hmC [85]. AMP-activated kinase (AMPK) phosphorylates TET2 and stabilizes this tumor suppressor protein. However, increase in blood glucose levels impairs AMPK activity, which leads to destabilization of TET2 and the subsequent dysregulation of 5mCs and 5hmCs [86].

8. Regulation of dNTP Pools

In humans, nucleotide levels are maintained by the nucleotide salvage and/or de novo synthesis of ribo- and deoxyribonucleotide triphosphates (rNTPs and dNTPs).

It is generally accepted that the levels and especially the relative balance of the cytosolic dNTP pools have great influence on the replication, repair, and stability of the nuclear genome [87–92]. The efficiency and fidelity of most, if not all, polymerases and many repair enzymes are affected by the level of substrate nucleotides [87]. Too low a concentration of a nucleotide results in poor incorporation frequency, and a level which is too high risks the misincorporation of the high-concentration nucleotide [93–95]. Therefore, it is of no surprise that the process of synthesizing dNTPs in the right concentrations is governed by a generous amount of regulation, feedback loops, and redundancy [96,97].

Mitochondrial dysfunction, due to mutations in the mitochondrial genome or a decrease in the mitochondrial DNA (mtDNA) copy number, is associated with a poor prognosis of many types of cancer [98–102], also reviewed by Chatterjee et al. in 2006 [103]. The accumulation of mutations in mtDNA or impeded ETC have even been associated with tumor aggressiveness [99,101,104–106]. We have previously shown a relationship between mitochondrial respiration and the regulation of cytosolic dNTP pools, and demonstrated a co-occurring decrease of chromosomal stability [51].

The de novo synthesis of nucleotides is split up into purine and pyrimidine synthesis, which go through two distinct pathways.

Despite having separate synthesis pathways, both purine and pyrimidine-based ribonucleotides occupy a central role in cellular metabolism. In addition to being basal components of DNA and RNA, they function as phosphate donors in the transport of cellular energy and participate in enzymatic reactions as well as intracellular and extracellular signaling [107].

Both the salvage and the de novo synthesis pathways utilize an activated sugar intermediate: 5-phosphoribosyl-1-pyrophosphate (PRPP). PRPP is generated by the action of PRPP synthetase and is utilized in both purine and pyrimidine synthesis [108]. The purine nucleotides are synthesized from PRPP, through inosine 5-monophosphate (IMP), and further into AMP and GMP, through two separate but allosterically regulated pathways. Pyrimidines, on the other hand, originate from the precursor pyrimidine nucleotide, UMP, which is used to synthesize all the cellular ribosyl and deoxyribosyl pyrimidines including UTP, CTP, dUMP, and dTTP [108]. A key catalytic enzyme in this process is the dihydroorotate dehydrogenase (DHODH) [109], located in the inner mitochondrial membrane and functionally codependent with the OXPHOS [110]. The oxidation of dihydroorotate by DHODH, to form orotate, is a bottleneck reaction of the de novo synthesis of pyrimidines and is electrochemically coupled with the reduction of ubiquinone to ubiquinol [56,111–113]. Mitochondrial respiration can modulate the nucleotide synthesis at two separate steps. A decrease of the mitochondrial respiration is therefore linked to an inhibition of the DHODH enzyme, which in turn modulates the synthesis of pyrimidines [51,114]. Furthermore, the activity of the RNR complex is regulated by the binding of ATP to its active site and inhibited by dATP. By affecting the levels of cytosolic ATP, the mitochondria can influence the activity of RNR, and hence the levels of dNTPs. Furthermore, RNR is allosterically regulated by the relative levels of individual NTPs and dNTPs, and so the de novo synthesis of dNTPs and their relative balance is highly dependent on the mitochondrial supply of pyrimidines and ATP [114–116].

The cytosolic pool of dNTPs, which supplies the replication of the nuclear genome, is cell cycle-regulated. Synthesis is initiated at the beginning of the S-phase, and stopped upon reaching G2. In the de novo pathway, this phase-dependent synthesis of dNTPs is mediated through the RNR—specifically, through the cell cycle regulation of expression and degradation of the RNR subunit RNR-R2 [117]. In the salvage pathway, the phase-dependent synthesis is controlled by the translational regulation of constituents of the nucleotide salvage pathway [118]. Outside of S-phase, a dNTP hydrolase called SAMHD1 (SAM and HD domain-containing deoxynucleoside triphosphate triphosphohydrolase 1) depletes the dNTP pools by its hydrolase activity to block viral replication, amongst other things [119]. In response to DNA damage, however, dNTP levels can increase by up to 4-fold [96]. In this case, both the RNR and SAMHD1 are then recruited to the site of damage to tightly regulate the amount of dNTPs supplied to the DNA repair machinery [96,120].

Not only replication of the nuclear genome requires a balanced dNTP pool. Unlike the replication of the nuclear genome, the replication of mitochondrial DNA is not regulated by the cell cycle, but is carried out continuously in both mitotic and post-mitotic cells and tissue. Imbalance of the mitochondrial dNTP pools affects the replication of mtDNA, resulting in the accumulation of point mutations and deletions [121,122].

The dNTP pool of the mitochondrial compartment is somewhat separate from the much larger pool supplying the nuclear genome [123,124]. However, cytosolic de novo synthesis of dNTP is essential for mtDNA maintenance, even in post-mitotic cells and tissue [125–127].

P53R2 is a protein that substitutes RNR-R2 in post-mitotic cells in response to DNA damage. P53R2 is transcribed by P53 and results, when forming the complex, in the activation of RNR and the de novo synthesis of dNTPs intended as substrates for DNA repair mechanisms [128]. Mutations of the RRM2B gene encoding P53R2 have been shown to induce mtDNA replication and repair deficiency in post-mitotic, but not dividing, human fibroblasts [125]. In humans, mutations in the gene encoding the RRM2B subunit have been correlated with severe mtDNA depletion of muscle tissue, and $RRM2b^{-/-}$ mice further display a severe decrease of mtDNA content in liver, kidney, and muscle [126].

It is important to realize that balanced dNTP pools for mtDNA maintenance do not need to be of mitochondrial origin. Imbalances of the nuclear dNTP pools resulting from genetic predisposition, age, or even just diet [129] have the potential to start a vicious cycle, whereby failure to maintain mtDNA integrity results in the decreased synthesis of pyrimidines and further dNTP pool imbalance.

Mitochondrial dysfunction is therefore not only a risk to the mitotic cell, but also fully differentiated post-mitotic cells [130], and is involved in the etiology of a wide array of pathologies, including cancer and Alzheimer's disease [131–133].

9. Conclusions

According to recent advancements, hallmarks of cancer include genomic instability, dysregulation of cellular energetics, and mitochondrial dysfunction, which also are common pathways important for cellular aging. Mitochondrial dysfunction is associated with a poor prognosis of many types of cancer, which could very well be linked to an imbalance of the cytosolic dNTP pools, as both of these conditions are related to one of the hallmarks of cancer—chromosomal instability. A better understanding of these pathological cellular processes would advance the development of therapeutic modalities in the prevention of cancer and at the same time help the understanding of biological aging.

Author Contributions: N.B.F., T.L.H., C.D., S.A., L.J.R. wrote the review.

References

1. Hanahan, D.; Weinberg, R.A. The hallmarks of cancer. *Cell* **2000**, *100*, 57–70. [CrossRef]
2. Hanahan, D.; Weinberg, R.A. Hallmarks of Cancer: The Next Generation. *Cell* **2011**, *144*, 646–674. [CrossRef] [PubMed]
3. López-Otín, C.; Blasco, M.A.; Partridge, L.; Serrano, M.; Kroemer, G. The hallmarks of aging. *Cell* **2013**, *153*, 1194–1217. [CrossRef]
4. Tubbs, A.; Nussenzweig, A. Endogenous DNA Damage as a Source of Genomic Instability in Cancer. *Cell* **2017**, *168*, 644–656. [CrossRef]
5. Sharma, P.; Sampath, H. Mitochondrial DNA Integrity: Role in Health and Disease. *Cells* **2019**, *8*, 100. [CrossRef] [PubMed]
6. Fan, P.; Xie, X.-H.; Chen, C.-H.; Peng, X.; Zhang, P.; Yang, C.; Wang, Y.-T. Molecular Regulation Mechanisms and Interactions Between Reactive Oxygen Species and Mitophagy. *DNA Cell Biol.* **2019**, *38*, 10–22. [CrossRef] [PubMed]
7. Aunan, J.R.; Cho, W.C.; Søreide, K. The Biology of Aging and Cancer: A Brief Overview of Shared and Divergent Molecular Hallmarks. *Aging Dis.* **2017**, *8*, 628. [CrossRef] [PubMed]
8. Burcham, P.C. Internal hazards: Baseline DNA damage by endogenous products of normal metabolism. *Mutat. Res./Genet. Toxicol. Environ. Mutagenesis* **1999**, *443*, 11–36. [CrossRef]
9. De Bont, R.; van Larebeke, N. Endogenous DNA damage in humans: A review of quantitative data. *Mutagenesis* **2004**, *19*, 169–185. [CrossRef]
10. Zeman, M.K.; Cimprich, K.A. Causes and consequences of replication stress. *Nat. Cell Biol.* **2014**, *16*, 2–9. [CrossRef] [PubMed]
11. White, R.R.; Vijg, J. Do DNA Double-Strand Breaks Drive Aging? *Mol. Cell* **2016**, *63*, 729–738. [CrossRef] [PubMed]
12. Qin, L.; Fan, M.; Candas, D.; Jiang, G.; Papadopoulos, S.; Tian, L.; Woloschak, G.; Grdina, D.J.; Li, J.J. CDK1 Enhances Mitochondrial Bioenergetics for Radiation-Induced DNA Repair. *Cell Rep.* **2015**, *13*, 2056–2063. [CrossRef]
13. Scheibye-Knudsen, M.; Mitchell, S.J.; Fang, E.F.; Iyama, T.; Ward, T.; Wang, J.; Dunn, C.A.; Singh, N.; Veith, S.; Hasan-Olive, M.M.; et al. A high-fat diet and NAD(+) activate Sirt1 to rescue premature aging in cockayne syndrome. *Cell Metab.* **2014**, *20*, 840–855. [CrossRef]
14. Fang, E.F.; Kassahun, H.; Croteau, D.L.; Scheibye-Knudsen, M.; Marosi, K.; Lu, H.; Shamanna, R.A.; Kalyanasundaram, S.; Bollineni, R.C.; Wilson, M.A.; et al. NAD(+) Replenishment Improves Lifespan and Healthspan in Ataxia Telangiectasia Models via Mitophagy and DNA Repair. *Cell Metab.* **2016**, *24*, 566–581. [CrossRef]
15. Fakouri, N.B.; Durhuus, J.A.; Regnell, C.E.; Angleys, M.; Desler, C.; Olive, M.H.; Martín-Pardillos, A.; Tsaalbi-Shtylik, A.; Thomsen, K.; Lauritzen, M.; et al. Rev1 contributes to proper mitochondrial function via the PARP-NAD+-SIRT1-PGC1α axis. *Sci. Rep.* **2017**, *7*, 12480. [CrossRef]
16. Rivera-Torres, J.; Acín-Perez, R.; Cabezas-Sánchez, P.; Osorio, F.G.; Gonzalez-Gómez, C.; Megias, D.; Cámara, C.; López-Otín, C.; Enríquez, J.A.; Luque-García, J.L.; et al. Identification of mitochondrial dysfunction in Hutchinson–Gilford progeria syndrome through use of stable isotope labeling with amino acids in cell culture. *J. Proteom.* **2013**, *91*, 466–477. [CrossRef] [PubMed]
17. Fang, E.F.; Scheibye-Knudsen, M.; Brace, L.E.; Kassahun, H.; SenGupta, T.; Nilsen, H.; Mitchell, J.R.; Croteau, D.L.; Bohr, V.A. Defective mitophagy in XPA via PARP-1 hyperactivation and NAD(+)/SIRT1 reduction. *Cell* **2014**, *157*, 882–896. [CrossRef]
18. Qian, W.; Choi, S.; Gibson, G.A.; Watkins, S.C.; Bakkenist, C.J.; Van Houten, B. Mitochondrial hyperfusion induced by loss of the fission protein Drp1 causes ATM-dependent G2/M arrest and aneuploidy through DNA replication stress. *J. Cell Sci.* **2012**, *125*, 5745–5757. [CrossRef] [PubMed]
19. Temelie, M.; Savu, D.I.; Moisoi, N. Intracellular and Intercellular Signalling Mechanisms following DNA Damage Are Modulated By PINK1. *Oxid. Med. Cell. Longev.* **2018**, *2018*, 1–15. [CrossRef]

20. Desler, C.; Hansen, T.L.; Frederiksen, J.B.; Marcker, M.L.; Singh, K.K.; Juel Rasmussen, L. Is There a Link between Mitochondrial Reserve Respiratory Capacity and Aging? *J. Aging Res.* **2012**, *2012*, 192503. [CrossRef]

21. Cosentino, C.; Grieco, D.; Costanzo, V. ATM activates the pentose phosphate pathway promoting anti-oxidant defence and DNA repair. *EMBO J.* **2011**, *30*, 546–555. [CrossRef] [PubMed]

22. Bozulic, L.; Surucu, B.; Hynx, D.; Hemmings, B.A. PKBα/Akt1 Acts Downstream of DNA-PK in the DNA Double-Strand Break Response and Promotes Survival. *Mol. Cell* **2008**, *30*, 203–213. [CrossRef]

23. Park, S.-J.; Gavrilova, O.; Brown, A.L.; Soto, J.E.; Bremner, S.; Kim, J.; Xu, X.; Yang, S.; Um, J.-H.; Koch, L.G.; et al. DNA-PK Promotes the Mitochondrial, Metabolic, and Physical Decline that Occurs During Aging. *Cell Metab.* **2017**, *25*, 1135–1146.e7. [CrossRef] [PubMed]

24. Matoba, S.; Kang, J.-G.; Patino, W.D.; Wragg, A.; Boehm, M.; Gavrilova, O.; Hurley, P.J.; Bunz, F.; Hwang, P.M. p53 regulates mitochondrial respiration. *Science* **2006**, *312*, 1650–1653. [CrossRef]

25. Bensaad, K.; Vousden, K.H. p53: New roles in metabolism. *Trends Cell Biol.* **2007**, *17*, 286–291. [CrossRef]

26. Hoshino, A.; Mita, Y.; Okawa, Y.; Ariyoshi, M.; Iwai-Kanai, E.; Ueyama, T.; Ikeda, K.; Ogata, T.; Matoba, S. Cytosolic p53 inhibits Parkin-mediated mitophagy and promotes mitochondrial dysfunction in the mouse heart. *Nat. Commun.* **2013**, *4*, 2308. [CrossRef] [PubMed]

27. Wang, D.B.; Kinoshita, C.; Kinoshita, Y.; Morrison, R.S. p53 and mitochondrial function in neurons. *Biochim. Biophys. Acta Mol. Basis Dis.* **2014**, *1842*, 1186–1197. [CrossRef]

28. Bai, P.; Nagy, L.; Fodor, T.; Liaudet, L.; Pacher, P. Poly(ADP-ribose) polymerases as modulators of mitochondrial activity. *Trends Endocrinol. Metab.* **2015**, *26*, 75–83. [CrossRef]

29. Luo, X.; Kraus, W.L. On PAR with PARP: Cellular stress signaling through poly(ADP-ribose) and PARP-1. *Genes Dev.* **2012**, *26*, 417–432. [CrossRef]

30. Krietsch, J.; Rouleau, M.; Pic, É.; Ethier, C.; Dawson, T.M.; Dawson, V.L.; Masson, J.-Y.; Poirier, G.G.; Gagné, J.-P. Reprogramming cellular events by poly(ADP-ribose)-binding proteins. *Mol. Asp. Med.* **2013**, *34*, 1066–1087. [CrossRef]

31. Davidovic, L.; Vodenicharov, M.; Affar, E.B.; Poirier, G.G. Importance of poly(ADP-ribose) glycohydrolase in the control of poly(ADP-ribose) metabolism. *Exp. Cell Res.* **2001**, *268*, 7–13. [CrossRef]

32. Bürkle, A.; Virag, L. Poly(ADP-ribose): PARadigms and PARadoxes. *Mol. Asp. Med.* **2013**, *34*, 1046–1065. [CrossRef]

33. Langelier, M.-F.; Planck, J.L.; Roy, S.; Pascal, J.M. Crystal structures of poly(ADP-ribose) polymerase-1 (PARP-1) zinc fingers bound to DNA: Structural and functional insights into DNA-dependent PARP-1 activity. *J. Biol. Chem.* **2011**, *286*, 10690–10701. [CrossRef] [PubMed]

34. Ali, A.A.E.; Timinszky, G.; Arribas-Bosacoma, R.; Kozlowski, M.; Hassa, P.O.; Hassler, M.; Ladurner, A.G.; Pearl, L.H.; Oliver, A.W. The zinc-finger domains of PARP1 cooperate to recognize DNA strand breaks. *Nat. Struct. Mol. Biol.* **2012**, *19*, 685–692. [CrossRef] [PubMed]

35. Gottschalk, A.J.; Timinszky, G.; Kong, S.E.; Jin, J.; Cai, Y.; Swanson, S.K.; Washburn, M.P.; Florens, L.; Ladurner, A.G.; Conaway, J.W.; et al. Poly(ADP-ribosyl)ation directs recruitment and activation of an ATP-dependent chromatin remodeler. *Proc. Natl. Acad. Sci. USA* **2009**, *106*, 13770–13774. [CrossRef] [PubMed]

36. Krishnakumar, R.; Kraus, W.L. The PARP side of the nucleus: Molecular actions, physiological outcomes, and clinical targets. *Mol. Cell* **2010**, *39*, 8–24. [CrossRef] [PubMed]

37. Fang, E.F.; Scheibye-Knudsen, M.; Chua, K.F.; Mattson, M.P.; Croteau, D.L.; Bohr, V.A. Nuclear DNA damage signalling to mitochondria in ageing. *Nat. Rev. Mol. Cell Biol.* **2016**, *17*, 308–321. [CrossRef] [PubMed]

38. Roos, W.P.; Thomas, A.D.; Kaina, B. DNA damage and the balance between survival and death in cancer biology. *Nat. Rev. Cancer* **2016**, *16*, 20–33. [CrossRef]

39. Maryanovich, M.; Zaltsman, Y.; Ruggiero, A.; Goldman, A.; Shachnai, L.; Zaidman, S.L.; Porat, Z.; Golan, K.; Lapidot, T.; Gross, A. An MTCH2 pathway repressing mitochondria metabolism regulates haematopoietic stem cell fate. *Nat. Commun.* **2015**, *6*, 7901. [CrossRef]

40. Feng, J.; Park, J.; Cron, P.; Hess, D.; Hemmings, B.A. Identification of a PKB/Akt hydrophobic motif Ser-473 kinase as DNA-dependent protein kinase. *J. Biol. Chem.* **2004**, *279*, 41189–41196. [CrossRef]

41. Matsuoka, S.; Ballif, B.A.; Smogorzewska, A.; McDonald, E.R.; Hurov, K.E.; Luo, J.; Bakalarski, C.E.; Zhao, Z.; Solimini, N.; Lerenthal, Y.; et al. ATM and ATR substrate analysis reveals extensive protein networks responsive to DNA damage. *Science* **2007**, *316*, 1160–1166. [CrossRef]

42. Park, J.; Feng, J.; Li, Y.; Hammarsten, O.; Brazil, D.P.; Hemmings, B.A. DNA-dependent protein kinase-mediated phosphorylation of protein kinase B requires a specific recognition sequence in the C-terminal hydrophobic motif. *J. Biol. Chem.* **2009**, *284*, 6169–6174. [CrossRef]

43. Toulany, M.; Maier, J.; Iida, M.; Rebholz, S.; Holler, M.; Grottke, A.; Jüker, M.; Wheeler, D.L.; Rothbauer, U.; Rodemann, H.P. Akt1 and Akt3 but not Akt2 through interaction with DNA-PKcs stimulate proliferation and post-irradiation cell survival of K-RAS-mutated cancer cells. *Cell Death Discov.* **2017**, *3*, 17072. [CrossRef] [PubMed]

44. Liu, Q.; Turner, K.M.; Yung, W.K.A.; Chen, K.; Zhang, W. Role of AKT signaling in DNA repair and clinical response to cancer therapy. *Neuro-Oncology* **2014**, *16*, 1313–1323. [CrossRef]

45. Stronach, E.A.; Chen, M.; Maginn, E.N.; Agarwal, R.; Mills, G.B.; Wasan, H.; Gabra, H. DNA-PK mediates AKT activation and apoptosis inhibition in clinically acquired platinum resistance. *Neoplasia* **2011**, *13*, 1069–1080. [CrossRef]

46. Robey, R.B.; Hay, N. Is Akt the "Warburg kinase"-Akt-energy metabolism interactions and oncogenesis. *Semin. Cancer Biol.* **2009**, *19*, 25–31. [CrossRef]

47. Brunet, A.; Bonni, A.; Zigmond, M.J.; Lin, M.Z.; Juo, P.; Hu, L.S.; Anderson, M.J.; Arden, K.C.; Blenis, J.; Greenberg, M.E. Akt promotes cell survival by phosphorylating and inhibiting a Forkhead transcription factor. *Cell* **1999**, *96*, 857–868. [CrossRef]

48. Kops, G.J.P.L.; de Ruiter, N.D.; De Vries-Smits, A.M.M.; Powell, D.R.; Bos, J.L.; Burgering, B.M.T. Direct control of the Forkhead transcription factor AFX by protein kinase B. *Nature* **1999**, *398*, 630–634. [CrossRef]

49. Webb, A.E.; Brunet, A. FOXO transcription factors: Key regulators of cellular quality control. *Trends Biochem. Sci.* **2014**, *39*, 159–169. [CrossRef] [PubMed]

50. Gray, M.W. Mitochondrial evolution. *Cold Spring Harb. Perspect. Biol.* **2012**, *4*, a011403. [CrossRef] [PubMed]

51. Lee, C.; Yen, K.; Cohen, P. Humanin: A harbinger of mitochondrial-derived peptides? *Trends Endocrinol. Metab.* **2013**, *24*, 222–228. [CrossRef] [PubMed]

52. Kim, K.H.; Son, J.M.; Benayoun, B.A.; Lee, C. The Mitochondrial-Encoded Peptide MOTS-c Translocates to the Nucleus to Regulate Nuclear Gene Expression in Response to Metabolic Stress. *Cell Metab.* **2018**, *28*, 516–524. [CrossRef]

53. Sulkowski, P.L.; Sundaram, R.K.; Oeck, S.; Corso, C.D.; Liu, Y.; Noorbakhsh, S.; Niger, M.; Boeke, M.; Ueno, D.; Kalathil, A.N.; et al. Krebs-cycle-deficient hereditary cancer syndromes are defined by defects in homologous-recombination DNA repair. *Nat. Genet.* **2018**, *50*, 1086–1092. [CrossRef]

54. Li, X.; Egervari, G.; Wang, Y.; Berger, S.L.; Lu, Z. Regulation of chromatin and gene expression by metabolic enzymes and metabolites. *Nat. Rev. Mol. Cell Biol.* **2018**, *19*, 563–578. [CrossRef] [PubMed]

55. Sivanand, S.; Rhoades, S.; Jiang, Q.; Lee, J.V.; Benci, J.; Zhang, J.; Yuan, S.; Viney, I.; Zhao, S.; Carrer, A.; et al. Nuclear Acetyl-CoA Production by ACLY Promotes Homologous Recombination. *Mol. Cell* **2017**, *67*, 252–265. [CrossRef] [PubMed]

56. Desler, C.; Munch-Petersen, B.; Stevnsner, T.; Matsui, S.-I.; Kulawiec, M.; Singh, K.K.; Rasmussen, L.J. Mitochondria as determinant of nucleotide pools and chromosomal stability. *Mutat. Res.* **2007**, *625*, 112–124. [CrossRef]

57. Rasmussen, A.K.; Chatterjee, A.; Rasmussen, L.J.; Singh, K.K. Mitochondria-mediated nuclear mutator phenotype in Saccharomyces cerevisiae. *Nucleic Acids Res.* **2003**, *31*, 3909–3917. [CrossRef]

58. Murphy, M.P. How mitochondria produce reactive oxygen species. *Biochem. J.* **2009**, *417*, 1–13. [CrossRef] [PubMed]

59. Sena, L.A.; Chandel, N.S. Physiological roles of mitochondrial reactive oxygen species. *Mol. Cell* **2012**, *48*, 158–167. [CrossRef] [PubMed]

60. Martínez-Reyes, I.; Diebold, L.P.; Kong, H.; Schieber, M.; Huang, H.; Hensley, C.T.; Mehta, M.M.; Wang, T.; Santos, J.H.; Woychik, R.; et al. TCA Cycle and Mitochondrial Membrane Potential Are Necessary for Diverse Biological Functions. *Mol. Cell* **2016**, *61*, 199–209. [CrossRef]

61. Westermann, B. Bioenergetic role of mitochondrial fusion and fission. *Biochim. Biophys. Acta Bioenerget.* **2012**, *1817*, 1833–1838. [CrossRef]

62. Brace, L.E.; Vose, S.C.; Stanya, K.; Gathungu, R.M.; Marur, V.R.; Longchamp, A.; Treviño-Villarreal, H.; Mejia, P.; Vargas, D.; Inouye, K.; et al. Increased oxidative phosphorylation in response to acute and chronic DNA damage. *NPJ Aging Mech. Dis.* **2016**, *2*, 16022. [CrossRef] [PubMed]

63. Youle, R.J.; van der Bliek, A.M. Mitochondrial fission, fusion, and stress. *Science* **2012**, *337*, 1062–1065. [CrossRef]

64. Sies, H.; Berndt, C.; Jones, D.P. Oxidative Stress. *Annu. Rev. Biochem.* **2017**, *86*, 715–748. [CrossRef]

65. Trifunovic, A.; Hansson, A.; Wredenberg, A.; Rovio, A.T.; Dufour, E.; Khvorostov, I.; Spelbrink, J.N.; Wibom, R.; Jacobs, H.T.; Larsson, N.-G. Somatic mtDNA mutations cause aging phenotypes without affecting reactive oxygen species production. *Proc. Natl. Acad. Sci. USA* **2005**, *102*, 17993–17998. [CrossRef]

66. Diebold, L.; Chandel, N.S. Mitochondrial ROS regulation of proliferating cells. *Free Radic. Biol. Med.* **2016**, *100*, 86–93. [CrossRef] [PubMed]

67. Maryanovich, M.; Gross, A. A ROS rheostat for cell fate regulation. *Trends Cell Biol.* **2013**, *23*, 129–134. [CrossRef] [PubMed]

68. Folmes, C.D.L.; Dzeja, P.P.; Nelson, T.J.; Terzic, A. Metabolic Plasticity in Stem Cell Homeostasis and Differentiation. *Cell Stem Cell* **2012**, *11*, 596–606. [CrossRef] [PubMed]

69. Nijnik, A.; Woodbine, L.; Marchetti, C.; Dawson, S.; Lambe, T.; Liu, C.; Rodrigues, N.P.; Crockford, T.L.; Cabuy, E.; Vindigni, A.; et al. DNA repair is limiting for haematopoietic stem cells during ageing. *Nature* **2007**, *447*, 686–690. [CrossRef]

70. Niedernhofer, L.J. DNA repair is crucial for maintaining hematopoietic stem cell function. *DNA Repair* **2008**, *7*, 523–529. [CrossRef] [PubMed]

71. Flach, J.; Bakker, S.T.; Mohrin, M.; Conroy, P.C.; Pietras, E.M.; Reynaud, D.; Alvarez, S.; Diolaiti, M.E.; Ugarte, F.; Forsberg, E.C.; et al. Replication stress is a potent driver of functional decline in ageing haematopoietic stem cells. *Nature* **2014**, *512*, 198–202. [CrossRef]

72. Drazic, A.; Myklebust, L.M.; Ree, R.; Arnesen, T. The world of protein acetylation. *Biochim. Biophys. Acta Proteins Proteom.* **2016**, *1864*, 1372–1401. [CrossRef] [PubMed]

73. Hauer, M.H.; Gasser, S.M. Chromatin and nucleosome dynamics in DNA damage and repair. *Genes Dev.* **2017**, *31*, 2204–2221. [CrossRef]

74. Zane, L.; Sharma, V.; Misteli, T. Common features of chromatin in aging and cancer: Cause or coincidence? *Trends Cell Biol.* **2014**, *24*, 686–694. [CrossRef] [PubMed]

75. Su, X.; Wellen, K.E.; Rabinowitz, J.D. Metabolic control of methylation and acetylation. *Curr. Opin. Chem. Biol.* **2016**, *30*, 52–60. [CrossRef] [PubMed]

76. Choudhary, C.; Weinert, B.T.; Nishida, Y.; Verdin, E.; Mann, M. The growing landscape of lysine acetylation links metabolism and cell signalling. *Nat. Rev. Mol. Cell Biol.* **2014**, *15*, 536–550. [CrossRef]

77. Ali, I.; Conrad, R.J.; Verdin, E.; Ott, M. Lysine Acetylation Goes Global: From Epigenetics to Metabolism and Therapeutics. *Chem. Rev.* **2018**, *118*, 1216–1252. [CrossRef] [PubMed]

78. Montgomery, D.C.; Sorum, A.W.; Guasch, L.; Nicklaus, M.C.; Meier, J.L. Metabolic Regulation of Histone Acetyltransferases by Endogenous Acyl-CoA Cofactors. *Chem. Biol.* **2015**, *22*, 1030–1039. [CrossRef]

79. Katada, S.; Imhof, A.; Sassone-Corsi, P. Connecting Threads: Epigenetics and Metabolism. *Cell* **2012**, *148*, 24–28. [CrossRef]

80. Lee, J.V.; Carrer, A.; Shah, S.; Snyder, N.W.; Wei, S.; Venneti, S.; Worth, A.J.; Yuan, Z.-F.; Lim, H.-W.; Liu, S.; et al. Akt-Dependent Metabolic Reprogramming Regulates Tumor Cell Histone Acetylation. *Cell Metab.* **2014**, *20*, 306–319. [CrossRef]

81. Kinnaird, A.; Zhao, S.; Wellen, K.E.; Michelakis, E.D. Metabolic control of epigenetics in cancer. *Nat. Rev. Cancer* **2016**, *16*, 694–707. [CrossRef]

82. Metzger, E.; Schüle, R. The expanding world of histone lysine demethylases. *Nat. Struct. Mol. Biol.* **2007**, *14*, 252–254. [CrossRef] [PubMed]

83. Forneris, F.; Binda, C.; Vanoni, M.A.; Mattevi, A.; Battaglioli, E. Histone demethylation catalysed by LSD1 is a flavin-dependent oxidative process. *FEBS Lett.* **2005**, *579*, 2203–2207. [CrossRef]

84. Metzger, E.; Imhof, A.; Patel, D.; Kahl, P.; Hoffmeyer, K.; Friedrichs, N.; Müller, J.M.; Greschik, H.; Kirfel, J.; Ji, S.; et al. Phosphorylation of histone H3T6 by PKCβI controls demethylation at histone H3K4. *Nature* **2010**, *464*, 792–796. [CrossRef]

85. He, Y.-F.; Li, B.-Z.; Li, Z.; Liu, P.; Wang, Y.; Tang, Q.; Ding, J.; Jia, Y.; Chen, Z.; Li, L.; et al. Tet-Mediated Formation of 5-Carboxylcytosine and Its Excision by TDG in Mammalian DNA. *Science* **2011**, *333*, 1303–1307. [CrossRef] [PubMed]

86. Wu, D.; Hu, D.; Chen, H.; Shi, G.; Fetahu, I.S.; Wu, F.; Rabidou, K.; Fang, R.; Tan, L.; Xu, S.; et al. Glucose-regulated phosphorylation of TET2 by AMPK reveals a pathway linking diabetes to cancer. *Nature* **2018**, *559*, 637–641. [CrossRef]

87. Pai, C.-C.; Kearsey, S.E. A Critical Balance: dNTPs and the Maintenance of Genome Stability. *Genes* **2017**, *8*, 57. [CrossRef]

88. Kunz, B.A. Mutagenesis and deoxyribonucleotide pool imbalance. *Mutat. Res.* **1988**, *200*, 133–147. [CrossRef]
89. Kunz, B.A.; Kohalmi, S.E.; Kunkel, T.A.; Mathews, C.K.; McIntosh, E.M.; Reidy, J.A. Deoxyribonucleoside triphosphate levels: A critical factor in the maintenance of genetic stability. *Mutat. Res. Toxicol.* **1994**, *318*, 1–64. [CrossRef]
90. Mathews, C.K. DNA precursor metabolism and genomic stability. *FASEB J.* **2006**, *20*, 1300–1314. [CrossRef] [PubMed]
91. Kumar, D.; Abdulovic, A.L.; Viberg, J.; Nilsson, A.K.; Kunkel, T.A.; Chabes, A. Mechanisms of mutagenesis in vivo due to imbalanced dNTP pools. *Nucleic Acids Res.* **2011**, *39*, 1360–1371. [CrossRef] [PubMed]
92. Reichard, P. Interactions between deoxyribonucleotide and DNA synthesis. *Annu. Rev. Biochem.* **1988**, *57*, 349–374. [CrossRef]
93. Meuth, M. The molecular basis of mutations induced by deoxyribonucleoside triphosphate pool imbalances in mammalian cells. *Exp. Cell Res.* **1989**, *181*, 305–316. [CrossRef]
94. Meuth, M. The genetic consequences of nucleotide precursor pool imbalance in mammalian cells. *Mutat. Res. Mol. Mech. Mutagen.* **1984**, *126*, 107–112. [CrossRef]
95. Haracska, L.; Prakash, S.; Prakash, L. Replication pastO6-Methylguanine by Yeast and Human DNA Polymerase η. *Mol. Cell. Biol.* **2000**, *20*, 8001–8007. [CrossRef]
96. Niida, H.; Shimada, M.; Murakami, H.; Nakanishi, M. Mechanisms of dNTP supply that play an essential role in maintaining genome integrity in eukaryotic cells. *Cancer Sci.* **2010**, *101*, 2505–2509. [CrossRef] [PubMed]
97. Niida, H.; Katsuno, Y.; Sengoku, M.; Shimada, M.; Yukawa, M.; Ikura, M.; Ikura, T.; Kohno, K.; Shima, H.; Suzuki, H.; et al. Essential role of Tip60-dependent recruitment of ribonucleotide reductase at DNA damage sites in DNA repair during G1 phase. *Genes Dev.* **2010**, *24*, 333–338. [CrossRef]
98. Tseng, L.-M.; Yin, P.-H.; Chi, C.-W.; Hsu, C.-Y.; Wu, C.-W.; Lee, L.-M.; Wei, Y.-H.; Lee, H.-C. Mitochondrial DNA mutations and mitochondrial DNA depletion in breast cancer. *Genes Chromosomes Cancer* **2006**, *45*, 629–638. [CrossRef]
99. Yu, M.; Zhou, Y.; Shi, Y.; Ning, L.; Yang, Y.; Wei, X.; Zhang, N.; Hao, X.; Niu, R. Reduced mitochondrial DNA copy number is correlated with tumor progression and prognosis in Chinese breast cancer patients. *IUBMB Life* **2007**, *59*, 450–457. [CrossRef] [PubMed]
100. Yamada, S.; Nomoto, S.; Fujii, T.; Kaneko, T.; Takeda, S.; Inoue, S.; Kanazumi, N.; Nakao, A. Correlation between copy number of mitochondrial DNA and clinico-pathologic parameters of hepatocellular carcinoma. *Eur. J. Surg. Oncol.* **2006**, *32*, 303–307. [CrossRef]
101. Matsuyama, W.; Nakagawa, M.; Wakimoto, J.; Hirotsu, Y.; Kawabata, M.; Osame, M. Mitochondrial DNA mutation correlates with stage progression and prognosis in non-small cell lung cancer. *Hum. Mutat.* **2003**, *21*, 441–443. [CrossRef] [PubMed]
102. Lièvre, A.; Chapusot, C.; Bouvier, A.-M.; Zinzindohoué, F.; Piard, F.; Roignot, P.; Arnould, L.; Beaune, P.; Faivre, J.; Laurent-Puig, P. Clinical value of mitochondrial mutations in colorectal cancer. *J. Clin. Oncol.* **2005**, *23*, 3517–3525. [CrossRef] [PubMed]
103. Chatterjee, A.; Mambo, E.; Sidransky, D. Mitochondrial DNA mutations in human cancer. *Oncogene* **2006**, *25*, 4663–4674. [CrossRef] [PubMed]
104. Simonnet, H. Low mitochondrial respiratory chain content correlates with tumor aggressiveness in renal cell carcinoma. *Carcinogenesis* **2002**, *23*, 759–768. [CrossRef]
105. Petros, J.A.; Baumann, A.K.; Ruiz-Pesini, E.; Amin, M.B.; Sun, C.Q.; Hall, J.; Lim, S.; Issa, M.M.; Flanders, W.D.; Hosseini, S.H.; et al. mtDNA mutations increase tumorigenicity in prostate cancer. *Proc. Natl. Acad. Sci. USA* **2005**, *102*, 719–724. [CrossRef] [PubMed]
106. Shidara, Y.; Yamagata, K.; Kanamori, T.; Nakano, K.; Kwong, J.Q.; Manfredi, G.; Oda, H.; Ohta, S. Positive contribution of pathogenic mutations in the mitochondrial genome to the promotion of cancer by prevention from apoptosis. *Cancer Res.* **2005**, *65*, 1655–1663. [CrossRef]
107. Ralevic, V.; Burnstock, G. Receptors for purines and pyrimidines. *Pharmacol. Rev.* **1998**, *50*, 413–492. [PubMed]
108. Smith, J.L. Enzymes of nucleotide synthesis. *Curr. Opin. Struct. Biol.* **1995**, *5*, 752–757. [CrossRef]
109. Fang, J.; Uchiumi, T.; Yagi, M.; Matsumoto, S.; Amamoto, R.; Takazaki, S.; Yamaza, H.; Nonaka, K.; Kang, D. Dihydro-orotate dehydrogenase is physically associated with the respiratory complex and its loss leads to mitochondrial dysfunction. *Biosci. Rep.* **2013**, *33*, e00021. [CrossRef]

110. Bader, B.; Knecht, W.; Fries, M.; Löffler, M. Expression, purification, and characterization of histidine-tagged rat and human flavoenzyme dihydroorotate dehydrogenase. *Protein Expr. Purif.* **1998**, *13*, 414–422. [CrossRef]

111. Löffler, M.; Jöckel, J.; Schuster, G.; Becker, C. Dihydroorotat-ubiquinone oxidoreductase links mitochondria in the biosynthesis of pyrimidine nucleotides. *Mol. Cell. Biochem.* **1997**, *174*, 125–129. [CrossRef]

112. Beuneu, C.; Auger, R.; Löffler, M.; Guissani, A.; Lemaire, G.; Lepoivre, M. Indirect inhibition of mitochondrial dihydroorotate dehydrogenase activity by nitric oxide. *Free Radic. Biol. Med.* **2000**, *28*, 1206–1213. [CrossRef]

113. Rawls, J.; Knecht, W.; Diekert, K.; Lill, R.; Löffler, M. Requirements for the mitochondrial import and localization of dihydroorotate dehydrogenase. *Eur. J. Biochem.* **2000**, *267*, 2079–2087. [CrossRef]

114. Uhlin, U.; Eklund, H. Structure of ribonucleotide reductase protein R1. *Nature* **1994**, *370*, 533–539. [CrossRef]

115. Jordan, A.; Reichard, P. Ribonucleotide reductases. *Annu. Rev. Biochem.* **1998**, *67*, 71–98. [CrossRef] [PubMed]

116. Kashlan, O.B.; Scott, C.P.; Lear, J.D.; Cooperman, B.S. A comprehensive model for the allosteric regulation of mammalian ribonucleotide reductase. Functional consequences of ATP- and dATP-induced oligomerization of the large subunit. *Biochemistry* **2002**, *41*, 462–474. [CrossRef]

117. Chabes, A.L.; Pfleger, C.M.; Kirschner, M.W.; Thelander, L. Mouse ribonucleotide reductase R2 protein: A new target for anaphase-promoting complex-Cdh1-mediated proteolysis. *Proc. Natl. Acad. Sci. USA* **2003**, *100*, 3925–3929. [CrossRef] [PubMed]

118. Munch-Petersen, B.; Cloos, L.; Jensen, H.K.; Tyrsted, G. Human thymidine kinase 1. Regulation in normal and malignant cells. *Adv. Enzyme Regul.* **1995**, *35*, 69–89. [CrossRef]

119. Goldstone, D.C.; Ennis-Adeniran, V.; Hedden, J.J.; Groom, H.C.T.; Rice, G.I.; Christodoulou, E.; Walker, P.A.; Kelly, G.; Haire, L.F.; Yap, M.W.; et al. HIV-1 restriction factor SAMHD1 is a deoxynucleoside triphosphate triphosphohydrolase. *Nature* **2011**, *480*, 379–382. [CrossRef]

120. Clifford, R.; Louis, T.; Robbe, P.; Ackroyd, S.; Burns, A.; Timbs, A.T.; Wright Colopy, G.; Dreau, H.; Sigaux, F.; Judde, J.G.; et al. SAMHD1 is mutated recurrently in chronic lymphocytic leukemia and is involved in response to DNA damage. *Blood* **2014**, *123*, 1021–1031. [CrossRef]

121. Song, S.; Wheeler, L.J.; Mathews, C.K. Deoxyribonucleotide pool imbalance stimulates deletions in HeLa cell mitochondrial DNA. *J. Biol. Chem.* **2003**, *278*, 43893–43896. [CrossRef]

122. López, L.C.; Akman, H.O.; García-Cazorla, A.; Dorado, B.; Martí, R.; Nishino, I.; Tadesse, S.; Pizzorno, G.; Shungu, D.; Bonilla, E.; et al. Unbalanced deoxynucleotide pools cause mitochondrial DNA instability in thymidine phosphorylase-deficient mice. *Hum. Mol. Genet.* **2009**, *18*, 714–722. [CrossRef] [PubMed]

123. Pontarin, G.; Gallinaro, L.; Ferraro, P.; Reichard, P.; Bianchi, V. Origins of mitochondrial thymidine triphosphate: Dynamic relations to cytosolic pools. *Proc. Natl. Acad. Sci. USA* **2003**, *100*, 12159–12164. [CrossRef] [PubMed]

124. Desler, C.; Munch-Petersen, B.; Rasmussen, L.J. The Role of Mitochondrial dNTP Levels in Cells with Reduced TK2 Activity. *Nucleosides Nucleotides Nucleic Acids* **2006**, *25*, 1171–1175. [CrossRef] [PubMed]

125. Pontarin, G.; Ferraro, P.; Bee, L.; Reichard, P.; Bianchi, V. Mammalian ribonucleotide reductase subunit p53R2 is required for mitochondrial DNA replication and DNA repair in quiescent cells. *Proc. Natl. Acad. Sci. USA* **2012**, *109*, 13302–13307. [CrossRef]

126. Bourdon, A.; Minai, L.; Serre, V.; Jais, J.-P.; Sarzi, E.; Aubert, S.; Chrétien, D.; de Lonlay, P.; Paquis-Flucklinger, V.; Arakawa, H.; et al. Mutation of RRM2B, encoding p53-controlled ribonucleotide reductase (p53R2), causes severe mitochondrial DNA depletion. *Nat. Genet.* **2007**, *39*, 776–780. [CrossRef] [PubMed]

127. Pontarin, G.; Ferraro, P.; Rampazzo, C.; Kollberg, G.; Holme, E.; Reichard, P.; Bianchi, V. Deoxyribonucleotide metabolism in cycling and resting human fibroblasts with a missense mutation in p53R2, a subunit of ribonucleotide reductase. *J. Biol. Chem.* **2011**, *286*, 11132–11140. [CrossRef] [PubMed]

128. Tanaka, H.; Arakawa, H.; Yamaguchi, T.; Shiraishi, K.; Fukuda, S.; Matsui, K.; Takei, Y.; Nakamura, Y. A ribonucleotide reductase gene involved in a p53-dependent cell-cycle checkpoint for DNA damage. *Nature* **2000**, *404*, 42–49. [CrossRef]

129. James, S.J.; Miller, B.J.; McGarrity, L.J.; Morris, S.M. The effect of folic acid and/or methionine deficiency on deoxyribonucleotide pools and cell cycle distribution in mitogen-stimulated rat lymphocytes. *Cell Prolif.* **1994**, *27*, 395–406. [CrossRef]

130. Micheli, V.; Camici, M.; G Tozzi, M.; L Ipata, P.; Sestini, S.; Bertelli, M.; Pompucci, G. Neurological Disorders of Purine and Pyrimidine Metabolism. *Curr. Top. Med. Chem.* **2011**, *11*, 923–947. [CrossRef]

131. Desler, C.; Marcker, M.L.; Singh, K.K.; Rasmussen, L.J. The importance of mitochondrial DNA in aging and cancer. *J. Aging Res.* **2011**, *2011*, 407536. [CrossRef] [PubMed]

132. Desler, C.; Frederiksen, J.H.; Angleys, M.; Maynard, S.; Keijzers, G.; Fagerlund, B.; Mortensen, E.L.; Osler, M.; Lauritzen, M.; Bohr, V.A.; et al. Increased deoxythymidine triphosphate levels is a feature of relative cognitive decline. *Mitochondrion* **2015**, *25*, 34–37. [CrossRef] [PubMed]

133. Maynard, S.; Hejl, A.-M.; Dinh, T.-S.T.; Keijzers, G.; Hansen, Å.M.; Desler, C.; Moreno-Villanueva, M.; Bürkle, A.; Rasmussen, L.J.; Waldemar, G.; et al. Defective mitochondrial respiration, altered dNTP pools and reduced AP endonuclease 1 activity in peripheral blood mononuclear cells of Alzheimer's disease patients. *Aging* **2015**, *7*, 793–815. [CrossRef] [PubMed]

8

Drug-Induced Mitochondrial Toxicity in the Geriatric Population: Challenges and Future Directions

Yvonne Will [1,*], Jefry E. Shields [1] and Kendall B. Wallace [2]

[1]   SCIENTIA LLC, Ledyard, CT 06339, USA; jefshields@yahoo.ca
[2]   Department of Biomedical Sciences, University of Minnesota Medical School, Duluth, MN 55455, USA; kwallace@d.umn.edu
*   Correspondence: yvonnewillrider@gmail.com

Abstract: Mitochondrial function declines with age, leading to a variety of age-related diseases (metabolic, central nervous system-related, cancer, etc.) and medication usage increases with age due to the increase in diseases. Drug-induced mitochondrial toxicity has been described for many different drug classes and can lead to liver, muscle, kidney and central nervous system injury and, in rare cases, to death. Many of the most prescribed medications in the geriatric population carry mitochondrial liabilities. We have demonstrated that, over the past decade, each class of drugs that demonstrated mitochondrial toxicity contained drugs with both more and less adverse effects on mitochondria. As patient treatment is often essential, we suggest using medication(s) with the best safety profile and the avoidance of concurrent usage of multiple medications that carry mitochondrial liabilities. In addition, we also recommend lifestyle changes to further improve one's mitochondrial function, such as weight loss, exercise and nutrition.

Keywords: drug-induced mitochondrial toxicity; polypharmacy; aging

1. Introduction

Known as the powerhouse of the cell, mitochondria are recognized for their ability to produce large amounts of a cell's energy currency, ATP (Adenosine Triphosphate), as well as being the only other organelle that contains DNA apart from the nucleus. Virtually all eukaryotic cells employ mitochondria to produce the majority of ATP needed to perform cellular functions (e.g., replication, protein synthesis, muscle contraction, etc.) and maintain cellular viability. The electron transport chain (ETC) and ATP synthase are interdependent systems in the mitochondria that generate ATP by coupling the electrochemical potential across the inner mitochondrial membrane created by the ETC to the phosphorylation of ADP by ATP synthase. The protein complexes comprising the ETC shuttle electrons down an energy gradient to ultimately reduce molecular oxygen to water, driving oxidative phosphorylation for ATP synthesis. Compromising the function of any of these protein complexes reduces the efficiency of ATP production and endangers the cell's ability to perform its function and can lead to cell death. Additionally, uncoupling the membrane potential from ATP synthesis through the loss of the inner mitochondrial membrane impermeability dissipates the harvested energy as heat and bypasses ATP synthesis and greatly impairs the cell's viability. Mitochondria contain their own DNA (mtDNA) and both inherited and acquired mutations in mtDNA have been linked to well over 100 mitochondrial syndromes such as Leber's hereditary optic neuropathy, mitochondrial myopathy, encephalomyopathy, lactic acidosis, stroke-like symptoms and myoclonic epilepsy with ragged red fibers [1]. MtDNA is susceptible to oxidative stress due to its proximity to the ETC and the fact that it does not contain histones or a repair mechanism.

As we age, mitochondrial function declines and it is described as the "mitochondrial theory of aging", leading to a variety of age-related diseases (Figure 1).

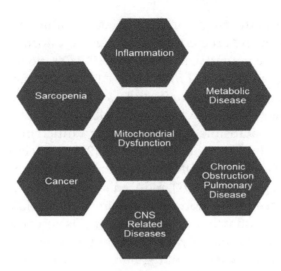

Figure 1. Mitochondrial dysfunction is implicated in many age-related diseases such as metabolic diseases (T2DM, obesity, cardiovascular and cerebrovascular disease, Non-Alcoholic Fatty Liver Disease (NAFDL)) [2–7], CNS-related diseases (Parkinson's, Alzheimer's and Huntington's disease, hearing loss, cataracts) [8–11], inflammation (osteoarthritis) [12], cancer [13,14], sarcopenia [15] and chronic obstructive pulmonary disease (COPD) [16].

These age-related diseases are often treated with multiple medications, some of which are known to cause drug-induced mitochondrial toxicity. In this review, we postulate that drug-induced mitochondrial dysfunction can increase in frequency and severity in the geriatric population due to two independent factors associated with aging, compromised mitochondrial function and polypharmacy.

2. The Mitochondrial Theory of Aging

The "Mitochondrial Theory of Aging" has gained considerable prominence in discussions of longevity, inherent vitality and the biology of mortality. First proposed in his book published in 1928, Raymond Pearl provided a lengthy account of the evidence leading him to posit that longevity is inversely proportional to "the rate of living"; by that, he is referring to the expenditure of energy. His theory is that one is born with a finite quantum of energy, the expenditure of which defines his or her mortality [17]. Although the tenants of this association may hold well for drosophila and perhaps other poikilotherms, in mammals this theory is essentially the antithesis for vitality. There is an abundance of evidence, much of which is current and clinical, demonstrating that energy expenditure is actually vital to delaying mortality and extending one's longevity [18–20]. This is all summarized in the pronouncements that exercise and diet are fundamental to a long and healthy life, perhaps delaying the natural biological regression that is associated with aging.

It is a well-established fact that mitochondrial numbers, function and bioenergetic capacity decline progressively with age [21,22]; Harman summarized this when he coined the term "Mitochondrial Clock" in 1972 [23], which is rooted in his seminal thesis dating from 1956 on the free radical theory of aging [24,25]. This theory is based on the demonstrated accumulation of oxidative damage to lipid, protein, and nucleic acids in aged tissues [26], which Harman attributed to the increased free radical generation observed with aging. The thought is that as biochemical efficiency and physiological function secede with age, the rate of free radical generation increases, leading to increased levels of oxidative damage. This line of thinking continues by prospecting that increased oxidative damage to the ETC within the mitochondrial compartment leads to a progressive loss of coupling efficiency and increased rates of free radical liberation from the electron transport chain. Accordingly, rather than being the consequence of aging, mitochondria are also implicated as the progenitor of the aging process [25]. It becomes quite apparent that the "Mitochondrial Theory of Aging" and the "Free Radical Theory of Aging" are closely intertwined, and it is subject to debate as to which is the cause and which is the consequence of aging (the chicken vs. egg conundrum).

Regardless of whether it is the cause or consequence, hallmarks of mitochondrial aging [19] include a decrease in the number and an increase in the size of mitochondria [27], a net decrease in the cellular mitochondrial membrane potential, a decreased ADP:O ratio (oxidative phosphorylation) and respiratory control index (RCI), and a loss of individual ETC enzyme activities [21,22]; the steady-state [ATP] concentration, however, tends to be unaffected.

Although each of these factors can individually contribute to the progressive loss of mitochondrial function with age, it is far more plausible that they reflect a much broader and concerted decline in homeostatic regulation directed from a molecular level [28]. Molecular hallmarks associated with mitochondrial aging include a decreased mtDNA copy number [29] accompanied by the accumulation of mutations to the mitochondrial genome [30,31], reduced abundance of both nuclear and mitochondrial encoded mRNA [22,32], decreased mitochondrial protein synthesis [33–36], and the dysregulation of the homeostatic balance between mitochondrial biogenesis, fission and mitophagy [19,28].

Ristow and Zarse [20] were first to apply the term "mitohormesis" to conceptualize the loss of the adaptive response of mitochondria by means of regulating mitochondrial homeostasis, contributing to cell and organismal senescence. This has been followed by a number of reviews suggesting that the age-related accumulation of defective mitochondria, accompanied by the loss of ability to clear these from the cell by way of mitophagy and replace them with healthy mitochondria through mitochondrial fission and biogenesis, underpins the mitochondrial theory of aging [19,28,37–39]. This loss of hormesis or mitochondrial homeostasis is equated to a progressive decline in the processes devoted to quality control (QC^{mt}) to sustain mitochondrial fidelity and capacity within the aging cell [19,28,40].

Two major surveillance mechanisms exist within the cell for sensing dysfunctional mitochondria: (1) bioenergetic or nutrient signaling and (2) mitochondrial proteostasis [19,28]. Nutrient sensing is largely by way of activating AMP kinase (AMPK), SIRT1, and the sestrins for a negative nutrient balance, and mTOR for nutrient surplus (Figure 2).

Figure 2. Flow diagram illustrating the interrelationships governing mitochondrial homeostasis in response to the loss of mitochondrial function, such as that which occurs with aging. The Sirt1-dependent regulation of both PGC1α and AMPK provides a well-controlled integration of the disposal of dysfunctional mitochondria (mitophagy) and their replacement with new, supposedly fully functional, mitochondria (biogenesis).

Pyridine nucleotide redox status (NAD$^+$/NADH) is a key factor linking the nutritional status of the cell to both free radical generation and mitochondrial homeostasis. Nutritional deficiency (i.e., mitochondrial dysfunction) is associated with a high NAD$^+$/NADH ratio and low rates of free radical generation. Under these same conditions, the accumulation of high [NAD$^+$] is also associated with high rates of mitochondrial proliferation (biogenesis) and disposal of defective mitochondria (mitophagy), both of which occur by way of the NAD$^+$-dependent activation of SIRT1. The activation of SIRT1 by NAD$^+$ stimulates mitochondrial biogenesis, both by stimulating the PGC1α-dependent activation of mitochondrial biogenesis combined with the AMPK-dependent inhibition of the negative regulator mTOR. The second surveillance pathway, mitochondrial proteostasis, actuates the unfolded protein response (UPR^{mt}) indigenous to mitochondria, where AMPK and mTOR are competing regulators. Collectively, these nutrient sensor pathways regulate both the disposal of defective mitochondria and their replenishment with supposedly fully functional mitochondria.

There is growing evidence that these various mitochondrial signaling pathways are compromised with aging. It may be as simple as the age-associated decrease of [NAD$^+$] [41,42] that is responsible for the lower rates of both mitochondrial biogenesis and mitophagy in aged tissues. Likewise, AMPK and the sirtuins are down-regulated with aging [43–45] as are the concentrations of PGC1α and the rate of mitophagic elimination of dysfunctional mitochondria [46]. These changes suggest loss of molecular mechanisms regulating quality control as being responsible for the ineffective nutrient sensing of mitochondria in aging tissues.

Regardless of the cause, the bioenergetic phenotype of mitochondria from most tissues of aged individuals is very different from that of young adults, which may be a significant factor accounting for the higher rates of drug-induced adverse events in geriatric populations. There is growing appreciation of the possibility that the decline in molecular regulation of mitochondrial hormesis is the primary factor that impedes the ability of aging mitochondria to withstand or adapt to external inputs [26,28,47]. It may be this loss of homeostatic regulation that underlies the sometimes-greater susceptibility of elderly patients to drug-induced adverse events.

3. Drug-Induced Mitochondrial Toxicity

Drug-induced mitochondrial toxicity has been studied in academic settings for well over 50 years. Indeed, many such studies relied on xenobiotic inhibitors, such as rotenone, antimycin and oligomycin, to deduce the function of the ETC, and uncouplers such as 2,4 dinitrophenol, to understand how mitochondria generate ATP. As a result, we should not be surprised that pharmaceutical xenobiotics intended to be therapeutics could also have deleterious 'side effects' on mitochondrial function. Drugs can inhibit mitochondrial function in many different ways such as through the inhibition of ETC protein complexes, inhibition of ATP synthase, inhibition of enzymes of the citric acid cycle, inhibition of various mitochondrial transporters, inhibition of the mitochondrial transcription and translational machinery, as well as through the uncoupling of the ETC from ATP synthase. However, most of these side effects were not detected in preclinical animal studies. This is due to the fact that in vivo toxicity studies are usually done in drug-naïve, young adult animals that have robust mitochondrial reserves; lack of sufficient genetic diversity to allow for idiosyncratic responses; absence of environmental factors; co-medication; insensitivity of histopathology for revealing mitochondrial failure. Much progress has been made in the past decade to develop a variety of high-throughput applicable organelle based and in vitro cell models preclinically [48]. Whereas, traditionally, cells were cultured in high glucose and were unresponsive to mitochondrial toxicity due to shifting to glycolysis for energy production, recently developed cell models grown in galactose can correctly identify potential drug-induced mitochondrial toxicity with greater sensitivity [49,50]. Drugs can also now be tested for potentially causing mitochondrial toxicity in 96- and 384-well formats using solid and soluble oxygen sensors [51,52].

Drug-induced mitochondrial toxicity has been recognized to cause organ toxicity to the liver, skeletal muscle, kidney, heart and the central nervous system. Drug classes identified to cause mitochondrial toxicity are anti-diabetic drugs (thiazolidinediones, fibrates, biguanides), cholesterol lowering drugs (statins), anti-depressants (SARIs), pain medications (NSAIDs), certain antibiotics (fluroquinolones, macrolide), and anti-cancer drugs (kinase inhibitors and anthracyclins) [48]. Most of these observations have been made through studies in isolated mitochondria and cell lines [48].

Over the past decade, our laboratories examined the effects of many different drug classes and found that in each drug class, some members of the class displayed greater potency for adverse effects in vitro than others and the rank order of toxicity observed mimicked the safety profile reported in patients. For example, the anti-diabetic drug Resulin (triglitazone), which was discontinued from the market for liver toxicity, caused greater mitochondrial toxicity when tested in isolated mitochondria than Actos (pioglitazone), which is on the market with a much better safety profile [53]. The same is true for the anti-depressant Zerzone (nefazadone), which belongs to the class of serotonin antagonist reuptake inhibitors. Whereas Zerzone was attrited due to liver toxicity caused at least in part by mitochondrial toxicity, Buspar (buspirone) is still on the market and is well tolerated [54]. Another class of anti-diabetic drugs is the biguanides. Phenformin was discontinued because it caused death by lactic acidosis which is considered a hallmark of mitochondrial toxicity. Glucophage (metformin), which causes much less mitochondrial toxicity is widely used in the clinic and only in rare occasions causes lactic acidosis in most likely already predisposed patients [55]. Table 1 provides additional examples of drugs and drug classes studied by our labs.

Table 1. Each drug class contains drugs with more and less observed mitochondrial toxicity.

Drug Class	Rank order of Toxicity Observed (High to Low)	Target Organ
Anti-diabetic (thiazolidinediones)	Trovan * (troglitazone), Avandia (rosiglitazone), Actos (pioglitazone)	Liver [53]
Cholesterol lowering (statins)	Baycol * (cerivastatin), Zocor (simvastatin), Lipitor (atorvastatin), Lescol (fluvastatin)	Muscle [53]
Anti-diabetic (biguanides)	Phenformin * (N-phenethylbiguanide), Buformin *(1-butylbiguanide), Glucophage (metformin)	Lactic acidosis [55]
Anti-depressant/anxiety (SARIs)	Zerzone * (nefazodone), Desyrel (trazodone), Buspar (buspirone)	Liver [54]
Anti-lipidemic (fibrates)	Lopid (gemfibrozil), Lipanor (ciprofibrate), Trilepix (fenofibrate)	Liver [53]
Pain medication (NSAIDs)	Avalanche * (celebrex), Mobic (meloxicam), Voltaran (dichlofenac), Felden (piroxicam), Aspirin (acetylsalicylic acid)	Liver, intestine [56]
Antibiotics (fluoroquinolones)	Trovan * (trovafloxicin), Levaquin (levafloxicin), Cetraxal (ciprofloxicin)	Liver [57]
Anti-cancer (topoisomerase inhibitors)	Adriamycin (doxorubicin)	Heart [58–61]

* withdrawn from the market.

4. Polypharmacy in the Geriatric Population

Geriatric patients are not only predisposed by having lower mitochondrial function due to age but are often also experiencing one or more of the age-related diseases mentioned above (Figure 1).

In addition, they are also often taking multiple medications (polypharmacy). In the United States, a 2010 and 2011 survey found that 87% of a representative sampling of 2206 adults aged 62 through 85, used at least one prescription medication and that more than one-third of the group were taking five or more prescription medications [62]. Additionally, it was found that 38% of those surveyed were using over-the-counter medications. A further study by Saraf et al. showed that following acute illness or injury, an average of 14 prescriptions were given to geriatric patients discharged from hospitals to skilled nursing facilities and that over one-third of these prescriptions included side-effects that could aggravate underlying geriatric conditions [63].

Of the most commonly used prescription and over-the-counter drugs in the US for older adults [64], many are known to cause mitochondrial toxicity such as the cholesterol lowering drugs (Zocor, Lipitor, Pravacol, Crestor), pain medication (Aspirin, Tylenol, Aleve) and heartburn medication (Prilosec). Table 2 lists references for mitochondrial dysfunction reported for these prescription and over-the-counter (OTC) medications.

It is important to note that most studies have been conducted using isolated mitochondria and cell systems and often these systems are not of human nature. Also, it is important to understand that the safety margin for a particular drug will depend on exposure (Cmax) [54,97] as well as other contributing mechanistic toxicities [98]. For example, Trovan and Serzone (troglitazone and nefazodone) not only have inhibitory effects on mitochondrial function, but also cause additional toxicities through inhibition of the bile salt efflux pump (BSEP) and the formation of reactive metabolites.

Cholesterol lowering statins are the most commonly prescribed drugs in the geriatric population. Almost 50% of the geriatric population was taking a statin in 2011–2014 versus only 20% in 1999–2002. Statins can cause myopathy in 10–15% of the patients. The adverse events range from mild myalgia and fatigue, to life threatening rhabdomyolysis. Baycol was removed from the market in 2001 because it caused death in 52 patients by rhabdomyolysis, which led to kidney failure [99]. Women, frail individuals and those with low body index as well as patients with increased alcohol consumption are at higher risk. Harper and Jacobson, 2010, noted that Zocor (simvastatin) has greater muscle toxicity and drug interactions and should be avoided if the patient has had adverse events and should be substituted with Lescol (fluvastatin) or Crestor (rosuvastatin) [100].

Mitochondrial toxicity has been postulated as a contributing, if not causal, factor of the observed muscle toxicity. It has been postulated that a deficit in CoQ10 is the cause. CoQ10 is an essential electron carrier in the ETC and the pathway for its synthesis has commonality with that of the cholesterol pathway. A decrease in circulatory CoQ10 levels of 27–50% has been reported [101]. However, since circulating CoQ10 is carried by low-density lipoproteins (LDL) the observed decrease may simply reflect the decrease in circulating levels of LDL [101]. Very few studies have actually examined the level of CoQ10 in muscle, probably due to the invasive nature of human muscle biopsies. While these studies did demonstrate significant decreases (30%) in muscle CoQ10 levels, they failed to demonstrate a decrease in ATP synthesis and no myopathic side effects were reported [102,103]. Since muscle toxicity seems to be patient specific and somewhat rare (the same is true for liver toxicity caused by troglitazone and nefazodone), it is most likely that patients will have either underlying mitochondrial dysfunction (for example, a silent mitochondrial disease) or have different levels of transporter expression (MCT4 in the case of statin accumulation) due to polymorphism in enzymes involved in statin metabolism [104].

Table 2. Most Commonly Used Prescription and Over-the-Counter Medications (OTC) in US Older Adults. Modified from [64].

Medication	Brand Name/Drug Name	% Prescribed	References	Mitochondrial Toxicity Reported
Pain medication (OTC)	Aspirin (acetylsalisylic acid)	40	[65–70]	Inhibition of Respiration, Uncoupling of Oxidative Phosphorylation, Opening of MPT Pore, Inhibition of ATPase, Alteration of Glutathione Status
Cholesterol lowering	Zocor (simvastatin)	22	[53,71–77]	Inhibition of Respiration, Uncoupling of oxidative Phosphorylation, Inhibition of ETC Complexes I, IV, V, Decrease in Membrane Potential, Increase Ca^{++} Release, Decrease ATP Levels
Blood pressure medication	Zestril (lisinopril)	20	No reports	
Diuretic	Microzide (hydrochlorothiazidine)	19	No reports	
Thyroid medication	Synthroid (levothyroxin)	15	No reports	
Heart medication	Lopressor (metoprolol)	15	No reports	
Heartburn (OTC)	Prilosec (omeprazole)	10	[78]	Inhibition of Carnitine/Acylcarnitie Transporter
Cholesterol lowering	Lipitor (atorvastatin)	9	[79–81]	Inhibits Mitochondrial Respiration in Pancreatic, Cardiomyocytes and Endothelial Cells
Pain medication (OTC)	Tylenol (acetaminophen)	9	[82–85]	Opening of MPT Pore, Formation of Reactive Oxygen Species, Depletion of mtDNA
Heart medication	Tenormin (atenolol)	8	No reports	
Diuretic	Lasix (furosemide)	7	[86–88]	Inhibition of Respiration, Uncoupling of Oxidative Phosphorylation
Blood thinner	Plavix (clopidogrel)	7	[89–91]	Inhibition of Respiration, Depletion of Glutathione, Induction of Oxidative Stress, Reduction in Membrane Potential
Blood thinner	Coumadin (warfarin)	6	No reports	
Heart medication	Coreg (carvedilol)	5	[92]	Mixed Reports of Mitochondrial Toxicity vs. Preventive Mode
Cholesterol lowering	Pravachol (pravastatin)	5	[93]	Opening MPT Pore, Inhibition of Respiration at High Concentrations
Cholesterol lowering	Crestor (rosuvastatin)	5	[94]	Mixed Reports of Mitochondrial Toxicity vs. Preventive Mode
Pain medication (OTC)	Aleve (naproxen)	5	[95,96]	Inhibition of Respiration, Inhibition of Ca^{++} Flux
Cholesterol lowering	Zetia (ezetimibe)	5	No reports	

Beyond the effect on CoQ10, statins have been reported to have direct effects on the ETC, especially the lipophilic statins, simvastatin and fluvastatin. In addition, statins have the ability to uncouple oxidative phosphorylation, inhibit fatty acid beta oxidation, induce mitochondrial permeability transition, and cause oxidative stress and decrease mtDNA levels by thus far unidentified mechanisms [105].

It has been reported that elderly patients taking cholesterol lowering drugs (Zocor, Lipitor, etc.) have shown drug–drug interactions (DDI), particularly with the anti-lipidemic drug Lopid (gemfibrozil [53,106]), but also with certain antibiotic classes, such as macrolides [107,108] and fluoroquinolones [109,110] and the heart medication, Nexteron (amiodarone) [64,111]. All of these drugs have been shown to cause mitochondrial toxicity by targeting a variety of, as well as multiple, mitochondrial mechanisms/targets.

While it is well documented that this is mainly due to changes in the drug metabolizing function in elderly patients, we hypothesize that polypharmacy with multiple drugs affecting mitochondrial function could contribute to the toxicities observed. We already spoke of the general mitochondrial decay with age and in age-related diseases.

How do we imagine an individual's lifestyle affects their mitochondrial health and energy production, or their response to medications that carry a potential mitochondrial liability (Table 3)? Differences in body mass index (BMI) have shown that obesity correlates with mitochondrial dysfunction [112]. Additionally, diets of high fat and high sucrose have been shown to be detrimental to mitochondrial function [113,114]. Mitochondria are also weakened by inactive lifestyles and can be revitalized with exercise [115,116]. Studies by DiNicolantonio et al. show deleterious effects on mitochondrial function when consuming large quantities of sugar-containing foods and drinks [117], while other labs have shown that imbibing red wine in moderation [118] and drinking green tea [119] have an advantageous effect on mitochondrial function. Even the choice of area of residency can lead to mitochondrial impairment. Lim et al. have studied the effects of incidental ingestion of pesticides/herbicides and have shown a correlation between the area of residence and increased exposure to exogenous agricultural chemicals which have adverse effects on mitochondrial function [120].

Table 3. Comparison of two geriatric people.

Variable	Patient 1	Patient 2
Age	75	75
Body Mass Index	18	28
Breakfast	Yogurt with granola, fresh fruit, poached egg, green tea	Eggs, bacon and potatoes
Exercise	1 h walk daily, swimming once a week	From the car to the house, around the grocery store
Lunch	Hummus and vegetables, banana, oat meal cookie	French fries and hot dogs, ice cream sundae
Medications	None	Zocor, Lopid, Prilosec, Voltaren (oral), Lasix, Nexteron
Dinner	Wild caught salmon and salad	Pasta with sausage and cheese
Drink Consumption	Red wine	Coke

Now, we imagine how different individuals with ideal vs. less than ideal lifestyles might tolerate mitochondrial insults from medications. "Patient 1" has a lifestyle that promotes mitochondrial health while "Patient 2's" lifestyle predisposes them to mitochondrial decay and toxicity in a number of ways. Taking medications that impair mitochondria is far more concerning for Patient 2 than for Patient 1. Patient 2's healthcare providers could examine their lifestyle and medication regiment and act in unison to come up with a medication plan that minimizes mitochondrial liabilities with the drugs they are prescribing for them, opting for drugs with the best safety profile. As mentioned previously, the combination of Zocor with Lopid should at least be substituted with Crestor. An improvement in Patient 2's diet could eliminate the daily use of Prilosec and Patient 2's pain medication of choice should be Aspirin or Tylenol in moderation.

The question arises if mitochondrial dysfunction/toxicity caused by these medications could be prevented or counteracted by natural compounds or drugs recently developed to treat mitochondrial diseases. A recent review by Rai et al., 2016, provides an overview of a variety of pharmaceuticals which either target mitochondria or maintain its homeostasis [121]. While the majority of these drugs target diseases caused by mutations (MELAS, LHON, MERFF, etc.), one therapy is being developed for improving skeletal muscle function in elderly patients. Elamipretide (MTP-131) has been shown to prevent peroxidation of cardiolipin by binding to the molecule and preventing its interaction with cytochorme c, which prevents the latter from functioning as a peroxidase rather than an electron carrier. The drug is currently in Phase III [121]. Another compound is Idebenone, which is based structurally upon CoQ10. Idebanone is currently being explored for LHON and MELAS [121], but not as a supplemental drug in statin therapy. There are a host of natural products and supplements that have been discussed to improve mitochondrial function such as resveratrol, curcumin, NAD and N-acetyl cysteine (NAC), but there is no clinical evidence of clear success.

5. Conclusions

As patient treatment is often essential, we suggest using medication(s) with the best safety profile and the avoidance of concurrent usage of multiple medications that carry mitochondrial liabilities. Our hope is that future therapies will be devoid of mitochondrial liabilities as screening paradigms can be deployed preclinically. In addition, we also recommend lifestyle changes to further improve one's mitochondrial function, such as weight loss, exercise and nutrition. Another major point is that the cause for mitochondrial dysfunction with age appears to be one of molecular homeostatic control of mitochondrial integrity or functional capacity, not simply an acute depletion of bioenergetic substrates, such as ATP. Consequently, bolus supplementation with mitochondrial cofactors has less potential than long-term lifestyle changes in extending vitality and drug tolerance in aging populations.

References

1.   Dimauro, S.; Davidzon, G. Mitochondrial DNA and disease. *Ann. Med.* **2005**, *37*, 222–232. [CrossRef]
2.   Blake, R.; Trounce, I.A. Mitochondrial dysfunction and complications associated with diabetes. *Biochim. Biophys. Acta* **2014**, *1840*, 1404–1412. [CrossRef] [PubMed]
3.   Peng, K.Y.; Watt, M.J.; Rensen, S.; Greve, J.W.; Huynh, K.; Jayawardana, K.S.; Meikle, P.J.; Meex, R.C.R. Mitochondrial dysfunction-related lipid changes occur in non-alcoholic fatty liver disease progression. *J. Lipid Res.* **2018**. [CrossRef] [PubMed]
4.   Bonora, M.; Wieckowski, M.R.; Sinclair, D.A.; Kroemer, G.; Pinton, P.; Galluzzi, L. Targeting mitochondria for cardiovascular disorders: Therapeutic potential and obstacles. *Nat. Rev. Cardiol.* **2019**, *16*, 33–55. [CrossRef]
5.   Hoppel, C.L.; Lesnefsky, E.J.; Chen, Q.; Tandler, B. Mitochondrial Dysfunction in Cardiovascular Aging. *Adv. Exp. Med. Biol.* **2017**, *982*, 451–464. [PubMed]
6.   Grimm, A.; Eckert, A. Brain aging and neurodegeneration: From a mitochondrial point of view. *J. Neurochem.* **2017**, *143*, 418–431. [CrossRef] [PubMed]
7.   Anupama, N.; Sindhu, G.; Raghu, K.G. Significance of mitochondria on cardiometabolic syndromes. *Fundam. Clin. Pharmacol.* **2018**, *32*, 346–356. [CrossRef] [PubMed]
8.   Macdonald, R.; Barnes, K.; Hastings, C.; Mortiboys, H. Mitochondrial abnormalities in Parkinson's disease and Alzheimer's disease: Can mitochondria be targeted therapeutically? *Biochem. Soc. Trans.* **2018**, *46*, 891–909. [CrossRef]
9.   Franco-Iborra, S.; Vila, M.; Perier, C. Mitochondrial Quality Control in Neurodegenerative Diseases: Focus on Parkinson's Disease and Huntington's Disease. *Front. Neurosci.* **2018**, *12*, 342. [CrossRef]
10.   Falah, M.; Houshmand, M.; Najafi, M.; Balali, M.; Mahmoudian, S.; Asghari, A.; Emamdjomeh, H.; Farhadi, M. The potential role for use of mitochondrial DNA copy number as predictive biomarker in presbycusis. *Ther. Clin. Risk Manag.* **2016**, *12*, 1573–1578. [CrossRef]

11. Leruez, S.; Marill, A.; Bresson, T.; de Saint Martin, G.; Buisset, A.; Muller, J.; Tessier, L.; Gadras, C.; Verny, C.; Gohier, P.; et al. A Metabolomics Profiling of Glaucoma Points to Mitochondrial Dysfunction, Senescence, and Polyamines Deficiency. *Investig. Ophthalmol. Vis. Sci.* **2018**, *59*, 4355–4361. [CrossRef]
12. Bolduc, J.A.; Collins, J.A.; Loeser, R.F. Reactive Oxygen Species, Aging and Articular Cartilage Homeostasis. *Free Radic. Biol. Med.* **2019**, *132*, 73–82. [CrossRef]
13. Ng Kee Kwong, F.; Nicholson, A.G.; Harrison, C.L.; Hansbro, P.M.; Adcock, I.M.; Chung, K.F. Is mitochondrial dysfunction a driving mechanism linking COPD to nonsmall cell lung carcinoma? *Eur. Respir. Rev.* **2017**, *26*. [CrossRef]
14. Zhu, Y.; Dean, A.E.; Horikoshi, N.; Heer, C.; Spitz, D.R.; Gius, D. Emerging evidence for targeting mitochondrial metabolic dysfunction in cancer therapy. *J. Clin. Investig.* **2018**, *128*, 3682–3691. [CrossRef]
15. Always, S.E.; Mohamed, J.S.; Myers, M.J. Mitochondria Initiate and Regulate Sarcopenia. *Exerc. Sport Sci. Rev.* **2017**, *45*, 58–69. [CrossRef]
16. Hara, H.; Kuwano, K.; Araya, J. Mitochondrial Quality Control in COPD and IPF. *Cells* **2018**, *7*, 86. [CrossRef]
17. Raymond, P. *The Rate of Living*; Johns Hopkins University: New York, NY, USA, 1928.
18. Lanza, I.R.; Nair, K.S. Mitochondrial function as a determinant of life span. *Pflugers Arch.* **2010**, *459*, 277–289. [CrossRef]
19. Lopez-Otin, C.; Galluzzi, L.; Freije, J.M.P.; Madeo, F.; Kroemer, G. Metabolic Control of Longevity. *Cell* **2016**, *166*, 802–821. [CrossRef]
20. Ristow, M.; Zarse, K. How increased oxidative stress promotes longevity and metabolic health: The concept of mitochondrial hormesis (mitohormesis). *Exp. Gerontol.* **2010**, *45*, 410–418. [CrossRef]
21. Conley, K.E.; Jubrias, S.A.; Esselman, P.C. Oxidative capacity and ageing in human muscle. *J. Physiol.* **2000**, *526*, 203–210. [CrossRef]
22. Short, K.R.; Bigelow, M.L.; Kahl, J.; Singh, R.; Coenen-Schimke, J.; Raghavakaimal, S.; Nair, K.S. Decline in skeletal muscle mitochondrial function with aging in humans. *Proc. Natl. Acad. Sci. USA* **2005**, *102*, 5618–5623. [CrossRef]
23. Harman, D. The biological clock: The mitochondria? *J. Am. Geriatr. Soc.* **1972**, *20*, 145–147. [CrossRef]
24. Harman, D. Aging: A theory based on free radical and radiation chemistry. *J. Gerontol.* **1956**, *11*, 298–300. [CrossRef]
25. Harman, D. Free radical theory of aging: Consequences of mitochondrial aging. *Age* **1983**, *6*, 86–94. [CrossRef]
26. Chistiakov, D.A.; Sobenin, I.A.; Revin, V.V.; Orekhov, A.N.; Bobryshev, Y.V. Mitochondrial aging and age-related dysfunction of mitochondria. *Biomed. Res. Int.* **2014**, *2014*, 238463. [CrossRef]
27. Tauchi, H.; Sato, T. Age changes in size and number of mitochondria of human hepatic cells. *J. Gerontol.* **1968**, *23*, 454–461. [CrossRef]
28. Lopez-Lluch, G. Mitochondrial activity and dynamics changes regarding metabolism in ageing and obesity. *Mech. Ageing Dev.* **2017**, *162*, 108–121. [CrossRef]
29. Welle, S.; Bhatt, K.; Shah, B.; Needler, N.; Delehanty, J.M.; Thornton, C.A. Reduced amount of mitochondrial DNA in aged human muscle. *J. Appl. Physiol. (1985)* **2003**, *94*, 1479–1484. [CrossRef]
30. Larsson, N.G. Somatic mitochondrial DNA mutations in mammalian aging. *Annu. Rev. Biochem.* **2010**, *79*, 683–706. [CrossRef]
31. Bratic, A.; Larsson, N.G. The role of mitochondria in aging. *J. Clin. Investig.* **2013**, *123*, 951–957. [CrossRef]
32. Lanza, I.R.; Short, D.K.; Short, K.R.; Raghavakaimal, S.; Basu, R.; Joyner, M.J.; McConnell, J.P.; Nair, K.S. Endurance exercise as a countermeasure for aging. *Diabetes* **2008**, *57*, 2933–2942. [CrossRef]
33. Bailey, P.J.; Webster, G.C. Lowered rates of protein synthesis by mitochondria isolated from organisms of increasing age. *Mech. Ageing Dev.* **1984**, *24*, 233–241. [CrossRef]
34. Marcus, D.L.; Ibrahim, N.G.; Freedman, M.L. Age-related decline in the biosynthesis of mitochondrial inner membrane proteins. *Exp. Gerontol.* **1982**, *17*, 333–341. [CrossRef]
35. Rooyackers, O.E.; Adey, D.B.; Ades, P.A.; Nair, K.S. Effect of age on in vivo rates of mitochondrial protein synthesis in human skeletal muscle. *Proc. Natl. Acad. Sci. USA* **1996**, *93*, 15364–15369. [CrossRef]
36. Rooyackers, O.E.; Kersten, A.H.; Wagenmakers, A.J. Mitochondrial protein content and in vivo synthesis rates in skeletal muscle from critically ill rats. *Clin. Sci. (Lond.)* **1996**, *91*, 475–481. [CrossRef]
37. Mammucari, C.; Rizzuto, R. Signaling pathways in mitochondrial dysfunction and aging. *Mech. Ageing Dev.* **2010**, *131*, 536–543. [CrossRef]

38. Vendelbo, M.H.; Nair, K.S. Mitochondrial longevity pathways. *Biochim. Biophys. Acta* **2011**, *1813*, 634–644. [CrossRef]

39. Palikaras, K.; Lionaki, E.; Tavernarakis, N. Coordination of mitophagy and mitochondrial biogenesis during ageing in *C. elegans*. *Nature* **2015**, *521*, 525–528. [CrossRef]

40. Tatsuta, T.; Langer, T. Quality control of mitochondria: Protection against neurodegeneration and ageing. *EMBO J.* **2008**, *27*, 306–314. [CrossRef]

41. Verdin, E. NAD(+) in aging, metabolism, and neurodegeneration. *Science* **2015**, *350*, 1208–1213. [CrossRef]

42. Gomes, A.P.; Price, N.L.; Ling, A.J.; Moslehi, J.J.; Montgomery, M.K.; Rajman, L.; White, J.P.; Teodoro, J.S.; Wrann, C.D.; Hubbard, B.P.; et al. Declining NAD(+) induces a pseudohypoxic state disrupting nuclear-mitochondrial communication during aging. *Cell* **2013**, *155*, 1624–1638. [CrossRef] [PubMed]

43. Lee, J.H.; Budanov, A.V.; Karin, M. Sestrins orchestrate cellular metabolism to attenuate aging. *Cell Metab.* **2013**, *18*, 792–801. [CrossRef] [PubMed]

44. Chang, H.C.; Guarente, L. SIRT1 mediates central circadian control in the SCN by a mechanism that decays with aging. *Cell* **2013**, *153*, 1448–1460. [CrossRef] [PubMed]

45. Guarente, L. Introduction: Sirtuins in aging and diseases. *Methods Mol. Biol.* **2013**, *1077*, 3–10. [PubMed]

46. Chabi, B.; Ljubicic, V.; Menzies, K.J.; Huang, J.H.; Saleem, A.; Hood, D.A. Mitochondrial function and apoptotic susceptibility in aging skeletal muscle. *Aging Cell* **2008**, *7*, 2–12. [CrossRef] [PubMed]

47. Weber, T.A.; Reichert, A.S. Impaired quality control of mitochondria: Aging from a new perspective. *Exp. Gerontol.* **2010**, *45*, 503–511. [CrossRef] [PubMed]

48. Will, Y.; Dykens, J. Mitochondrial toxicity assessment in industry–a decade of technology development and insight. *Expert Opin. Drug Metab. Toxicol.* **2014**, *10*, 1061–1067. [CrossRef]

49. Swiss, R.; Will, Y. Assessment of mitochondrial toxicity in HepG2 cells cultured in high-glucose- or galactose-containing media. *Curr. Protoc. Toxicol.* **2011**, *49*, 2.20.1–2.20.14. [CrossRef]

50. Kamalian, L.; Chadwick, A.E.; Bayliss, M.; French, N.S.; Monshouwer, M.; Snoeys, J.; Park, B.K. The utility of HepG2 cells to identify direct mitochondrial dysfunction in the absence of cell death. *Toxicol. In Vitro* **2015**, *29*, 732–740. [CrossRef]

51. Hynes, J.; Swiss, R.L.; Will, Y. High-Throughput Analysis of Mitochondrial Oxygen Consumption. *Methods Mol. Biol.* **2018**, *1782*, 71–87.

52. Nadanaciva, S.; Rana, P.; Beeson, G.C.; Chen, D.; Ferrick, D.A.; Beeson, C.C.; Will, Y. Assessment of drug-induced mitochondrial dysfunction via altered cellular respiration and acidification measured in a 96-well platform. *J. Bioenerg. Biomembr.* **2012**, *44*, 421–437. [CrossRef]

53. Nadanaciva, S.; Dykens, J.A.; Bernal, A.; Capaldi, R.A.; Will, Y. Mitochondrial impairment by PPAR agonists and statins identified via immunocaptured OXPHOS complex activities and respiration. *Toxicol. Appl. Pharmacol.* **2007**, *223*, 277–287. [CrossRef]

54. Dykens, J.A.; Jamieson, J.D.; Marroquin, L.D.; Nadanaciva, S.; Xu, J.J.; Dunn, M.C.; Smith, A.R.; Will, Y. In vitro assessment of mitochondrial dysfunction and cytotoxicity of nefazodone, trazodone, and buspirone. *Toxicol. Sci.* **2008**, *103*, 335–345. [CrossRef]

55. Dykens, J.A.; Jamieson, J.; Marroquin, L.; Nadanaciva, S.; Billis, P.A.; Will, Y. Biguanide-induced mitochondrial dysfunction yields increased lactate production and cytotoxicity of aerobically-poised HepG2 cells and human hepatocytes in vitro. *Toxicol. Appl. Pharmacol.* **2008**, *233*, 203–210. [CrossRef]

56. Nadanaciva, S.; Aleo, M.D.; Strock, C.J.; Stedman, D.B.; Wang, H.; Will, Y. Toxicity assessments of nonsteroidal anti-inflammatory drugs in isolated mitochondria, rat hepatocytes, and zebrafish show good concordance across chemical classes. *Toxicol. Appl. Pharmacol.* **2013**, *272*, 272–280. [CrossRef]

57. Nadanaciva, S.; Dillman, K.; Gebhard, D.F.; Shrikhande, A.; Will, Y. High-content screening for compounds that affect mtDNA-encoded protein levels in eukaryotic cells. *J. Biomol. Screen.* **2010**, *15*, 937–948. [CrossRef]

58. Solem, L.E.; Henry, T.R.; Wallace, K.B. Disruption of mitochondrial calcium homeostasis following chronic doxorubicin administration. *Toxicol. Appl. Pharmacol.* **1994**, *129*, 214–222. [CrossRef]

59. Palmeira, C.M.; Serrano, J.; Kuehl, D.W.; Wallace, K.B. Preferential oxidation of cardiac mitochondrial DNA following acute intoxication with doxorubicin. *Biochim. Biophys. Acta* **1997**, *1321*, 101–106. [CrossRef]

60. Wallace, K.B. Doxorubicin-induced cardiac mitochondrionopathy. *Pharmacol. Toxicol.* **2003**, *93*, 105–115. [CrossRef]

61. Sardao, V.A.; Oliveira, P.J.; Holy, J.; Oliveira, C.R.; Wallace, K.B. Doxorubicin-induced mitochondrial dysfunction is secondary to nuclear p53 activation in H9c2 cardiomyoblasts. *Cancer Chemother. Pharmacol.* **2009**, *64*, 811–827. [CrossRef]

62. Qato, D.M.; Wilder, J.; Schumm, L.P.; Gillet, V.; Alexander, G.C. Changes in Prescription and Over-the-Counter Medication and Dietary Supplement Use among Older Adults in the United States, 2005 vs 2011. *JAMA Intern. Med.* **2016**, *176*, 473–482. [CrossRef]

63. Saraf, A.A.; Petersen, A.W.; Simmons, S.F.; Schnelle, J.F.; Bell, S.P.; Kripalani, S.; Myers, A.P.; Mixon, A.S.; Long, E.A.; Jacobsen, J.M.; et al. Medications associated with geriatric syndromes and their prevalence in older hospitalized adults discharged to skilled nursing facilities. *J. Hosp. Med.* **2016**, *11*, 694–700. [CrossRef]

64. Merel, S.E.; Paauw, D.S. Common Drug Side Effects and Drug-Drug Interactions in Elderly Adults in Primary Care. *J. Am. Geriatr. Soc.* **2017**, *65*, 1578–1585. [CrossRef]

65. Chatterjee, S.S.; Stefanovich, V. Influence of anti-inflammatory agents on rat liver mitochondrial ATPase. *Arzneimittel-Forschung* **1976**, *26*, 499–502.

66. Nulton-Persson, A.C.; Szweda, L.I.; Sadek, H.A. Inhibition of cardiac mitochondrial respiration by salicylic acid and acetylsalicylate. *J. Cardiovasc. Pharmacol.* **2004**, *44*, 591–595. [CrossRef]

67. Raza, H.; John, A. Implications of altered glutathione metabolism in aspirin-induced oxidative stress and mitochondrial dysfunction in HepG2 cells. *PLoS ONE* **2012**, *7*, e36325. [CrossRef]

68. Deschamps, D.; Fisch, C.; Fromenty, B.; Berson, A.; Degott, C.; Pessayre, D. Inhibition by salicylic acid of the activation and thus oxidation of long chain fatty acids. Possible role in the development of Reye's syndrome. *J. Pharmacol. Exp. Ther.* **1991**, *259*, 894–904.

69. Oh, K.W.; Qian, T.; Brenner, D.A.; Lemasters, J.J. Salicylate enhances necrosis and apoptosis mediated by the mitochondrial permeability transition. *Toxicol. Sci.* **2003**, *73*, 44–52. [CrossRef]

70. Zimmerman, H.J. Effects of aspirin and acetaminophen on the liver. *Arch. Intern. Med.* **1981**, *141*, 333–342. [CrossRef]

71. Bonifacio, A.; Mullen, P.J.; Mityko, I.S.; Navegantes, L.C.; Bouitbir, J.; Krahenbuhl, S. Simvastatin induces mitochondrial dysfunction and increased atrogin-1 expression in H9c2 cardiomyocytes and mice in vivo. *Arch. Toxicol.* **2016**, *90*, 203–215. [CrossRef]

72. Fisar, Z.; Hroudova, J.; Singh, N.; Koprivova, A.; Maceckova, D. Effect of Simvastatin, Coenzyme Q10, Resveratrol, Acetylcysteine and Acetylcarnitine on Mitochondrial Respiration. *Folia Biol.* **2016**, *62*, 53–66.

73. van Diemen, M.P.J.; Berends, C.L.; Akram, N.; Wezel, J.; Teeuwisse, W.M.; Mik, B.G.; Kan, H.E.; Webb, A.; Beenakker, J.W.M.; Groeneveld, G.J. Validation of a pharmacological model for mitochondrial dysfunction in healthy subjects using simvastatin: A randomized placebo-controlled proof-of-pharmacology study. *Eur. J. Pharmacol.* **2017**, *815*, 290–297. [CrossRef]

74. Busanello, E.N.B.; Figueira, T.R.; Marques, A.C.; Navarro, C.D.C.; Oliveira, H.C.F.; Vercesi, A.E. Facilitation of Ca(2+) -induced opening of the mitochondrial permeability transition pore either by nicotinamide nucleotide transhydrogenase deficiency or statins treatment. *Cell Biol. Int.* **2018**, *42*, 742–746. [CrossRef]

75. Sirvent, P.; Bordenave, S.; Vermaelen, M.; Roels, B.; Vassort, G.; Mercier, J.; Raynaud, E.; Lacampagne, A. Simvastatin induces impairment in skeletal muscle while heart is protected. *Biochem. Biophys. Res. Commun.* **2005**, *338*, 1426–1434. [CrossRef]

76. Sirvent, P.; Mercier, J.; Vassort, G.; Lacampagne, A. Simvastatin triggers mitochondria-induced Ca2+ signaling alteration in skeletal muscle. *Biochem. Biophys. Res. Commun.* **2005**, *329*, 1067–1075. [CrossRef]

77. Wagner, B.K.; Kitami, T.; Gilbert, T.J.; Peck, D.; Ramanathan, A.; Schreiber, S.L.; Golub, T.R.; Mootha, V.K. Large-scale chemical dissection of mitochondrial function. *Nat. Biotechnol.* **2008**, *26*, 343–351. [CrossRef]

78. Tonazzi, A.; Giangregorio, N.; Console, L.; Indiveri, C. Mitochondrial carnitine/acylcarnitine translocase: Insights in structure/function relationships. Basis for drug therapy and side effects prediction. *Mini Rev. Med. Chem.* **2015**, *15*, 396–405. [CrossRef]

79. Urbano, F.; Bugliani, M.; Filippello, A.; Scamporrino, A.; Di Mauro, S.; Di Pino, A.; Scicali, R.; Noto, D.; Rabuazzo, A.M.; Averna, M.; et al. Atorvastatin but Not Pravastatin Impairs Mitochondrial Function in Human Pancreatic Islets and Rat beta-Cells. Direct Effect of Oxidative Stress. *Sci. Rep.* **2017**, *7*, 11863. [CrossRef]

80. Godoy, J.C.; Niesman, I.R.; Busija, A.R.; Kassan, A.; Schilling, J.M.; Schwarz, A.; Alvarez, E.A.; Dalton, N.D.; Drummond, J.C.; Roth, D.M.; et al. Atorvastatin, but not pravastatin, inhibits cardiac Akt/mTOR signaling and disturbs mitochondrial ultrastructure in cardiac myocytes. *FASEB J.* **2019**, *33*, 1209–1225. [CrossRef]

81. Broniarek, I.; Jarmuszkiewicz, W. Atorvastatin affects negatively respiratory function of isolated endothelial mitochondria. *Arch. Biochem. Biophys.* **2018**, *637*, 64–72. [CrossRef]

82. Hinson, J.A.; Reid, A.B.; McCullough, S.S.; James, L.P. Acetaminophen-induced hepatotoxicity: Role of metabolic activation, reactive oxygen/nitrogen species, and mitochondrial permeability transition. *Drug Metab. Rev.* **2004**, *36*, 805–822. [CrossRef]

83. Masubuchi, Y.; Suda, C.; Horie, T. Involvement of mitochondrial permeability transition in acetaminophen-induced liver injury in mice. *J. Hepatol.* **2005**, *42*, 110–116. [CrossRef]

84. Prill, S.; Bavli, D.; Levy, G.; Ezra, E.; Schmalzlin, E.; Jaeger, M.S.; Schwarz, M.; Duschl, C.; Cohen, M.; Nahmias, Y. Real-time monitoring of oxygen uptake in hepatic bioreactor shows CYP450-independent mitochondrial toxicity of acetaminophen and amiodarone. *Arch. Toxicol.* **2016**, *90*, 1181–1191. [CrossRef]

85. Moles, A.; Torres, S.; Baulies, A.; Garcia-Ruiz, C.; Fernandez-Checa, J.C. Mitochondrial-Lysosomal Axis in Acetaminophen Hepatotoxicity. *Front. Pharmacol.* **2018**, *9*, 453. [CrossRef]

86. Manuel, M.A.; Weiner, M.W. Effects of ethacrynic acid and furosemide on isolated rat kidney mitochondria: Inhibition of electron transport in the region of phosphorylation site II. *J. Pharmacol. Exp. Ther.* **1976**, *198*, 209.

87. Orita, Y.; Fukuhara, Y.; Yanase, M.; Ando, A.; Okada, N.; Abe, H. Effect of furosemide on mitochondrial electron transport system and oxidative phosphorylation. *Arzneimittel-Forschung* **1983**, *33*, 1446–1450.

88. Wong, S.G.W.; Card, J.W.; Racz, W.J. The role of mitochondrial injury in bromobenzene and furosemide induced hepatotoxicity. *Toxicol. Lett.* **2000**, *116*, 171–181. [CrossRef]

89. Tai, Y.K.; Cheong, Y.M.; Almsherqi, Z.A.; Chia, S.H.; Deng, Y.; McLachlan, C.S. High dose clopidogrel decreases mice liver mitochondrial respiration function in vitro. *Int. J. Cardiol.* **2009**, *133*, 250–252. [CrossRef]

90. Maseneni, S.; Donzelli, M.; Brecht, K.; Krahenbuhl, S. Toxicity of thienopyridines on human neutrophil granulocytes and lymphocytes. *Toxicology* **2013**, *308*, 11–19. [CrossRef]

91. Zahno, A.; Bouitbir, J.; Maseneni, S.; Lindinger, P.W.; Brecht, K.; Krahenbuhl, S. Hepatocellular toxicity of clopidogrel: Mechanisms and risk factors. *Free Radic. Biol. Med.* **2013**, *65*, 208–216. [CrossRef]

92. Felix, L.; Oliveira, M.M.; Videira, R.; Maciel, E.; Alves, N.D.; Nunes, F.M.; Alves, A.; Almeida, J.M.; Domingues, M.R.; Peixoto, F.P. Carvedilol exacerbate gentamicin-induced kidney mitochondrial alterations in adult rat. *Exp. Toxicol. Pathol.* **2017**, *69*, 83–92. [CrossRef]

93. Busanello, E.N.B.; Marques, A.C.; Lander, N.; de Oliveira, D.N.; Catharino, R.R.; Oliveira, H.C.F.; Vercesi, A.E. Pravastatin Chronic Treatment Sensitizes Hypercholesterolemic Mice Muscle to Mitochondrial Permeability Transition: Protection by Creatine or Coenzyme Q10. *Front. Pharmacol.* **2017**, *8*, 185. [CrossRef]

94. Westwood, F.R.; Scott, R.C.; Marsden, A.M.; Bigley, A.; Randall, K. Rosuvastatin: Characterization of induced myopathy in the rat. *Toxicol. Pathol.* **2008**, *36*, 345–352. [CrossRef]

95. van Leeuwen, J.S.; Unlu, B.; Vermeulen, N.P.; Vos, J.C. Differential involvement of mitochondrial dysfunction, cytochrome P450 activity, and active transport in the toxicity of structurally related NSAIDs. *Toxicol. In Vitro* **2012**, *26*, 197–205. [CrossRef]

96. Moreno-Sanchez, R.; Bravo, C.; Vasquez, C.; Ayala, G.; Silveira, L.H.; Martinez-Lavin, M. Inhibition and uncoupling of oxidative phosphorylation by nonsteroidal anti-inflammatory drugs: Study in mitochondria, submitochondrial particles, cells, and whole heart. *Biochem. Pharmacol.* **1999**, *57*, 743–752. [CrossRef]

97. Porceddu, M.; Buron, N.; Roussel, C.; Labbe, G.; Fromenty, B.; Borgne-Sanchez, A. Prediction of liver injury induced by chemicals in human with a multiparametric assay on isolated mouse liver mitochondria. *Toxicol. Sci.* **2012**, *129*, 332–345. [CrossRef]

98. Aleo, M.D.; Luo, Y.; Swiss, R.; Bonin, P.D.; Potter, D.M.; Will, Y. Human drug-induced liver injury severity is highly associated with dual inhibition of liver mitochondrial function and bile salt export pump. *Hepatology* **2014**, *60*, 1015–1022. [CrossRef]

99. Mendes, P.; Robles, P.G.; Mathur, S. Statin-induced rhabdomyolysis: A comprehensive review of case reports. *Physiother. Can.* **2014**, *66*, 124–132. [CrossRef]

100. Harper, C.R.; Jacobson, T.A. Evidence-based management of statin myopathy. *Curr. Atheroscler. Rep.* **2010**, *12*, 322–330. [CrossRef]

101. Hargreaves, I.P.; Duncan, A.J.; Heales, S.J.; Land, J.M. The effect of HMG-CoA reductase inhibitors on coenzyme Q10: Possible biochemical/clinical implications. *Drug Saf.* **2005**, *28*, 659–676. [CrossRef]

102. Paiva, H.; Thelen, K.M.; Van Coster, R.; Smet, J.; De Paepe, B.; Mattila, K.M.; Laakso, J.; Lehtimaki, T.; von Bergmann, K.; Lutjohann, D.; et al. High-dose statins and skeletal muscle metabolism in humans: A randomized, controlled trial. *Clin. Pharmacol. Ther.* **2005**, *78*, 60–68. [CrossRef]

103. Avis, H.J.; Hargreaves, I.P.; Ruiter, J.P.; Land, J.M.; Wanders, R.J.; Wijburg, F.A. Rosuvastatin lowers coenzyme Q10 levels, but not mitochondrial adenosine triphosphate synthesis, in children with familial hypercholesterolemia. *J. Pediatr.* **2011**, *158*, 458–462. [CrossRef]

104. Neergheen, V.; Dyson, A.; Wainwright, L.; Hargreaves, I.P. Statin and Fibrate-induced Dichotomy of Mitochondrial Function. In *Mitochondrial Dysfunction Caused by Drugs and Environmental Toxicants*; Will, Y., Dykens, J., Eds.; Wiley: New York, NY, USA, 2018; pp. 459–473.

105. Hargreaves, I.P.; Al Shahrani, M.; Wainwright, L.; Heales, S.J. Drug-Induced Mitochondrial Toxicity. *Drug Saf.* **2016**, *39*, 661–674. [CrossRef]

106. Johnson, T.E.; Zhang, X.; Shi, S.; Umbenhauer, D.R. Statins and PPARalpha agonists induce myotoxicity in differentiated rat skeletal muscle cultures but do not exhibit synergy with co-treatment. *Toxicol. Appl. Pharmacol.* **2005**, *208*, 210–221. [CrossRef]

107. Salimi, A.; Eybagi, S.; Seydi, E.; Naserzadeh, P.; Kazerouni, N.P.; Pourahmad, J. Toxicity of macrolide antibiotics on isolated heart mitochondria: A justification for their cardiotoxic adverse effect. *Xenobiotica* **2016**, *46*, 82–93. [CrossRef]

108. Mathis, A.; Wild, P.; Boettger, E.C.; Kapel, C.M.; Deplazes, P. Mitochondrial ribosome as the target for the macrolide antibiotic clarithromycin in the helminth Echinococcus multilocularis. *Antimicrob. Agents Chemother.* **2005**, *49*, 3251–3255. [CrossRef]

109. Ding, L.; Zang, L.; Zhang, Y.; Zhang, Y.; Wang, X.; Ai, W.; Ding, N.; Wang, H. Joint toxicity of fluoroquinolone and tetracycline antibiotics to zebrafish (Danio rerio) based on biochemical biomarkers and histopathological observation. *J. Toxicol. Sci.* **2017**, *42*, 267–280. [CrossRef]

110. Kaur, K.; Fayad, R.; Saxena, A.; Frizzell, N.; Chanda, A.; Das, S.; Chatterjee, S.; Hegde, S.; Baliga, M.S.; Ponemone, V.; et al. Fluoroquinolone-related neuropsychiatric and mitochondrial toxicity: A collaborative investigation by scientists and members of a social network. *J. Community Support. Oncol.* **2016**, *14*, 54–65. [CrossRef]

111. Finsterer, J.; Zarrouk-Mahjoub, S. Mitochondrial toxicity of cardiac drugs and its relevance to mitochondrial disorders. *Expert Opin. Drug Metab. Toxicol.* **2015**, *11*, 15–24. [CrossRef]

112. De Mello, A.H.; Costa, A.B.; Engel, J.D.G.; Rezin, G.T. Mitochondrial dysfunction in obesity. *Life Sci.* **2018**, *192*, 26–32. [CrossRef]

113. Miotto, P.M.; LeBlanc, P.J.; Holloway, G.P. High-Fat Diet Causes Mitochondrial Dysfunction as a Result of Impaired ADP Sensitivity. *Diabetes* **2018**, *67*, 2199–2205. [CrossRef]

114. Jorgensen, W.; Rud, K.A.; Mortensen, O.H.; Frandsen, L.; Grunnet, N.; Quistorff, B. Your mitochondria are what you eat: A high-fat or a high-sucrose diet eliminates metabolic flexibility in isolated mitochondria from rat skeletal muscle. *Physiol. Rep.* **2017**, *5*. [CrossRef] [PubMed]

115. Gram, M.; Dahl, R.; Dela, F. Physical inactivity and muscle oxidative capacity in humans. *Eur. J. Sport Sci.* **2014**, *14*, 376–383. [CrossRef]

116. Kim, Y.; Triolo, M.; Hood, D.A. Impact of Aging and Exercise on Mitochondrial Quality Control in Skeletal Muscle. *Oxid. Med. Cell. Longev.* **2017**, *2017*, 3165396. [CrossRef]

117. DiNicolantonio, J.J.; Berger, A. Added sugars drive nutrient and energy deficit in obesity: A new paradigm. *Open Heart* **2016**, *3*, e000469. [CrossRef]

118. Chen, W.J.; Du, J.K.; Hu, X.; Yu, Q.; Li, D.X.; Wang, C.N.; Zhu, X.Y.; Liu, Y.J. Protective effects of resveratrol on mitochondrial function in the hippocampus improves inflammation-induced depressive-like behavior. *Physiol. Behav.* **2017**, *182*, 54–61. [CrossRef] [PubMed]

119. Assuncao, M.; Andrade, J.P. Protective action of green tea catechins in neuronal mitochondria during aging. *Front. Biosci.* **2015**, *20*, 247–262.

120. Lim, S.; Ahn, S.Y.; Song, I.C.; Chung, M.H.; Jang, H.C.; Park, K.S.; Lee, K.U.; Pak, Y.K.; Lee, H.K. Chronic exposure to the herbicide, atrazine, causes mitochondrial dysfunction and insulin resistance. *PLoS ONE* **2009**, *4*, e5186. [CrossRef]

121. Rai, P.K.; Russell, O.M.; Lightowlers, R.N.; Turnbull, D.M. Potential compounds for the treatment of mitochondrial disease. *Br. Med. Bull.* **2015**, *116*, 5–18. [CrossRef]

9

Incomplete Healing as a Cause of Aging: The Role of Mitochondria and the Cell Danger Response

Robert K. Naviaux

The Mitochondrial and Metabolic Disease Center, Departments of Medicine, Pediatrics, Pathology, University of California, San Diego School of Medicine, San Diego, CA 92103, USA; Naviaux@ucsd.edu

Abstract: The rate of biological aging varies cyclically and episodically in response to changing environmental conditions and the developmentally-controlled biological systems that sense and respond to those changes. Mitochondria and metabolism are fundamental regulators, and the cell is the fundamental unit of aging. However, aging occurs at all anatomical levels. At levels above the cell, aging in different tissues is qualitatively, quantitatively, and chronologically distinct. For example, the heart can age faster and differently than the kidney and vice versa. Two multicellular features of aging that are universal are: (1) a decrease in physiologic reserve capacity, and (2) a decline in the functional communication between cells and organ systems, leading to death. Decreases in reserve capacity and communication impose kinetic limits on the rate of healing after new injuries, resulting in dyssynchronous and incomplete healing. Exercise mitigates against these losses, but recovery times continue to increase with age. Reinjury before complete healing results in the stacking of incomplete cycles of healing. Developmentally delayed and arrested cells accumulate in the three stages of the cell danger response (CDR1, 2, and 3) that make up the healing cycle. Cells stuck in the CDR create physical and metabolic separation—buffer zones of reduced communication—between previously adjoining, synergistic, and metabolically interdependent cells. Mis-repairs and senescent cells accumulate, and repeated iterations of incomplete cycles of healing lead to progressively dysfunctional cellular mosaics in aging tissues. Metabolic cross-talk between mitochondria and the nucleus, and between neighboring and distant cells via signaling molecules called metabokines regulates the completeness of healing. Purinergic signaling and sphingolipids play key roles in this process. When viewed against the backdrop of the molecular features of the healing cycle, the incomplete healing model provides a new framework for understanding the hallmarks of aging and generates a number of testable hypotheses for new treatments.

Keywords: cell danger response; healing cycle; mitochondria; purinergic signaling; metabokines; sphingolipids; integrated cell stress response; de-emergence; crabtree effect; pasteur effect

1. Introduction

Some of the oldest [1], and the most recent [2,3] scientific publications on the biology of aging have focused on nutrition and metabolism as prime drivers. Mitochondria are located at the hub of the wheel of cellular metabolism. The mitochondrial proteome is transcriptionally and post-transcriptionally regulated according to tissue-specific needs [4], consists of about 1300 proteins [5], responds to injury [6], food quality [7], exercise [8], environmental pollution [9], and coordinates the cell danger response (CDR) [10]. The CDR is a term that was coined in 2014 [10], but includes elements of inflammation and healing that have been studied since before the time of Hippocrates (c. 460–370 BCE) [11]. The CDR is an evolutionarily conserved, multi-system response of multicellular organisms that is used to manage and heal from threat or injury. The CDR is a graded response that consists of nested layers that range from the molecular control of electron utilization and cellular oxygen consumption, through changes in the microbiome, mast cells and immune system, to the autonomic nervous system, enteric nervous system, and neuroendocrine circuits that are needed for whole-body integration of the response. When analyzed at the molecular and single-cell level, a widely-studied component of the CDR is known as the integrated cell stress response (ICSR) [12–14].

2. Defining Cellular Stress

In this paper, the word "stress" has a specific scientific meaning. Stress is any force, condition, chemical, pathogen or other stimulus that acts to perturb cellular function, requiring the expenditure of energy and resources to return the cell to its pre-stimulus or to a new steady state. Remarkably, psychological stresses, particularly early life stresses (ELS), regulate some of the same metabolic and gene expression networks used to defend the cell from microbial pathogens, physical injury, poisoning, and adversity of many other types [15–17]. In the case of major depressive disorder, innate immune/pro-inflammatory gene expression is increased, while adaptive immune/anti-inflammatory/pro-resolving gene expression is decreased [18]. Greater stresses stimulate proportionately more nucleotide and metabolite release through cell membrane channels [19], leading to greater metabokine and purinergic signaling [20,21]. Learning and development emerge from both conscious stresses and subconscious chemical stresses encountered throughout life. Stresses lead to metabolic memories that help cells and tissues improve future responses to previously encountered conditions [22]. Transient increases in the mitochondrial and cellular sources of reactive oxygen species (ROS) such as superoxide and hydrogen peroxide, reactive nitrogen species (RNS) such as nitric oxide (NO) and peroxynitrite (ONO_2^-), reactive aldehydes (RAs), and dissolved oxygen itself, help to regulate cellular redox. Redox, in turn, regulates the efflux of metabolites from the cell via membrane channels and transporters that contain redox-responsive cysteine disulfide residues [23]. Pulses of dissolved oxygen occur with a carbohydrate-rich meal because of the transient inhibitory effect of glucose on mitochondria produced by the Crabtree effect [24]. ROS, insulin, and IL1β are also stimulated naturally by every meal and can vary in magnitude according to the nutrient content of the meal [25]. As the dissolved oxygen concentration rises within the cell, glycolysis becomes inhibited by the Pasteur effect, creating a natural brake on an unchecked inhibition of mitochondrial oxphos from the meal-associated glucose and the Crabtree effect. However, glucose, oxygen, ROS, RNS, and RAs are only a part of the multi-faceted metabolic signaling network that is used to control cellular reactivity, epigenetic marking, and gene expression. Over 100 chemosensory G-protein coupled receptors respond to metabokines and peptides released after stress and injury and regulate the healing cycle [11].

3. The Healing Cycle

The mitochondrial responses that initiate and maintain the CDR are used to control cellular bioenergetics, oxygen utilization, redox signaling, and metabolism needed for healing [6] and regeneration [26] after injury or threat. The stages of the CDR are illustrated in Figure 1. Wakeful activity with nutrient intake, followed by restorative sleep are essential parts of health. These activities stimulate an integrated mix of three metabolic states that are controlled locally by metabolic signaling, and systemically by the central nervous system (CNS). Healthy whole-body function requires the coordination and use of cell-specific (1) glycolysis, (2) aerobic glycolysis, and (3) oxidative phosphorylation for energy and metabolism (Figure 1). Chemical activity associated with nutrient intake, brain activity, and basal metabolism, and added physical activity from natural child play or adult exercise lead to the graded release of extracellular ATP and related nucleotides, and to glutamate release [27,28] through stress-gated P2X7-pannexin and other channels in the cell membrane [19]. Once outside the cell, ATP and related nucleotides participate in purinergic signaling. Receptor binding to ATP and ADP leads to IP3-gated intracellular calcium release [29] and contextual changes in gene expression through autocrine and paracrine signaling pathways [30]. After extracellular metabolism by CD73 and CD39, ATP is converted to ADP, AMP, and to adenosine that acts to inhibit excess chemical stimulation and plays a key role in initiating and maintaining sleep by binding to P1/Adenosine /ADORA A2AR and A1R receptors [31]. This is illustrated as the restorative sleep cycle in Figure 1.

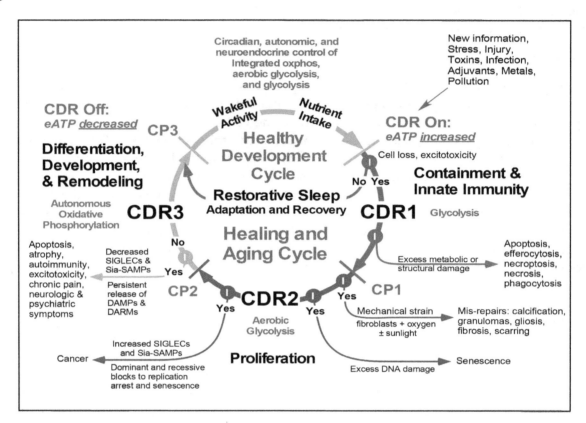

Figure 1. The metabolic features of the health and healing cycles. Abbreviations: CDR—cell danger response, eATP—extracellular ATP, CP1-3—checkpoints 1, 2, and 3, DAMP—damage-associated molecular pattern, DARM—damage-associated reactive metabolites, SIGLEC—sialic acid binding immunoglobulin-type lectin, e.g., CD33-related SIGLECs (CD33r-SIGLECs), Sia-SAMP—sialoglycan self-associated molecular pattern.

When the stress is of sufficient magnitude to cause cell death, more ATP is released and acts as a pro-inflammatory damage-associated molecular pattern (DAMP). Increased extracellular ATP triggers entry into the CDR1 stage of the healing cycle (Figure 1). Once the CDR is triggered, three different metabolic stages must be activated in sequence to heal. Healing cannot occur without activation of this metabolically-controlled cycle. CDR1 is characterized by the upregulation of anaerobic glycolysis and a reallocation of cellular resources for defense, damage containment, innate immunity, and repair at the expense of normal differentiated tissue function. Gap junctions between cells are decreased or lost as the tissue structure is disrupted by injury, and cell-autonomous functions become primary and metabolic cooperation between neighboring cells is decreased or suspended. Platelets and neutrophils are recruited to sites of injury or infection. CDR2 uses aerobic glycolysis to support stem cell recruitment and cell division needed for biomass replacement of cells lost in CDR1. If cell loss is not replaced, then age-related atrophy and sarcopenia occur. If excessive DNA damage is sustained by a cell in CDR2, replicative senescence occurs [32]. If the blocks to senescence are broken, then cancer can occur. If oxygen levels are high and significant mechanical strain is present, tissue fibrosis or wound scarring is stimulated (Figure 1). Fibrosis is one of several different types of mis-repairs that contribute to the symptoms of aging [33–35] (Figures 1–3).

In CDR3, cell-autonomous, aerobic metabolism by mitochondrial oxidative phosphorylation is gradually restored as new cells born in CDR2 take up residence in the recovering tissue and establish new tissue-specific contacts and gap junctions needed to extinguish the gene expression programs used for defense and growth in CDR1 and CDR2, and to restore normal differentiated cell, tissue, and organ function. If damage-associated molecular pattern (DAMP) and damage-associated reactive metabolite (DARM) release persists [36] or if ROS production is extinguished prematurely [37], autoimmunity can develop [38]. The adaptive immune response is regulated in CDR3. Persistent DAMP and DARM release can stimulate excitotoxicity in cells still in the CDR1 and CDR2 stages within a dyssynchronous mosaic of healing cells. With the completion of CDR3, the concentration of metabokines and DAMPS in the extracellular space is actively reduced to levels compatible with restoration of cell specialization and reintegration of cells back into a metabolically optimized cellular network. Re-integration and re-specialization are necessary for cells that have recently exited the CDR in order to re-establish their responsiveness to circadian patterns of wakeful activity and restorative sleep (Figure 1).

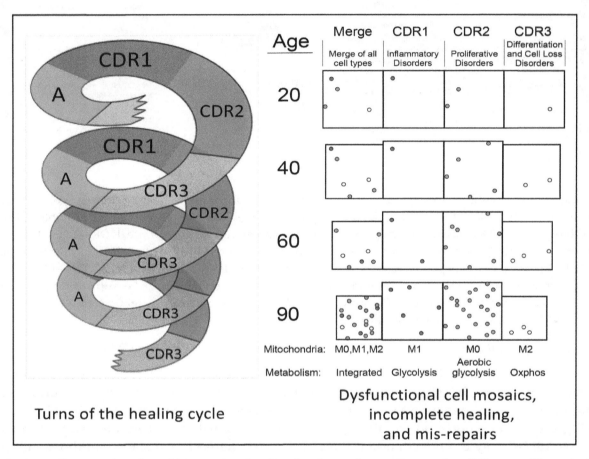

Figure 2. Repeated cycles of incomplete healing lead to aging and age-related disease. The spiral represents sequential turns of the healing cycle throughout life. Colored cells in the boxes on the right represent cells that have been delayed or arrested in a stage of the healing cycle. The decreased size of some boxes represents the loss in tissue volume from cell loss and atrophy. In this example, most arrested or delayed cells in the merge on the right after 60 and 90 years are in CDR2 (green). This will create an increased risk of proliferative disorders such as diabetes, heart disease, and cancer. Color code: CDR1 cells—red; CDR2 cells—green; CDR3 cells—yellow. Abbreviations: A—wakeful activity and nutrient intake. M1—mitochondria adapted for cell defense, reactive oxygen, nitrogen, and aldehyde production; M0—mitochondria adapted for cell growth and Warburg metabolism; M2—mitochondria adapted for oxidative phosphorylation (oxphos).

The sequence and stages of the healing cycle are highly conserved and tightly choreographed. Once pathological stress or cell death occurs, the same stages of the healing cycle are activated and restore normal function after any recoverable injury (Figure 2). Inevitably, some cells fail to complete the healing cycle and are left behind with each turn of the cycle. These arrested or delayed cells are unable to return to a normal metabolism and the gene expression pattern that is needed for peak differentiated cell and organ function (Figure 2). As non-specialized cells and mis-repairs such as fibrosis accumulate in incomplete stages of the healing cycle, the peak performance of tissues is degraded over time, and the risk for age-related disease is increased.

Figure 3. The hallmarks of aging as natural products of incomplete healing and the cell danger response [3,39]. Black font: hallmarks that oppose aging. Red font: hallmarks that promote aging. Abbreviations: CDR—cell danger response, ICSR—integrated cell stress response, DDR—DNA damage response, BMR—basal metabolic rate, T°—basal body temperature, HIF1α—hypoxia inducible factor 1α, PARP—poly ADP ribose polymerase, NAD+—nicotinamide adenine dinucleotide, ADPR—adenosine diphosphate ribose, SAM—S-adenosyl methionine, AcCoA—acetyl CoA, α-KG—alpha ketoglutarate, SAH—S-adenosyl homocysteine, PPi—pyrophosphate, NUDIX—nucleoside diphosphate X hydrolases, e.g., NUDT5, ECM—extracellular matrix.

4. Three Functionally-Polarized Forms of Mitochondria Are Used by the CDR

For over 60 years, mitochondria have been thought of as "damaged" or "dysfunctional" if they shift from energy production by oxidative phosphorylation to ROS production or shift from burning carbon skeletons to CO_2 and water to synthesizing new carbon skeletons for export as building blocks needed for cell growth. Yet mitochondria shift regularly and necessarily between these states throughout life. A simplified way of understanding the alternative differentiation states of mitochondria is to see the organelles as the metabolic gate-keepers of the electrons harvested by breaking down the carbon–carbon bonds in food. In this scheme, electrons can be used in mitochondria: (1) to fully reduce oxygen (O_2) to water (H_2O) while capturing the released chemical energy to make ATP by oxidative phosphorylation in the third stage of the cell danger response, CDR3 and in health, (2) to partially reduce oxygen to superoxide radicals (O_2^-) and hydrogen peroxide (H_2O_2) while relying on anaerobic glycolysis for ATP synthesis in CDR1 and cell defense, or (3) to use the electrons to synthesize new carbon–carbon bonds to produce and export building blocks such as citrate for cell membrane lipid synthesis or orotic acid for pyrimidine synthesis, while still consuming oxygen to make water and making ATP by aerobic glycolysis in CDR2 and cell growth (Figure 1).

A new nomenclature was introduced in 2017 to describe these three, functionally-polarized forms of mitochondria of the CDR [11,29]. All three "species" of mitochondria co-exist in different proportions in cells throughout development and aging in all multicellular organisms. The transition between states is determined by the interaction between nutrition and metabolism, the developmental and chronological age of the organism, the recent state of cell danger signaling and healing, and ambient environmental conditions. The naming of the differentiation states of mitochondria was based on the recognition that the pro-inflammatory state of macrophages known as M1 macrophages corresponded with the ROS producing capacity of their mitochondria and energy production by glycolysis [40]. The anti-inflammatory/pro-resolving M2 macrophages were found to contain mitochondria adapted for oxidative phosphorylation (oxphos). M0 macrophages are not yet committed to a fully M1 or M2 phenotype and contain mitochondria that are intermediate between M1 and M2. In the healing cycle, three different mitochondrial differentiation states are used to meet the specialized needs of each stage of the CDR. M1 mitochondria are used in CDR1. M0 mitochondria are used in CDR2, and M2 mitochondria are used in CDR3 (Figures 1 and 2, Table 1).

In vitro protocols have recently been developed that distinguish between M1, M0, and M2 macrophages experimentally based on mitochondrial phenotypes [41]. M1 mitochondria consume small amounts of oxygen, have a low spare respiratory capacity (SRC, or physiologic reserve capacity), can use fatty acids for ROS production and NLRP3 assembly [42], are not dependent on glutamine, and the cells containing M1 mitochondria produce large amounts of lactic acid. In contrast, M2 mitochondria consume more oxygen at baseline, can use both glucose oxidized to pyruvate and fatty acids for oxphos, have a higher SRC, are dependent on glutamine for the fully differentiated phenotype, and the cells produce small amounts of acid. M0, uncommitted or multipotential mitochondria have a low basal oxygen consumption similar to M1, shunt some glucose down the pentose phosphate pathway (PPP) for NADPH and building block production, have an SRC that is intermediate between M2 and M1 organelles, and produce small amounts of extracellular acid, similar to M2 [41] (Table 1).

Table 1. Phenotypic characteristics of animal cell mitochondria.

No.	Trait	Mitochondrial Phenotype [40,41,43]		
		M0	M1	M2
1	Cellular energy metabolism	Aerobic glycolysis	Glycolysis	Oxidative phosphorylation
2	Mitochondrial DNA copy number	Intermediate	Low	High
3	Predominant morphology	Intermediate	Punctate	Filamentous
4	Cell replicative potential	High (Warburg)	Intermediate	Low
5	Cell multilineage regenerative potential	High	Low	Low
6	Cell differentiation potential	Low	Intermediate	High
7	Cell cancer potential	High	Intermediate	Low
8	Inflammatory potential	Intermediate	High	Low
9	Cell susceptibility to killing by apoptosis	Low	Intermediate	High
10	Inducible organellar quality control	Intermediate	Low	High
11	Baseline oxygen consumption	Low	Low	High
12	Stressed (uncoupled) oxygen consumption above baseline (spare respiratory capacity)	Intermediate	Low	High
13	ROS production	Intermediate	High	Low
14	NLRP3 inflammasome assembly	Low	High	Low
15	Lactate release from cells	Intermediate	High	Low
16	Pentose phosphate pathway (PPP)	High—NADPH for biosynthesis and cell growth	Intermediate— NADPH for NOX	Intermediate— NADPH for redox

Table 1. *Cont.*

No.	Trait	Mitochondrial Phenotype [40,41,43]		
		M0	M1	M2
17	Use of fatty acid oxidation (FAO)	Fatty acid synthesis for growth > FAO	For ROS and NLRP3 activation	For oxphos
18	Use of glucose	Glycolysis and PPP	Glycolysis and lactate release	PPP and pyruvate for oxphos
19	Use of glutamine	High: citrate for ATP citrate lyase and Acetyl-CoA	Low	High: oxphos via alpha-ketoglutarate
20	Stage of greatest use in the healing cycle and cell danger response	CDR2	CDR1	CDR3

M0, M1, and M2 mitochondrial phenotypes also occur in solid tissues and can be recognized in part by morphological criteria. Mitochondria can be described informally as being distributed along a spaghetti (filamentous) and meatball (punctate) gradient. M2 mitochondria are filamentous and interconnected, and predominate in post-mitotic or slowly regenerating tissues. M1 mitochondria are punctate, and M0 mitochondria are intermediate in form, with both short filaments and punctate organelles reminiscent of the coccobacillary forms of their proteobacterial ancestors [44]. Mitochondrial fusion–fission dynamics naturally regulate the balance between fused and elongated mitochondria, and fragmented/fissioned mitochondria according the growth and metabolic characteristics of the cell [45]. M0, uncommitted, or stem-like mitochondria predominate in cells that survive after exposure to chemotherapeutic agents or toxins [46]. M2 mitochondria under these conditions are depleted by DRP1-dependent fission/fragmentation, and conversion to M1 organelles prior to cell removal by apoptosis. Similar transitions in mitochondrial structure and function are readily demonstrated in brain astroglia before and after treatment with pro-inflammatory triggers such as lipopolysaccharide (LPS) and interferon gamma (IFN-γ) [43].

The total mitochondrial biomass is decreased naturally after triggering the cell danger response (CDR) with toxins [46], physical injury [6], infection, or any trigger that activates the healing cycle [11]. Mitochondrial biomass can also be reduced experimentally by the dominant-negative expression of the D1135A allele of the mitochondrial polymerase gamma (POLG1) to deplete mitochondrial DNA copy numbers by about 50% [47]. This mouse model mimics the mitochondrial defects that are a well-established hallmark of aging [48]. The phenotypes of aging found in this model included increased NFkB and matrix metalloproteinase 9 (MMP9) expression, increased inflammation, age spots, wrinkled skin, and premature hair loss. These transcriptional and anatomical signs of aging were reversed within 1 month of treatment in mice by unblocking mtDNA synthesis and restoring normal mtDNA copy numbers [47].

5. The Importance of Nucleotides and Purinergic Signaling

Of an estimated 1300 mitochondrial protein coding genes, 1158 are catalogued in MitoCarta v2.0 [5]. Only 13 mitochondrial proteins are encoded by mitochondrial DNA (mtDNA). The remaining 1145 are encoded by nuclear genes that are subject to tissue-specific gene expression programs. At least 789 mitochondrial proteins (68% of 1158) are enzymes with catalytic functions that have been assigned enzyme commission (EC) numbers, or encode subunits of multi-protein enzyme complexes such as those in respiratory chain complexes I, II, III, IV, and V, or are transporters, or kinases that use ATP (Table S1). At least 433 (55% of 789) of these proteins are regulated by the availability of purine and pyrimidine nucleotides such as ATP, GTP, UTP, NAD(P)+, or FAD either as substrates, or as allosteric regulators (Table S1). No other single class of molecules regulates more of the mitochondrial proteome than the nucleotides. In addition, an unknown fraction of nuclear mitochondrial genes is regulated transcriptionally and post-transcriptionally by purinergic signaling via the 12 G-protein coupled receptors (GPCRs; 4 P1R and 8 P2YR) and seven ionotropic receptors (P2XR) that are widely distributed in all tissues [49]. Some purinergic receptors are also expressed in intracellular compartments such as mitochondria, lysosomes, and the nucleus [50]. For example, P2X6 receptors are translocated to the nucleus in an age-dependent manner, interact with mRNA splicing factor 3A1, decrease mRNA processing, and contribute to aging [51].

6. The Importance of Nutrition in Healing and Aging

Different stages in child development, human aging, and athletic performance have different specific nutrients and calories that produce the best outcomes at each stage [52–54]. Based on measured differences in mitochondrial substrate preferences between M1, M0, and M2 organelles (Table 1), it is hypothesized that each stage of the healing cycle—CDR 1, 2, and 3 in Figure 1, and even certain chronic illnesses stuck in one of the three stages of the CDR [11]—will also have different stage-specific nutritional needs for optimal outcomes. Both chemical mass action from substrate supply and metabolite signaling via metabokines [11] are likely to be important mechanistically. Some of the broadest clues that connect nutrition with aging, mitochondria, and healing come from studies of caloric restriction [3]. Natural aging results in a reduction in the rate of turnover of mitochondria (mitochondrial biogenesis, or "mitochondriogenesis"), and a decrease in mitochondrial protein synthesis, standing mitochondrial biomass, respiratory reserve capacity, and oxphos function [55] (Figure 3). Caloric restriction, on the other hand, stimulates mitochondrial turnover through pathways associated with AMPK-stimulated autophagy and mitophagy [56]. This leads to improved mitochondrial quality control, oxphos function, and reserve capacity, but does not increase overall mitochondrial biomass measured as mtDNA copy number [57]. Caloric restriction also leads to a decrease in circulating thyroid hormone, decreased resting energy expenditure (REE), and a decrease in circulating anabolic hormones such as IGFI, insulin, human growth hormone, and testosterone [58]. From an evolutionary point of view, this hypometabolic response allows fewer calories to be consumed while opposing weight loss during periods of seasonal hardship.

Caloric restriction is a classical trigger of a reversible, stress-resistant, non-reproductive stage in the nematode *Caenorhabditis elegans* called dauer. Dauer has been the source of discovery of many longevity genes and has stimulated a productive discussion of the difference between lifespan and healthspan extension [59]. Dauer permits animals to live for up to 4 months under harsh conditions instead of their normal lifespan of 2 weeks. However, longevity in dauer comes at the cost of much reduced function and many changes associated with altered sensory anatomy [60], repetitive behaviors [61] and metabolism [62]. When calories are restored to animals in dauer, they exit the stage and re-enter their normal life-cycle, picking up where they left off, as if little or no biological aging had occurred during the time they spent in dauer [63].

More specific changes in nutrient supply also play an important role in aging and healing. Dietary supplementation with branch chain amino acids at a level of 1.5 g/kg/day, corresponding to about 1% of daily calorie intake in mice, has been shown to extend lifespan by about 10% [64]. This effect required normal production of nitric oxide (NO) by endothelial nitric oxide synthase (eNOS) [64]. The selective addition of a stoichiometric mix of essential amino acids (EAAs) including branch chain amino acids, also has anti-cancer effects by promoting growth inhibition and apoptosis in transformed but not in normal cells [65]. EAAs also promoted wound healing by moderating inflammation in the early stages, and maintaining TGFβ needed for tissue remodeling in the later stages of healing [66]. This later effect is in what would be called CDR3 in the model presented here (Figure 1). Interestingly, TGF β (DAF-7) signaling also plays a key role in recovery from dauer and the re-establishment of normal development in *C. elegans* [67].

7. Progressively Dysfunctional Cellular Mosaics

The number of nucleated cells in a 70-kg adult male is about 5×10^{12}. Non-nucleated red blood cells are 5-times more abundant (2.5×10^{13}), but make up just 6.5% of the total mass of an adult [68]. The total number of human cells in an adult is 3.0×10^{13}. There are also 3.8×10^{13} bacterial cells in a typical adult body [68]. Cells die every day and must be replaced. It is estimated that an adult turns over about 1×10^{10} (10 billion; about 10 grams of) cells/day by apoptosis [69]. This is equivalent to about 1 in 500 nucleated cells/day removed by apoptosis. The distribution of cell turnover is highly heterogeneous. Most spontaneous, or physiologic cell death with replacement occurs in short-lived cells such as those in bone marrow, intestines, skin, and hair follicles whose function is tolerant to spatial changes in tissue architecture produced by continuous cell growth and use-dependent removal or exit of cells from the compartment of origin. These rapidly dividing and structurally malleable tissues can turn over several times per year, with nearly 100% of the cells in these compartments turning over in a few days to weeks or months. Other tissues turn over more slowly. Adipose tissue is replaced at a rate of 10% of the cells per year [70], turning over completely in about 10 years. Skeletal muscle turns over at a rate of 6.6% per year [71]. Muscle fiber loss accelerates after age 60, leading to sarcopenia [72]. The kidneys weigh about 150 grams each, shed about 1.7×10^6 epithelial cells/day into the urine [73], and replace this loss and other losses by cell division and remodeling from recruited stem cells [74]. The adult liver weighs about 1400 grams and consists of about 2.4×10^{11} cells and replaces about 1.8% per year as a young adult, but fewer as liver size decreases with age [75]. Heart cells are replaced at a rate of 1% per year at age 25, falling to 0.45% per year at age 75 [76], and pancreatic islet β-cells are long-lived and not replaced after age 30 years [77].

Exposure to physical injury, toxins, or infection adds pathological cell death to the basal level of physiologic cell death described above. When a cell dies physiologically by apoptosis, the inflammatory reactions associated with CDR1 are avoided. Instead, the tissue skips to CDR2 and CDR3 to replace the lost cell and restore normal metabolism and tissue-specific gene expression patterns (Figure 1). The number of cells that die pathologically during a typical viral or bacterial infection will be dependent on the type of microbial pathogen and the severity of the infection, but the exact cell numbers lost in the course of a typical infection are not known. An average child has 5–6 recognized viral or bacterial infections each year for the first 5 years of life, then 2–3 per year throughout adult life [78]. Pathological cell death caused by infection, toxins, or injury will trigger inflammation and entry into the healing cycle by activating CDR1. As a thought experiment, one can imagine a systemic viral infection that might kill 1×10^{10} cells (about 10 grams, or 2 teaspoons), a number equal to the basal loss per day by apoptosis. Somatic DNA mutation rates are about 2.7×10^{-5} per typical 10,000 bp, protein-coding locus per cell division [79]. In this example, one turn of the healing cycle would result in 270,000 cells (10^{10} cells replaced $\times 2.7 \times 10^{-5}$ mutations/gene/division = 270,000 cells) sustaining a mutation that marks that cell as different from neighboring cells in the tissue. Mitotic recombination errors and chromosomal microaneuploidy [80], mobilization of retroelements [81] and endogenous retroviruses [82] in recruited stem cells, and reactivation and suppression cycles of latent DNA virus infections [83] will contribute to genetic variation produced by repetitive activation of the CDR over a lifetime. In addition to DNA mutations, there will also be an even larger number of induced and stochastic changes in transcription, post-transcriptional, and metabolic features that lead to changes in cell development.

With each turn of the healing cycle, cells such as neutrophils move out of capillaries and into tissues, releasing ROS via activated NADPH oxidases such as NOX2. Over time, this cyclic process creates tides of reactive oxygen, metabolic, innate immune, and inflammatory defenses that rise with injury and fall during wellness, ebbing and flowing with each turn of the healing cycle. Sialic acid binding immunoglobulin-type lectins (SIGLECs) include the CD33-related molecules expressed on neutrophils, natural killer (NK), macrophages, and T-cells that modulate ROS production, innate immune cell, and adaptive T-cell activity upon binding to sia-SAMPs (sialoglycan self-associated molecular patterns) [84]. Across species, the number of CD33r-SIGLEC genes is associated with healthy aging in the "wellderly", and decreased numbers accelerate age-related symptoms in mouse models [85]. Many cancers emerge from hypersialated cellular fields that have the effect of dampening the immune response by engaging inhibitory SIGLECs such as Siglec-9 [86]. The ceaseless tides or waves of innate immune cell migration into and out of tissue compartments continues throughout life with each turn of the healing cycle (Figures 1 and 2), and contributes to the progressively dysfunctional mosaics illustrated in Figure 2.

In the brain, a compensatory system of glial–lymphatic (glymphatic) tidal flows occurs by regulated changes in cell volume that are controlled by circadian changes in metabolism [87]. This daily cycle of glympahtic flow helps to remove aggregates of tau and beta amyloid that would otherwise accumulate as the byproducts of CDR activation both from normal learning and from microglial and synaptosomal innate immune activation that increase progressively with aging. Interestingly, a number of molecules that regulate mTOR and other metabolic aspects of the CDR, have recently been found to slow the aging process and extend longevity, while simultaneously protecting against age-related markers of Alzheimer dementia in animal models [88]. These "geroneuroprotecting" drugs were plant-based natural products similar to curcumin and polyphenols such as fisetin. The healing cycle-promoting properties of these drugs prevented the accumulation of tau and beta amyloid markers of Alzheimer dementia even though the drugs were not directed at the protein markers specifically [88].

The importance of innate immune activation and healing in aging is underscored by a recent discovery in Werner syndrome. Werner syndrome is a recessively inherited adult progeria syndrome caused by mutations in the Werner helicase (WRN). In addition to genomic instability caused by WRN mutations, the protein was recently found to play a key role in innate immunity as a transcriptional coactivator of the NFkB-dependent expression of the chemokine IL8 [89]. Werner mutations inhibit NFkB- and IL8-dependent ROS production. ROS production is not only an essential component of an effective CDR1 (Figure 1), but is important for NRF2 induction of long-term anti-oxidant and detoxification defenses [90]. In addition, the WRN protein is important for HIF1 stabilization [91] needed for tissue regeneration [26] during CDR2 (Figure 1).

With each turn of the healing cycle, the induced combination of transcriptional and metabolic changes and the DNA damage response will result in some injured and newly replaced cells being unable to complete the normal stages of the cycle. Perhaps 0.1–1 million cells of the 10^{10} cells that must be replaced after pathological cell death may be left behind, stuck or delayed in one of the three stages, CDR1, CDR2, and CDR3. An even larger number of cells whose function was transiently changed by injury, but were not killed, will contribute to the cells that are left behind in stages of the healing cycle. This process is illustrated as progressively dysfunctional mosaics on the right of the spiral in Figure 2. The ecogenetic interaction of inherited genotype of a given individual with the particular environmental insult (nutritional stress, pathogen, toxin, or physical injury) will determine how many cells are delayed or lost in the three different stages of the CDR. Examples of aging cellular mosaics are illustrated at age 20, 40, 60, and 90 years (Figure 2). Delayed and arrested cells that are incompletely differentiated create physical and metabolic separation—buffer zones—that act like control rods in a nuclear reactor that absorb signals and inhibit communication between previously adjoining, synergistic, and metabolically interdependent cells. Loss of cellular connectivity through functional gap junctions decreases the physiologic reserve capacity and increases vulnerability to stress-related cell death [92].

The propagation of calcium waves from cell to cell in a tissue via the inositol trisphosphate (IP3)-gated release of intracellular calcium stores is a common example of the cooperative response to neuroendocrine signaling, and is highly dependent on fully differentiated mitochondrial function [93]. CD38 increases with age [94] and is used by the cell to synthesize cyclic adenosine diphosphate ribose (cADPR) from NAD+ and nicotinic acid adenine dinucleotide phosphate (NAADP) from NADP+ as IP3-responsive calcium signaling declines [95]. cADPR and NAADP are intracellular ligands that stimulate IP3-independent release of calcium from the endoplasmic reticulum (ER) and lysosomes, respectively [29]. NAD+ and NADP+ are depleted by CD38 in the course of aging [94].

Cellular depletion of NAD+ and NADH leads to a decrease in mitonuclear communication [96], and to progressive declines in mitochondrial electron transport that contribute to aging [97]. Supplementation with the NAD+ precursor, nicotinamide riboside (NR), in animal models improves cell differentiation, restores laminin scaffolding and a more normal cellular mosaic in tissues, attenuates senescent cell formation, and increases longevity by about 10% [98]. In a recent study of the effect of transplanted senescent cells, the authors found that ≥ 1 senescent cell among 10,000 total cells in the body (0.01%), or ≥ 1 in 350 normal cells in a specific tissue (≥0.28%) was enough to produce a dysfunctional cellular mosaic and measurable functional defects such as decreased grip strength and exercise capacity [99].

8. De-Emergence as a Cause of Dysfunction

Complex living systems are comprised of at least seven discrete subsystems: (1) molecules; monomers, metabolites, and other building blocks, (2) polymers requiring energy for synthesis, such as proteins, polysaccharides, nucleic acids, and lipids made of amino acid, monosaccharide, nucleotide, acetyl and isoprene monomers, respectively, (3) polymers that assemble spontaneously such as charged and neutral lipids and hydrophobic proteins that form membranes, lipid droplets, and other lowered free energy structures in aqueous matrices, (4) organelles, (5) cells, (6) tissues, (7) organs. Many of the phenotypes associated with normal development, health, disease, and aging are emergent properties that depend on the function, arrangement, and interaction of the subsystems, but are qualitatively, quantitatively, and chronologically distinct from any single subsystem. For example, long-term memory is an emergent property that requires new protein synthesis that alters several aspects of all the subsystems that make up the brain, but knowledge of any one of the subsystems is insufficient to explain long-term memory. Other emergent properties of health include the ability to walk, talk, think, eat, excrete, mount an immune response, reproduce, detect and respond to a toxin or injury, and to heal. Aging degrades each of these abilities. If health is thought of as a collection of emergent phenotypes, then illness and aging can be thought of the gradual fading away, or de-emergence of the emergent properties that results from the degradation of metabolic and cellular order and the interactions of the subsystems that define health and resilience to environmental change. The images of progressively dysfunctional cellular mosaics shown in Figure 2 illustrate just one level—the cellular level—of the problem. Dysfunctional mosaics occur in every one of the seven subsystems, and mis-repairs accumulate at each level with each turn of the healing cycle.

9. The Hallmarks of Aging Emerge as a Result of Incomplete Healing

The molecular, cellular [2,3,48] and gene expression hallmarks [39] of aging can be organized according to their usage during the healing cycle and the stages of the multisystem CDR [10,11,29] (Figure 3). These hallmarks have been identified in studies of aging that have led naturally to an improved molecular understanding of mitochondrial stress [13,17,100], the integrated cell stress response (ICSR) [12,101,102], and the CDR [10,11,29,103]. Each trait associated with these hallmarks arises naturally from the activation of a molecular feature needed in the healing cycle, followed by the failure to extinguish this normal function or gene expression state of the CDR once it is no longer needed. Persistence of an aging hallmark after a turn of the healing cycle (Figure 2) can also occur in five other ways: (1) when a cell sustains too much genetic damage and becomes senescent, (2) when a cell that has been removed is not replaced and leads to tissue atrophy, (3) when a cell is replaced but fails to re-specialize according to the differentiated needs of the tissue, (4) when a mis-repair such as fibrosis or scarring [104] cannot be removed by remodeling, and (5) when genetic and metabolic changes bypass senescence and lead to cancer (Figure 1). The legacy of each of these events is to add to the dysfunctional mosaic illustrated in Figure 2.

Brain, muscle, nerve, and endocrine tissues are particularly susceptible to the incomplete replacement of lost cells once they have died and have been removed because of their limited regeneration capacity and the high degree of spatial organization required for optimal organ function. The function of these tissues is highly dependent on the spatial organization and metabolic complementarity of the cellular mosaic. This complementarity can only be achieved through cell specialization and chemical cooperativity between neighboring cells, which in turn, depends on the relative position and architecture of layers and columns of cells that must remain fixed over long periods of time. The cost of removing a cell from a chain of connected cells in the cerebral cortex or any other part of the brain has a high price that cannot easily be repaid by recruiting stem cells from another location. However, the cost of converting a cell to the hypersecretory phenotype of a senescent cell [105] is even higher, since just one senescent cell in 350 normal cells is enough to decrease the function of a tissue [99]. The smaller collective volume of cells that occurs in most tissues with age is illustrated in Figure 2. The decreasing volume of tissues in the columns labeled "Merge" and "CDR3" represents the effect of cell loss (atrophy) that occurs with incomplete progress through the healing cycle (Figures 1 and 2). In the example illustrated in Figure 2, more cells have accumulated in CDR2 (illustrated in green) by the ages of 60 and 90 years. Accumulation of cells in CDR2 will increase the risk of diseases such as diabetes, heart disease, and cancer because cells arrested or delayed in CDR2 maintain their proliferative capacity [11] (Figure 1). Proliferative capacity is maintained in part because cells in CDR2 contain more multipotential M0 mitochondria adapted for Warburg metabolism (Table 1). Inherited mutations in the RECQL4 helicase, which interacts with p53 and POLG in mitochondria, increase aerobic glycolysis associated with CDR2, lead to an increased risk of cancer, and to a form of progeria known as Rothmund–Thomson syndrome [106–108].

10. Conclusions

A new model is presented that reframes aging as the result of repeated cycles of incomplete healing. In this model, cycles of incomplete healing stack over time, leading to cellular mosaics that become progressively dysfunctional with age (Figure 2). Cells that accumulate in one of the three stages of the cell danger response (CDR) lead to specific risks of age-related disease. The accumulation of cells in CDR1 leads to chronic inflammatory and pain syndromes, and to susceptibility to chronic viral, bacterial, and fungal infections that require adaptive T-cell immunity for eradication [11]. The accumulation of cells in CDR2 leads to diabetes, heart disease, congestive heart failure, peripheral vascular disease, fibrotic disorders, and cancer risk. The accumulation of cells in CDR3 leads to autoimmune disorders, immune suppression or deficiency, neuropathic pain syndromes, behavioral and mental health disorders, or neurodevelopmental and neurodegenerative disease [11]. It is currently unknown what drugs, devices, or procedures can unblock arrested cells in the mosaic and permit the completion of the healing cycle. However, specific nutritional interventions such as nicotinamide riboside or essential amino acids have been found to facilitate healing [66], longevity [98] or both [64,66] in animal models. A prediction of the incomplete healing model is that differentiation checkpoints exist at each stage of the CDR (Figure 1) and that the molecular signals that are used naturally by cells to facilitate completion of healing may provide fresh clues for both preventing and treating age-related symptoms and disease. One procedure that is well-known to improve physical and psychological well-being, decrease mortality, and decrease the risk of age-related disease, is exercise [109,110]. The effects of exercise are multifaceted, but the increase in autophagy and remodeling of the mitochondrial network, leading to adaptive improvements in quality control and increased reserve capacity, may play key roles [111]. The search for geroneuroprotectants [88] and chemical exercise mimetics [112] has already begun. However, a deeper understanding of the role of natural metabolites as signaling molecules—metabokines [11]—and molecules regulated by exercise—exerkines and exosomes [113–115]—that regulate the completion of the healing cycle holds promise for preventing, slowing, and perhaps reversing [47] some of the effects of aging. Interventions that exploit purinergic [20] and sphingolipid [116] signaling pathways may be particularly powerful since over half of all mitochondrial proteins are regulated by ATP, NAD+, and related nucleotides (Table S1), and many of the molecular hallmarks of aging trace to or regulate the interplay between purines, mitochondria, sphingolipids [117,118], and the nucleus [119].

Acknowledgments: RKN thanks the many families with primary mitochondrial disease, autism spectrum disorder (ASD), and myalgic encephalomyelitis/chronic fatigue syndrome (ME/CFS) who have helped make this research possible. RKN thanks Scott McAvoy from the UCSD Digital Media Lab for preparing the art work for the healing spiral in Figure 2, and Vamsi Mootha, Sarah Calvo, and Jonathan Monk for the bioinformatic analysis of mitochondrial proteins and enzymes.

References

1.   McCay, C.M.; Crowell, M.F. Prolonging the life span. *Sci. Mon.* **1934**, *39*, 405–414.
2.   Finkel, T. The metabolic regulation of aging. *Nat. Med.* **2015**, *21*, 1416–1423. [CrossRef] [PubMed]
3.   Lopez-Otin, C.; Galluzzi, L.; Freije, J.M.P.; Madeo, F.; Kroemer, G. Metabolic Control of Longevity. *Cell* **2016**, *166*, 802–821. [CrossRef]
4.   Pagliarini, D.J.; Calvo, S.E.; Chang, B.; Sheth, S.A.; Vafai, S.B.; Ong, S.E.; Walford, G.A.; Sugiana, C.; Boneh, A.; Chen, W.K.; et al. A mitochondrial protein compendium elucidates complex I disease biology. *Cell* **2008**, *134*, 112–123. [CrossRef]
5.   Calvo, S.E.; Clauser, K.R.; Mootha, V.K. MitoCarta2.0: An updated inventory of mammalian mitochondrial proteins. *Nucleic Acids Res.* **2016**, *44*, D1251–D1257. [CrossRef] [PubMed]
6.   Naviaux, R.K.; Le, T.P.; Bedelbaeva, K.; Leferovich, J.; Gourevitch, D.; Sachadyn, P.; Zhang, X.M.; Clark, L.; Heber-Katz, E. Retained features of embryonic metabolism in the adult MRL mouse. *Mol. Genet. Metab.* **2009**, *96*, 133–144. [CrossRef] [PubMed]
7.   Ma, S.; Huang, Q.; Tominaga, T.; Liu, C.; Suzuki, K. An 8-Week Ketogenic Diet Alternated Interleukin-6, Ketolytic and Lipolytic Gene Expression, and Enhanced Exercise Capacity in Mice. *Nutrients* **2018**, *10*, 1696. [CrossRef]
8.   Ogborn, D.I.; McKay, B.R.; Crane, J.D.; Safdar, A.; Akhtar, M.; Parise, G.; Tarnopolsky, M.A. Effects of age and unaccustomed resistance exercise on mitochondrial transcript and protein abundance in skeletal muscle of men. *Am. J. Physiol. Regul. Integr. Comp. Physiol.* **2015**, *308*, R734–R741. [CrossRef] [PubMed]
9.   Winckelmans, E.; Nawrot, T.S.; Tsamou, M.; Den Hond, E.; Baeyens, W.; Kleinjans, J.; Lefebvre, W.; Van Larebeke, N.; Peusens, M.; Plusquin, M.; et al. Transcriptome-wide analyses indicate mitochondrial responses to particulate air pollution exposure. *Environ. Health A Glob. Access Sci. Source* **2017**, *16*, 87. [CrossRef] [PubMed]
10. Naviaux, R.K. Metabolic features of the cell danger response. *Mitochondrion* **2014**, *16*, 7–17. [CrossRef]
11. Naviaux, R.K. Metabolic features and regulation of the healing cycle-A new model for chronic disease pathogenesis and treatment. *Mitochondrion* **2018**. [CrossRef] [PubMed]
12. Quiros, P.M.; Prado, M.A.; Zamboni, N.; D'Amico, D.; Williams, R.W.; Finley, D.; Gygi, S.P.; Auwerx, J. Multi-omics analysis identifies ATF4 as a key regulator of the mitochondrial stress response in mammals. *J. Cell Biol.* **2017**, *216*, 2027–2045. [CrossRef] [PubMed]
13. Nikkanen, J.; Forsstrom, S.; Euro, L.; Paetau, I.; Kohnz, R.A.; Wang, L.; Chilov, D.; Viinamaki, J.; Roivainen, A.; Marjamaki, P.; et al. Mitochondrial DNA Replication Defects Disturb Cellular dNTP Pools and Remodel One-Carbon Metabolism. *Cell Metab.* **2016**, *23*, 635–648. [CrossRef]
14. Silva, J.M.; Wong, A.; Carelli, V.; Cortopassi, G.A. Inhibition of mitochondrial function induces an integrated stress response in oligodendroglia. *Neurobiol. Dis.* **2009**, *34*, 357–365. [CrossRef]
15. Cameron, J.L.; Eagleson, K.L.; Fox, N.A.; Hensch, T.K.; Levitt, P. Social Origins of Developmental Risk for Mental and Physical Illness. *J. Neurosci. Off. J. Soc. Neurosci.* **2017**, *37*, 10783–10791. [CrossRef] [PubMed]
16. Fredrickson, B.L.; Grewen, K.M.; Algoe, S.B.; Firestine, A.M.; Arevalo, J.M.; Ma, J.; Cole, S.W. Psychological well-being and the human conserved transcriptional response to adversity. *PLoS ONE* **2015**, *10*, e0121839. [CrossRef] [PubMed]
17. Picard, M.; McManus, M.J.; Gray, J.D.; Nasca, C.; Moffat, C.; Kopinski, P.K.; Seifert, E.L.; McEwen, B.S.; Wallace, D.C. Mitochondrial functions modulate neuroendocrine, metabolic, inflammatory, and transcriptional responses to acute psychological stress. *Proc. Natl. Acad. Sci. USA* **2015**, *112*, E6614–E6623. [CrossRef] [PubMed]
18. Leday, G.G.R.; Vertes, P.E.; Richardson, S.; Greene, J.R.; Regan, T.; Khan, S.; Henderson, R.; Freeman, T.C.; Pariante, C.M.; Harrison, N.A.; et al. Replicable and Coupled Changes in Innate and Adaptive Immune Gene Expression in Two Case-Control Studies of Blood Microarrays in Major Depressive Disorder. *Biol. Psychiatry* **2018**, *83*, 70–80. [CrossRef] [PubMed]

19. Burnstock, G.; Knight, G.E. Cell culture: Complications due to mechanical release of ATP and activation of purinoceptors. *Cell Tissue Res.* **2017**. [CrossRef]

20. Burnstock, G. The therapeutic potential of purinergic signalling. *Biochem. Pharmacol.* **2018**, *151*, 157–165. [CrossRef]

21. Burnstock, G. Short- and long-term (trophic) purinergic signalling. *Philos. Trans. R. Soc. Lond.* **2016**, *371*, 20150422. [CrossRef]

22. De la Fuente, I.M. Elements of the cellular metabolic structure. *Front. Mol. Biosci.* **2015**, *2*, 16. [CrossRef] [PubMed]

23. Jindrichova, M.; Kuzyk, P.; Li, S.; Stojilkovic, S.S.; Zemkova, H. Conserved ectodomain cysteines are essential for rat P2X7 receptor trafficking. *Purinergic Signal.* **2012**, *8*, 317–325. [CrossRef] [PubMed]

24. Sussman, I.; Erecinska, M.; Wilson, D.F. Regulation of cellular energy metabolism: The Crabtree effect. *Biochim. Biophys. Acta* **1980**, *591*, 209–223. [CrossRef]

25. Dror, E.; Dalmas, E.; Meier, D.T.; Wueest, S.; Thevenet, J.; Thienel, C.; Timper, K.; Nordmann, T.M.; Traub, S.; Schulze, F.; et al. Postprandial macrophage-derived IL-1beta stimulates insulin, and both synergistically promote glucose disposal and inflammation. *Nat. Immunol.* **2017**, *18*, 283–292. [CrossRef]

26. Heber-Katz, E. Oxygen, Metabolism, and Regeneration: Lessons from Mice. *Trends Mol. Med.* **2017**, *23*, 1024–1036. [CrossRef] [PubMed]

27. Barros-Barbosa, A.R.; Oliveira, A.; Lobo, M.G.; Cordeiro, J.M.; Correia-de-Sa, P. Under stressful conditions activation of the ionotropic P2X7 receptor differentially regulates GABA and glutamate release from nerve terminals of the rat cerebral cortex. *Neurochem. Int.* **2018**, *112*, 81–95. [CrossRef]

28. Xiong, Y.; Teng, S.; Zheng, L.; Sun, S.; Li, J.; Guo, N.; Li, M.; Wang, L.; Zhu, F.; Wang, C.; et al. Stretch-induced Ca(2+) independent ATP release in hippocampal astrocytes. *J. Physiol.* **2018**, *596*, 1931–1947. [CrossRef]

29. Naviaux, R.K. Antipurinergic therapy for autism-An in-depth review. *Mitochondrion* **2017**. [CrossRef]

30. Sakaki, H.; Tsukimoto, M.; Harada, H.; Moriyama, Y.; Kojima, S. Autocrine regulation of macrophage activation via exocytosis of ATP and activation of P2Y11 receptor. *PLoS ONE* **2013**, *8*, e59778. [CrossRef] [PubMed]

31. Huang, Z.L.; Zhang, Z.; Qu, W.M. Roles of adenosine and its receptors in sleep-wake regulation. *Int. Rev. Neurobiol.* **2014**, *119*, 349–371. [PubMed]

32. He, S.; Sharpless, N.E. Senescence in Health and Disease. *Cell* **2017**, *169*, 1000–1011. [CrossRef] [PubMed]

33. Wang-Michelitsch, J.; Michelitsch, T.M. Misrepair accumulation theory: A theory for understanding aging, cancer development, longevity, and adaptation. *arXiv* **2015**, arXiv:1505.07016.

34. Wang-Michelitsch, J.; Michelitsch, T.M. Tissue fibrosis: A principal proof for the central role of Misrepair in aging. *arXiv* **2015**, arXiv:1505.01376.

35. Wang, J.; Michelitsch, T.; Wunderlin, A.; Mahadeva, R. Aging as a consequence of misrepair–a novel theory of aging. *arXiv* **2009**, arXiv:0904.0575.

36. Zhao, R.; Liang, D.; Sun, D. Blockade of Extracellular ATP Effect by Oxidized ATP Effectively Mitigated Induced Mouse Experimental Autoimmune Uveitis (EAU). *PLoS ONE* **2016**, *11*, e0155953. [CrossRef]

37. Hultqvist, M.; Olsson, L.M.; Gelderman, K.A.; Holmdahl, R. The protective role of ROS in autoimmune disease. *Trends Immunol.* **2009**, *30*, 201–208. [CrossRef]

38. Alvarez, K.; Vasquez, G. Damage-associated molecular patterns and their role as initiators of inflammatory and auto-immune signals in systemic lupus erythematosus. *Int. Rev. Immunol.* **2017**, *36*, 259–270. [CrossRef] [PubMed]

39. Frenk, S.; Houseley, J. Gene expression hallmarks of cellular ageing. *Biogerontology* **2018**, *19*, 547–566. [CrossRef]

40. Chen, W.; Sandoval, H.; Kubiak, J.Z.; Li, X.C.; Ghobrial, R.M.; Kloc, M. The phenotype of peritoneal mouse macrophages depends on the mitochondria and ATP/ADP homeostasis. *Cell. Immunol.* **2018**, *324*, 1–7. [CrossRef] [PubMed]

41. Liu, P.S.; Ho, P.C. Determining Macrophage Polarization upon Metabolic Perturbation. *Methods Mol. Biol.* **2019**, *1862*, 173–186. [PubMed]

42. Van den Bossche, J.; O'Neill, L.A.; Menon, D. Macrophage Immunometabolism: Where Are We (Going)? *Trends Immunol.* **2017**, *38*, 395–406. [CrossRef] [PubMed]

43. Motori, E.; Puyal, J.; Toni, N.; Ghanem, A.; Angeloni, C.; Malaguti, M.; Cantelli-Forti, G.; Berninger, B.; Conzelmann, K.K.; Gotz, M.; et al. Inflammation-induced alteration of astrocyte mitochondrial dynamics requires autophagy for mitochondrial network maintenance. *Cell Metab.* **2013**, *18*, 844–859. [CrossRef]

44. Roger, A.J.; Munoz-Gomez, S.A.; Kamikawa, R. The Origin and Diversification of Mitochondria. *Curr. Biol.* **2017**, *27*, R1177–R1192. [CrossRef] [PubMed]

45. Chen, H.; Chan, D.C. Mitochondrial Dynamics in Regulating the Unique Phenotypes of Cancer and Stem Cells. *Cell Metab.* **2017**, *26*, 39–48. [CrossRef] [PubMed]

46. Giedt, R.J.; Fumene Feruglio, P.; Pathania, D.; Yang, K.S.; Kilcoyne, A.; Vinegoni, C.; Mitchison, T.J.; Weissleder, R. Computational imaging reveals mitochondrial morphology as a biomarker of cancer phenotype and drug response. *Sci. Rep.* **2016**, *6*, 32985. [CrossRef]

47. Singh, B.; Schoeb, T.R.; Bajpai, P.; Slominski, A.; Singh, K.K. Reversing wrinkled skin and hair loss in mice by restoring mitochondrial function. *Cell Death Dis.* **2018**, *9*, 735. [CrossRef] [PubMed]

48. Atamna, H.; Tenore, A.; Lui, F.; Dhahbi, J.M. Organ reserve, excess metabolic capacity, and aging. *Biogerontology* **2018**, *19*, 171–184. [CrossRef] [PubMed]

49. Verkhratsky, A.; Burnstock, G. Biology of purinergic signalling: Its ancient evolutionary roots, its omnipresence and its multiple functional significance. *BioEssays News Rev. Mol. Cell. Dev. Biol.* **2014**, *36*, 697–705. [CrossRef]

50. Burnstock, G. Intracellular expression of purinoceptors. *Purinergic Signal.* **2015**, *11*, 275–276. [CrossRef] [PubMed]

51. Diaz-Hernandez, J.I.; Sebastian-Serrano, A.; Gomez-Villafuertes, R.; Diaz-Hernandez, M.; Miras-Portugal, M.T. Age-related nuclear translocation of P2X6 subunit modifies splicing activity interacting with splicing factor 3A1. *PLoS ONE* **2015**, *10*, e0123121. [CrossRef]

52. Dietz, W.H. Critical periods in childhood for the development of obesity. *Am. J. Clin. Nutr.* **1994**, *59*, 955–959. [CrossRef]

53. Das, J.K.; Salam, R.A.; Thornburg, K.L.; Prentice, A.M.; Campisi, S.; Lassi, Z.S.; Koletzko, B.; Bhutta, Z.A. Nutrition in adolescents: Physiology, metabolism, and nutritional needs. *Ann. N. Y. Acad. Sci.* **2017**, *1393*, 21–33. [CrossRef]

54. Desbrow, B.; Burd, N.A.; Tarnopolsky, M.; Moore, D.R.; Elliott-Sale, K.J. Nutrition for Special Populations: Young, Female, and Masters Athletes. *Int. J. Sport Nutr. Exerc. Metab.* **2019**, 1–8. [CrossRef]

55. Lopez-Lluch, G.; Irusta, P.M.; Navas, P.; de Cabo, R. Mitochondrial biogenesis and healthy aging. *Exp. Gerontol.* **2008**, *43*, 813–819. [CrossRef] [PubMed]

56. Weir, H.J.; Yao, P.; Huynh, F.K.; Escoubas, C.C.; Goncalves, R.L.; Burkewitz, K.; Laboy, R.; Hirschey, M.D.; Mair, W.B. Dietary Restriction and AMPK Increase Lifespan via Mitochondrial Network and Peroxisome Remodeling. *Cell Metab.* **2017**, *26*, 884–896 e885. [CrossRef]

57. Rabol, R.; Svendsen, P.F.; Skovbro, M.; Boushel, R.; Haugaard, S.B.; Schjerling, P.; Schrauwen, P.; Hesselink, M.K.; Nilas, L.; Madsbad, S.; et al. Reduced skeletal muscle mitochondrial respiration and improved glucose metabolism in nondiabetic obese women during a very low calorie dietary intervention leading to rapid weight loss. *Metabolism* **2009**, *58*, 1145–1152. [CrossRef]

58. Muller, M.J.; Enderle, J.; Pourhassan, M.; Braun, W.; Eggeling, B.; Lagerpusch, M.; Gluer, C.C.; Kehayias, J.J.; Kiosz, D.; Bosy-Westphal, A. Metabolic adaptation to caloric restriction and subsequent refeeding: The Minnesota Starvation Experiment revisited. *Am. J. Clin. Nutr.* **2015**, *102*, 807–819. [CrossRef] [PubMed]

59. Ewald, C.Y.; Castillo-Quan, J.I.; Blackwell, T.K. Untangling Longevity, Dauer, and Healthspan in Caenorhabditis elegans Insulin/IGF-1-Signalling. *Gerontology* **2018**, *64*, 96–104. [CrossRef] [PubMed]

60. Albert, P.S.; Riddle, D.L. Developmental alterations in sensory neuroanatomy of the Caenorhabditis elegans dauer larva. *J. Comp. Neurol.* **1983**, *219*, 461–481. [CrossRef] [PubMed]

61. Lee, D.; Lee, H.; Kim, N.; Lim, D.S.; Lee, J. Regulation of a hitchhiking behavior by neuronal insulin and TGF-beta signaling in the nematode Caenorhabditis elegans. *Biochem. Biophys. Res. Commun.* **2017**, *484*, 323–330. [CrossRef] [PubMed]

62. Lant, B.; Storey, K.B. An overview of stress response and hypometabolic strategies in Caenorhabditis elegans: Conserved and contrasting signals with the mammalian system. *Int. J. Biol. Sci.* **2010**, *6*, 9–50. [CrossRef] [PubMed]

63. Androwski, R.J.; Flatt, K.M.; Schroeder, N.E. Phenotypic plasticity and remodeling in the stress-induced Caenorhabditis elegans dauer. *Wiley Interdiscip. Rev. Dev. Biol.* **2017**, *6*, e278. [CrossRef]

64. D'Antona, G.; Ragni, M.; Cardile, A.; Tedesco, L.; Dossena, M.; Bruttini, F.; Caliaro, F.; Corsetti, G.; Bottinelli, R.; Carruba, M.O.; et al. Branched-chain amino acid supplementation promotes survival and supports cardiac and skeletal muscle mitochondrial biogenesis in middle-aged mice. *Cell Metab.* **2010**, *12*, 362–372. [CrossRef]

65. Bonfili, L.; Cecarini, V.; Cuccioloni, M.; Angeletti, M.; Flati, V.; Corsetti, G.; Pasini, E.; Dioguardi, F.S.; Eleuteri, A.M. Essential amino acid mixtures drive cancer cells to apoptosis through proteasome inhibition and autophagy activation. *FEBS J.* **2017**, *284*, 1726–1737. [CrossRef] [PubMed]

66. Corsetti, G.; Romano, C.; Pasini, E.; Marzetti, E.; Calvani, R.; Picca, A.; Flati, V.; Dioguardi, F.S. Diet enrichment with a specific essential free amino acid mixture improves healing of undressed wounds in aged rats. *Exp. Gerontol.* **2017**, *96*, 138–145. [CrossRef]

67. Fielenbach, N.; Antebi, A.C. elegans dauer formation and the molecular basis of plasticity. *Genes Dev.* **2008**, *22*, 2149–2165. [CrossRef]

68. Sender, R.; Fuchs, S.; Milo, R. Revised Estimates for the Number of Human and Bacteria Cells in the Body. *PLoS Biol.* **2016**, *14*, e1002533. [CrossRef]

69. Renehan, A.G.; Booth, C.; Potten, C.S. What is apoptosis, and why is it important? *BMJ* **2001**, *322*, 1536–1538. [CrossRef]

70. Spalding, K.L.; Arner, E.; Westermark, P.O.; Bernard, S.; Buchholz, B.A.; Bergmann, O.; Blomqvist, L.; Hoffstedt, J.; Naslund, E.; Britton, T.; et al. Dynamics of fat cell turnover in humans. *Nature* **2008**, *453*, 783–787. [CrossRef]

71. Spalding, K.L.; Bhardwaj, R.D.; Buchholz, B.A.; Druid, H.; Frisen, J. Retrospective birth dating of cells in humans. *Cell* **2005**, *122*, 133–143. [CrossRef] [PubMed]

72. Doherty, T.J. Invited review: Aging and sarcopenia. *J. Appl. Physiol.* **2003**, *95*, 1717–1727. [CrossRef]

73. Prescott, L.F. The normal urinary excretion rates of renal tubular cells, leucocytes and red blood cells. *Clin. Sci.* **1966**, *31*, 425–435. [PubMed]

74. Rinkevich, Y.; Montoro, D.T.; Contreras-Trujillo, H.; Harari-Steinberg, O.; Newman, A.M.; Tsai, J.M.; Lim, X.; Van-Amerongen, R.; Bowman, A.; Januszyk, M.; et al. In vivo clonal analysis reveals lineage-restricted progenitor characteristics in mammalian kidney development, maintenance, and regeneration. *Cell Rep.* **2014**, *7*, 1270–1283. [CrossRef] [PubMed]

75. Kim, I.H.; Kisseleva, T.; Brenner, D.A. Aging and liver disease. *Curr. Opin. Gastroenterol.* **2015**, *31*, 184–191. [CrossRef] [PubMed]

76. Bergmann, O.; Bhardwaj, R.D.; Bernard, S.; Zdunek, S.; Barnabe-Heider, F.; Walsh, S.; Zupicich, J.; Alkass, K.; Buchholz, B.A.; Druid, H.; et al. Evidence for cardiomyocyte renewal in humans. *Science* **2009**, *324*, 98–102. [CrossRef]

77. Perl, S.; Kushner, J.A.; Buchholz, B.A.; Meeker, A.K.; Stein, G.M.; Hsieh, M.; Kirby, M.; Pechhold, S.; Liu, E.H.; Harlan, D.M.; et al. Significant human beta-cell turnover is limited to the first three decades of life as determined by in vivo thymidine analog incorporation and radiocarbon dating. *J. Clin. Endocrinol. Metab.* **2010**, *95*, E234–E239. [CrossRef] [PubMed]

78. Fox, J.P.; Hall, C.E.; Cooney, M.K.; Luce, R.E.; Kronmal, R.A. The Seattle virus watch. II. Objectives, study population and its observation, data processing and summary of illnesses. *Am. J. Epidemiol.* **1972**, *96*, 270–285. [CrossRef] [PubMed]

79. Milholland, B.; Dong, X.; Zhang, L.; Hao, X.; Suh, Y.; Vijg, J. Differences between germline and somatic mutation rates in humans and mice. *Nat. Commun.* **2017**, *8*, 15183. [CrossRef]

80. Peterson, S.E.; Westra, J.W.; Paczkowski, C.M.; Chun, J. Chromosomal mosaicism in neural stem cells. *Methods Mol. Biol.* **2008**, *438*, 197–204.

81. Muotri, A.R.; Chu, V.T.; Marchetto, M.C.; Deng, W.; Moran, J.V.; Gage, F.H. Somatic mosaicism in neuronal precursor cells mediated by L1 retrotransposition. *Nature* **2005**, *435*, 903–910. [CrossRef]

82. Romer, C.; Singh, M.; Hurst, L.D.; Izsvak, Z. How to tame an endogenous retrovirus: HERVH and the evolution of human pluripotency. *Curr. Opin. Virol.* **2017**, *25*, 49–58. [CrossRef]

83. Harris, S.A.; Harris, E.A. Herpes Simplex Virus Type 1 and Other Pathogens are Key Causative Factors in Sporadic Alzheimer's Disease. *J. Alzheimer's Dis. JAD* **2015**, *48*, 319–353. [CrossRef]

84. Bornhofft, K.F.; Goldammer, T.; Rebl, A.; Galuska, S.P. Siglecs: A journey through the evolution of sialic acid-binding immunoglobulin-type lectins. *Dev. Comp. Immunol.* **2018**, *86*, 219–231. [CrossRef]

85. Schwarz, F.; Pearce, O.M.; Wang, X.; Samraj, A.N.; Laubli, H.; Garcia, J.O.; Lin, H.; Fu, X.; Garcia-Bingman, A.; Secrest, P.; et al. Siglec receptors impact mammalian lifespan by modulating oxidative stress. *Elife* **2015**, *4*. [CrossRef]

86. Stanczak, M.A.; Siddiqui, S.S.; Trefny, M.P.; Thommen, D.S.; Boligan, K.F.; von Gunten, S.; Tzankov, A.; Tietze, L.; Lardinois, D.; Heinzelmann-Schwarz, V.; et al. Self-associated molecular patterns mediate cancer immune evasion by engaging Siglecs on T cells. *J. Clin. Investig.* **2018**, *128*, 4912–4923. [CrossRef]

87. Bower, N.I.; Hogan, B.M. Brain drains: New insights into brain clearance pathways from lymphatic biology. *J. Mol. Med.* **2018**, *96*, 383–390. [CrossRef]

88. Schubert, D.; Currais, A.; Goldberg, J.; Finley, K.; Petrascheck, M.; Maher, P. Geroneuroprotectors: Effective Geroprotectors for the Brain. *Trends Pharmacol. Sci.* **2018**, *39*, 1004–1007. [CrossRef]

89. Mizutani, T.; Ishizaka, A.; Furuichi, Y. The Werner Protein Acts as a Coactivator of Nuclear Factor kappaB (NF-kappaB) on HIV-1 and Interleukin-8 (IL-8) Promoters. *J. Biol. Chem.* **2015**, *290*, 18391–18399. [CrossRef]

90. Huang, Y.; Li, W.; Su, Z.Y.; Kong, A.N. The complexity of the Nrf2 pathway: Beyond the antioxidant response. *J. Nutr. Biochem.* **2015**, *26*, 1401–1413. [CrossRef]

91. Li, B.; Iglesias-Pedraz, J.M.; Chen, L.Y.; Yin, F.; Cadenas, E.; Reddy, S.; Comai, L. Downregulation of the Werner syndrome protein induces a metabolic shift that compromises redox homeostasis and limits proliferation of cancer cells. *Aging Cell* **2014**, *13*, 367–378. [CrossRef]

92. Blanc, E.M.; Bruce-Keller, A.J.; Mattson, M.P. Astrocytic gap junctional communication decreases neuronal vulnerability to oxidative stress-induced disruption of Ca2+ homeostasis and cell death. *J. Neurochem.* **1998**, *70*, 958–970. [CrossRef] [PubMed]

93. Duchen, M.R. Mitochondria and calcium: From cell signalling to cell death. *J. Physiol.* **2000**, *529 Pt 1*, 57–68. [CrossRef]

94. Camacho-Pereira, J.; Tarrago, M.G.; Chini, C.C.S.; Nin, V.; Escande, C.; Warner, G.M.; Puranik, A.S.; Schoon, R.A.; Reid, J.M.; Galina, A.; et al. CD38 Dictates Age-Related NAD Decline and Mitochondrial Dysfunction through an SIRT3-Dependent Mechanism. *Cell Metab.* **2016**, *23*, 1127–1139. [CrossRef]

95. Igwe, O.J.; Filla, M.B. Aging-related regulation of myo-inositol 1,4,5-trisphosphate signal transduction pathway in the rat striatum. *Brain Res. Mol. Brain Res.* **1997**, *46*, 39–53. [CrossRef]

96. Gomes, A.P.; Price, N.L.; Ling, A.J.; Moslehi, J.J.; Montgomery, M.K.; Rajman, L.; White, J.P.; Teodoro, J.S.; Wrann, C.D.; Hubbard, B.P.; et al. Declining NAD(+) induces a pseudohypoxic state disrupting nuclear-mitochondrial communication during aging. *Cell* **2013**, *155*, 1624–1638. [CrossRef]

97. Chini, C.C.S.; Tarrago, M.G.; Chini, E.N. NAD and the aging process: Role in life, death and everything in between. *Mol. Cell. Endocrinol.* **2017**, *455*, 62–74. [CrossRef] [PubMed]

98. Zhang, H.; Ryu, D.; Wu, Y.; Gariani, K.; Wang, X.; Luan, P.; D'Amico, D.; Ropelle, E.R.; Lutolf, M.P.; Aebersold, R.; et al. NAD(+) repletion improves mitochondrial and stem cell function and enhances life span in mice. *Science* **2016**, *352*, 1436–1443. [CrossRef] [PubMed]

99. Xu, M.; Pirtskhalava, T.; Farr, J.N.; Weigand, B.M.; Palmer, A.K.; Weivoda, M.M.; Inman, C.L.; Ogrodnik, M.B.; Hachfeld, C.M.; Fraser, D.G.; et al. Senolytics improve physical function and increase lifespan in old age. *Nat. Med.* **2018**, *24*, 1246–1256. [CrossRef] [PubMed]

100. Go, Y.M.; Fernandes, J.; Hu, X.; Uppal, K.; Jones, D.P. Mitochondrial network responses in oxidative physiology and disease. *Free Radic. Biol. Med.* **2018**, *116*, 31–40. [CrossRef]

101. Salminen, A.; Kaarniranta, K.; Kauppinen, A. Integrated stress response stimulates FGF21 expression: Systemic enhancer of longevity. *Cell Signal.* **2017**, *40*, 10–21. [CrossRef] [PubMed]

102. Pakos-Zebrucka, K.; Koryga, I.; Mnich, K.; Ljujic, M.; Samali, A.; Gorman, A.M. The integrated stress response. *EMBO Rep.* **2016**, *17*, 1374–1395. [CrossRef] [PubMed]

103. Naviaux, R.K. Oxidative shielding or oxidative stress? *J. Pharmacol. Exp. Ther.* **2012**, *342*, 608–618. [CrossRef] [PubMed]

104. Wang-Michelitsch, J.; Michelitsch, T. Aging as a process of accumulation of Misrepairs. *arXiv* **2015**, arXiv:1503.07163.

105. Hernandez-Segura, A.; de Jong, T.V.; Melov, S.; Guryev, V.; Campisi, J.; Demaria, M. Unmasking Transcriptional Heterogeneity in Senescent Cells. *Curr. Biol.* **2017**, *27*, 2652–2660 e2654. [CrossRef] [PubMed]

106. Kumari, J.; Hussain, M.; De, S.; Chandra, S.; Modi, P.; Tikoo, S.; Singh, A.; Sagar, C.; Sepuri, N.B.; Sengupta, S. Mitochondrial functions of RECQL4 are required for the prevention of aerobic glycolysis-dependent cell invasion. *J. Cell Sci.* **2016**, *129*, 1312–1318. [CrossRef] [PubMed]

107. Gupta, S.; De, S.; Srivastava, V.; Hussain, M.; Kumari, J.; Muniyappa, K.; Sengupta, S. RECQL4 and p53 potentiate the activity of polymerase gamma and maintain the integrity of the human mitochondrial genome. *Carcinogenesis* **2014**, *35*, 34–45. [CrossRef]

108. Croteau, D.L.; Singh, D.K.; Hoh Ferrarelli, L.; Lu, H.; Bohr, V.A. RECQL4 in genomic instability and aging. *Trends Genet.* **2012**, *28*, 624–631. [CrossRef]

109. Hupin, D.; Roche, F.; Gremeaux, V.; Chatard, J.C.; Oriol, M.; Gaspoz, J.M.; Barthelemy, J.C.; Edouard, P. Even a low-dose of moderate-to-vigorous physical activity reduces mortality by 22% in adults aged >/=60 years: A systematic review and meta-analysis. *Br. J. Sports Med.* **2015**, *49*, 1262–1267. [CrossRef]

110. Gries, K.J.; Raue, U.; Perkins, R.K.; Lavin, K.M.; Overstreet, B.S.; D'Acquisto, L.J.; Graham, B.; Finch, W.H.; Kaminsky, L.A.; Trappe, T.A.; et al. Cardiovascular and Skeletal Muscle Health with Lifelong Exercise. *J. Appl. Physiol.* **2018**. [CrossRef]

111. Radak, Z.; Torma, F.; Berkes, I.; Goto, S.; Mimura, T.; Posa, A.; Balogh, L.; Boldogh, I.; Suzuki, K.; Higuchi, M.; et al. Exercise effects on physiological function during aging. *Free Radic. Biol. Med.* **2019**, *132*, 33–41. [CrossRef]

112. Fan, W.; Evans, R.M. Exercise Mimetics: Impact on Health and Performance. *Cell Metab.* **2017**, *25*, 242–247. [CrossRef]

113. Yu, M.; Tsai, S.F.; Kuo, Y.M. The Therapeutic Potential of Anti-Inflammatory Exerkines in the Treatment of Atherosclerosis. *Int. J. Mol. Sci.* **2017**, *18*, 1260. [CrossRef]

114. Whitham, M.; Parker, B.L.; Friedrichsen, M.; Hingst, J.R.; Hjorth, M.; Hughes, W.E.; Egan, C.L.; Cron, L.; Watt, K.I.; Kuchel, R.P.; et al. Extracellular Vesicles Provide a Means for Tissue Crosstalk during Exercise. *Cell Metab.* **2018**, *27*, 237–251 e234. [CrossRef]

115. Safdar, A.; Tarnopolsky, M.A. Exosomes as Mediators of the Systemic Adaptations to Endurance Exercise. *Cold Spring Harb. Perspect. Med.* **2018**, *8*, a029827. [CrossRef]

116. Jesko, H.; Stepien, A.; Lukiw, W.J.; Strosznajder, R.P. The Cross-Talk Between Sphingolipids and Insulin-Like Growth Factor Signaling: Significance for Aging and Neurodegeneration. *Mol. Neurobiol.* **2018**. [CrossRef]

117. Trayssac, M.; Hannun, Y.A.; Obeid, L.M. Role of sphingolipids in senescence: Implication in aging and age-related diseases. *J. Clin. Investig.* **2018**, *128*, 2702–2712. [CrossRef]

118. Jazwinski, S.M. Mitochondria to nucleus signaling and the role of ceramide in its integration into the suite of cell quality control processes during aging. *Ageing Res. Rev.* **2015**, *23*, 67–74. [CrossRef]

119. Fakouri, N.B.; Hansen, T.L.; Desler, C.; Anugula, S.; Rasmussen, L.J. From powerhouse to perpetrator—mitochondria in health and disease. *Biology* **2019**, (in press).

10

Cardiovascular Manifestations of Mitochondrial Disease

Jason Duran, Armando Martinez and Eric Adler *

Department of Cardiology, University of California San Diego Medical Center, La Jolla, CA 92037, USA;
jaduran@ucsd.edu (J.D.); arm021@ucsd.edu (A.M.)
* Correspondence: eradler@ucsd.edu

Abstract: Genetic mitochondrial cardiomyopathies are uncommon causes of heart failure that may not be seen by most physicians. However, the prevalence of mitochondrial DNA mutations and somatic mutations affecting mitochondrial function are more common than previously thought. In this review, the pathogenesis of genetic mitochondrial disorders causing cardiovascular disease is reviewed. Treatment options are presently limited to mostly symptomatic support, but preclinical research is starting to reveal novel approaches that may lead to better and more targeted therapies in the future. With better understanding and clinician education, we hope to improve clinician recognition and diagnosis of these rare disorders in order to improve ongoing care of patients with these diseases and advance research towards discovering new therapeutic strategies to help treat these diseases.

Keywords: mitochondrial; genetic mutations; cardiovascular disease; heart failure; cardiomyopathy

1. Introduction

Mitochondrial diseases affect nearly 1 in 5000–10,000 births [1–3] and genetic mutations in mitochondrial DNA (mtDNA) are even more commonly found, with studies on umbilical cord blood reporting mutations in as many as 1 in 200 samples [3,4]. Although relatively common, mitochondrial diseases have a wide array of clinical presentations and their dysfunction affects a wide variety of organs and tissues [5] including the heart [6]. As such the diagnosis of a mitochondrial disorder can be complex and easily overlooked. Thus, physician exposure to mitochondrial disorders is quite limited despite its relatively common incidence.

Normal mitochondria serve to supply energy in the form of adenosine triphosphate (ATP), generate and regulate radical oxygen species (ROS), buffer cytosolic calcium ions, and regulate cellular apoptosis via the mitochondrial permeability pore complex [1]. Mitochondria are more richly expressed in tissues with high energy demand, including the heart, brain, skeletal muscle and endocrine system, and their dysfunction will disproportionately affect these systems [7]. Tissues that are more metabolically active will typically have greater vulnerability to defects in mtDNA [8] and they will be affected earlier and more severely than less metabolic tissues [9]. Cardiomyopathy is common and usually increases mortality, with one study reporting that 17% of infants and children hospitalized with an array of mitochondrial diseases had cardiac manifestations, and patients with cardiomyopathy had markedly increased mortality (71%) compared to those without a cardiac phenotype (26%) [10]. Mitochondrial mutations can have variable expression in tissues, and cells can exhibit heteroplasmy in which a single cell can have a mixed population mitochondria with either wild-type or mutant-type mtDNA [8].

The variability of expression of a mutation to mtDNA coupled with the wide variety of symptoms and characteristics of each disorder can make these diseases difficult to identify and diagnose. The diagnostic gold standard of mitochondrial disorders continues to be muscle biopsy, however this is only achieved if physicians are aware of mitochondrial disorders and thinking about them in their differential when diagnosing a patient. In this review, we discuss the pathophysiology of mitochondrial disorders and seek to provide a comprehensive clinical resource on mitochondrial cardiomyopathies and their treatment options. We begin by discussing mitochondrial dysfunction in normal aging, followed by a review of primary (congenital) and secondary mitochondrial disorders with cardiovascular phenotypes. We seek to improve physician recognition and identification of patients with mitochondrial disorders so that we can improve future recognition, diagnosis and treatments of these diseases.

2. Mitochondrial Dysfunction in Normal Aging

The heart is one of the most metabolically active tissues in the human body, relying heavily on mitochondrial ATP production to maintain the high energy demand of individually contracting cardiac myocytes. Cardiac aging, or senescence, is coupled with a decline in mitochondrial function, increased production of reactive oxygen species (ROS) and suppressed mitophagy [11,12]. The mitochondrial free radical theory of aging supposes that, with time, free radicals produced as unwanted byproducts of normal mitochondrial metabolism from the respiratory chain on the inner mitochondrial membrane build up in the cell where they are converted to hydrogen peroxide by superoxide dismutase. These hydrogen peroxides are then converted by the Fenton reaction to damaging free radicals that are toxic to nearly all molecules in the cell [12,13]. On the microscopic level, it has been well-established that cells progressively accumulate damage to peptides and lipid molecules with time [14].

In addition to damaging proteins and lipids, free radicals also produces mutations in mitochondrial DNA. Over time, and especially in highly metabolic cells like cardiomyocytes that have high cellular concentrations of mitochondria, ROS-induced molecular damage leads to progressive accumulation of mitochondrial DNA mutations [15–17]. This ultimately leads to increasingly greater mitochondrial dysfunction, and, in damaged cells, dysfunctional mitochondria divide and produce more dysfunctional mitochondria that contain greater number of mtDNA mutations [11,17]. Over time, this leads to progressive cellular dysfunction at the organellar level. In metabolically active and mitochondria-rich cells like cardiomyocytes, the cumulation of damaged peptides, lipids and organelles is more pronounced and has a more pronounced contribution to cellular dysfunction and aging [11].

Maintaining protein homeostasis is also central to the normal function of any cell. When peptides get damaged or degraded, the ability to continue normal cellular function relies on the ability to break down and dispose of damage proteins. The cell must also then replace these damage peptides with normally functioning new proteins [11]. The limited ability to remove damaged proteins or replace them can be damaging to normal cell function [18]. Experimental mechanisms that enhance protein homeostasis include reducing insulin-like growth factor-1 (IGF-1) signaling [19,20], caloric restriction or inhibiting mammalian target of rapamycin (mTOR) signaling with rapamycin treatment [21,22]. As the cellular proteome ages, damaged proteins start to build up, protein degradation slows, and cells progressively accumulate more damaged molecules and become progressively more dysfunctional. This is consistent with experimental results that have demonstrated increased levels of protein ubiquitination in the aging heart, [21] but without increased rates of protein turnover [11,21]. On the cellular level, these microscopic changes lead to changes on the organellar and cellular level, with increasingly dysfunctional autophagy with age.

3. Primary Mitochondrial Disorders

3.1. Mitochondrial Encephalopathy with Lactic Acidosis and Stroke-Like Episodes (MELAS)

First described by Pavlakis et al. in 1984, [23] MELAS has a reported prevalence of 0.18 per 100,000 [24]. Typically presenting in childhood, with 76–80% presenting before 20 years old, the disease rapidly progresses after presentation [25,26]. It has a wide-ranging phenotype that includes stroke-like symptoms (weakness, aphasia, vision loss), encephalopathy (manifesting often as seizures or dementia), lactic acidosis and myopathy [24,26,27]. Additional symptoms include coma, vomiting, fever, headaches, ataxia, external opthalmoplegia, diabetes, hearing impairment, developmental delay, and short stature (Table 1) [26,27].

Cardiac dysfunction has been reported to occur in approximately 30–32% of cases, [24,28] with both hypertrophic and dilated cardiomyopathies having been reported [29]. Conduction abnormalities have also been reported, most notably Wolff–Parkinson–White syndrome [26,30]. The most common genetic mutation involved is A3243G, which has been reported in up to 80% of MELAS presentations [25]. Other mutations that have been identified include T3271C, A3252G, T9957C, 14787del4, G14453A, A13084T, A13045C, A12770G, A11084G, T3949C, G3946A, G3697A, G3376A, T3308C, A13514G, G13513A, G3697, and it is likely several others have yet to be identified (Table 2) [31,32].

Studies have shown treatment with nitric oxide (NO) precursors increase NO production and reportedly reduce stroke-like symptoms [33,34]. One study found plasma lactate decreased significantly after citrulline supplementation [35]. Though no studies have looked directly at the effects of NO precursor therapy on cardiac manifestations, some have theorized they may work by increasing NO production and decreasing cellular damage in cardiac tissue [36]. One case report found improvement in seizure control and reduction in stroke-like episodes after initiation of a ketogenic diet [37]. Reports have shown possible benefits from creatine, CoQ10, and lipoic acid therapy including improvement in symptoms of body composition, strength, and lactate level [38].

Table 1. Summary of mitochondrial disorders with cardiac phenotypes.

Disease	Incidence Age at Onset/Death	Primary Phenotype	Cardiac Manifestations	Genetic Mutations	Treatments
MELAS	0.18/100,000 <20 years Rapid progression to death after onset	• Stroke-like symptoms • Encephalopathy • Lactic Acidemia • Myopathy	30% of cases: • HCM, DCM • Conduction abnormalities (WPW)	A324G (80% of cases)	• Nitric oxide precursors • Citrulline supplementation • Ketogenic diet • Creatine, CoQ10, lipoic acid therapy
Leigh Syndrome	1/32,000–40,000 <1–2 years Median age of death 2.4 years	• Encephalopathy with cognitive and behavioral dysfunction • Seizures • Hypotonia/Ataxia • Oculomotor dysfunction • Respiratory dysfunction	20% of cases: • HCM • Pericardial effusions • Conduction abnormalities	Mutations to SURF1 gene G13513A (WPW and HCM)	• High dose biotin • Thiamine for SLC19A3 • CoQ10
MERRF	0.9 or <1/100,000 10–20 years Progression to death within 2–15 years of onset (median 8.4 years)	• Myoclonus • Lactic acidosis • Cerebellar ataxia • Muscle weakness • Ragged red fibers	• DCM • HCM • Conduction abnormalities (WPW, SVT, RBBB)	A8344G (83–90% of cases and 53% of cases with cardiac involvement)	• Treatment of seizures with antiepileptic drugs
MIDD	6/100,000 (~1% of patients with diabetes) <35 years	• Diabetes (type I or II) • Bilateral neurosensory hearing loss	• LVH (55%) • HCM (15–30%) • Conduction abnormalities (WPW, SSS, Afib)	A3243G	• Treatment of diabetes • Cochlear implantation • CoQ10
NARP	1/12,000–40,000 3–12 months	• Neuropathy • Ataxia • Retinitis Pigmentosa • Deafness • Myoclonic epilepsy	• DCM • HCM • Conduction abnormalities (WPW)	Point mutations at 8993 MT-ATP6 gene (most commonly T8993G, then T8993C)	• Experimental: mitochondrially targeted obligate heterodimeric zinc finger nucleases to target mitochondrial DNA with the NARP T8993G mutation
GRACILE	1/47,000 (in Finland, may be lower worldwide) Onset in utero 50% die within first 4 months of life, remainder die by 4 years	• Growth restriction • Aminoaciduria • Cholestasis • Iron overload • Early death	• Prolonged QT • Reduced levels of complex III in myocardial tissues post mortem	homozygous point mutation A232G within the BCS1L gene	• Symptomatic/palliative care (usually lethal in first months of life).

Table 1. Cont.

Disease	Incidence Age at Onset/Death	Primary Phenotype	Cardiac Manifestations	Genetic Mutations	Treatments
MNGIE	* Only 100 cases ever reported Mean age of onset 18 years Mean age of death 35 years	• Chronic intestinal dysmotility • Leukoencephalopathy • Failure to thrive • Ptosis • Ophthalmoparesis • Peripheral neuropathy	• LVH • Conduction abnormalities (prolonged QT, SVT, sudden cardiac death)	Loss of function mutations to thymidine phosphorylase (TP) gene, chromosome 22q13.32-qter	• Allogeneic hematopoietic stem cell transplantation • Platelet transfusion • Hemodialysis or peritoneal dialysis • Experimental gene therapies aimed to restore thymidine phosphorylase activity
Barth Syndrome	1:300,000–400,000 <1 year Most die within first 4 years of life	• DCM • Skeletal myopathy (proximal) • Neutropenia • Growth retardation	• DCM • Cardiac abnormalities in utereo • Endocardial fibroelastosis • LV noncompaction • Conduction abnormalities (prolonged WT, SVT, WPW, VT)	G4.5 gene (TAZ gene) on Xq28	• Treatment of heart failure • Cardiac transplantation
LHON	1/31,000–50,000 2–87 years	• Acute/subacute painless vision loss • Dystonia • Peripheral neuropathy	• LV hypertrebeculation • Prolonged QT • WPW	90% caused by G11778A (ND4 gene), G3460A (ND1 gene), and the T14484C (NG6 gene) which all cause dysfunction in complex I	• EPI-743: experimental drug targeting glutathione production • Idebenone (antioxidant that can slow vision loss)
Pearson Syndrome	1/1,000,000 Presents in infancy most deaths by 3 years of age	• Transfusion-dependent anemia (presenting finding) • Severe Infections • Liver, Kidney, Pancreas and CNS abnormalities	• Increased wall thickness • Depolarization abnormalities • Prolonged QT	Large deletions ranging from 4.9–14 kb	• Treatment of anemia with transfusions, EPO, GCSF • Treatment of pancreatic insufficiency with enzyme replacement
Kearns-Sayre Syndrome	1–3/100,000	• Progressive external ophthalmoplegia (ptosis, weakness of eye muscles) • Retinopathy • Ataxia • Elevated CSF proteins	• Conduction abnormalities (AV block requiring PPM) • Cardiac arrest	Large deletions ranging from 1000 to 10,000 base pairs	• ECG screening • PPM implantation for AV block
CPEO	1–3/100,000	• Loss of motor function of the eye and eyelid • Spectrum of disorders with PS and KSS	• HCM • Arrhythmias	Large mtDNA deletions similar to PS or KSS AD: mutations to nuclear-encoded genes ANT1, C10orf2 and POLG	• Symptomatic/supportive care

Table 1. Cont.

Disease	Incidence Age at Onset/Death	Primary Phenotype	Cardiac Manifestations	Genetic Mutations	Treatments
Freiderich's Ataxia	1–47:1,000,000 Presents in childhood Mean life expectancy 40 years	• Progressive ataxia/areflexia • Progressive and life-threatening cardiomyopathy (2/3 patients die from cardiovascular causes)	• HCM • DCM	Expansion of DNA triplet intron repeat GAA in the frataxin (FXN) gene	• Idebenone (antioxidant), reduces cardiac hypertrophy

Abbreviations: hypertrophic cardiomyopathy (HCM), dilated cardiomyopathy (DCM), Wolff-Parkinson-White syndrome (WPW), supraventricular tachycardia (SVT), right bundle branch block (RBBB), left ventricular hypertrophy (LVH), sick sinus syndrome (SSS), atrial fibrillation (Afib), ventricular tachyarrhythmias, permanent pacemaker (PPM), autosomal dominant (AD).

Table 2. Genetic mutations associated with mitochondrial disorders.

Disease	Mutations
MELAS	A324G (80% of cases), T3271C, A3252G, T9957C, 14787del4, G14453A, A13084T, A13045C, A12770G, A11084G, T3949C, G3946A, G3697A, G3376A, T3308C, A13514G, G13513A, G3697
Leigh Syndrome	Mutations to SURF1 gene, G13513A (WPW and HCM), 312del10/insAT, T8993C, T8993G, C688T, 772delCC, 751C>T, 845delCT, 868insT, G385A, G618C, T751C, A8344G, A3243G, G13513A, and C1177A.
MERRF	A8344G, T8356C, G8363A
MIDD	A3243G, point mutations at 568 and 8281
NARP	Point mutations at 8993, mutations to MT-ATP6 gene (most commonly T8993G, then T8993C), G8839C, G8989C, 8618insT, T9185C, and a 2 bp microdeletion 9127e9128 del AT
GRACILE	Homozygous point mutation A232G within the BCS1L gene
MNGIE	Loss of function mutations to thymidine phosphorylase (TP) gene, chromosome 22q13.32-qter
Barth Syndrome	G4.5 gene (TAZ gene) on Xq28
LHON	90% caused by G11778A (ND4 gene), G3460A (ND1 gene), and the T14484C (NG6 gene) which all cause dysfunction in complex I
Pearson Syndrome	Large deletions ranging from 4.9–14 kb
Kearns-Sayre Syndrome	Large deletions ranging from 1000 to 10,000 base pairs
CPEO	Large mtDNA deletions similar to PS or KSS, AD form: mutations to nuclear-encoded genes ANT1, C10orf2 and POLG
Freiderich's Ataxia	Expansion of DNA triplet intron repeat GAA in the frataxin (FXN) gene

*Principal mutations of each disorder are bolded (that most frequently attributed to each disease).

3.2. Leigh Syndrome

Leigh Syndrome (LS), or subacute necrotizing encephalomyelopathy, was first described by Dr. Denis Leigh, a British neuropsychiatrist, in 1951 [39]. It is a mitochondrial disorder that causes symmetric necrotic lesions in subcortical areas of the brain, particularly the brain stem and basal ganglia. Prevalence is thought to be between 1 per 32,000 and 1 per 40,000 [40,41]. Symptom onset occurs early in life, with initial presentation in infancy or adolescence, and with a majority of presentations before age 1 and 81% by age 2 [42,43]. Initial presentation is often some combination of signs and symptoms of progressive encephalopathy with cognitive and behavioral dysfunction, seizures, hypotonia, oculomotor abnormalities, ataxia, and respiratory dysfunction (Table 1) [40,42,44].

Patients often present with late-stage disease, with 39% of patients dying by the age of 21 years, at a median age of 2.4 years [42,43]. Atypical and slowly progressing presentations have also been described with more rare mutations. Lactate levels are often elevated and diagnosis is usually confirmed by radiologic findings of characteristic bilateral symmetric subcortical hypodensities on computed tomography (CT) or hyperintense signal abnormalities on T2-weighted magnetic resonance imaging (MRI) [42,45,46]. Cardiac manifestations can occur in up to 18–21% of cases, including cardiomyopathy, pericardial effusion, and conduction abnormalities [42,43,47,48]. Of those, hypertrophic cardiomyopathy was found in 50% of patients with cardiac manifestations (Table 1) [43]. One particular study associated the G13513A mutation with development of Wolff–Parkinson–White and hypertrophic cardiomyopathy [48]. One of the major identified causes of LS is Cytochrome c oxidase (COX) deficiency secondary to mutations in the SURF1 gene [49,50]. Over 35 other gene mutations have been identified in association with LS, some of the more studied mutations include 312del10/insAT, T8993C, T8993G, C688T, 772delCC, 751C>T, 845delCT, 868insT, G385A, G618C, T751C, A8344G, A3243G, G13513A, and C1177A (Table 2) [49–54].

As with other mitochondrial disorders, treatment options for LS are limited. One case series showed improvement in life-expectancy with Thiamine therapy in patients whose LS was secondary to a SLC19A3 mutation [31]. High dose biotin should be administered to every patient with suspected LS, given similarities with biotin-responsive basal ganglia disease. Some case reports have shown positive results for treating with Coenxyme Q10.

3.3. Myoclonic Epilepsy with Ragged Red Fibers (MERRF)

In 1921 Dr. Ramsey Hunt, an American neurologist, first published in the journal *Brain* a syndrome afflicting 6 patients that resembled Freidrich's ataxia which he described as "dyssynergia cereballaris myoclonica." It was not until 1973 that Tsairis et al. discovered mitochondrial abnormalities in a family with this disorder, and not until 1980 until Dr. Fukuhara discovered these symptoms associated with ragged red muscle fibers [55]. Finally in 1990 Schoffner et al. first identified a mitochondrial mutation associated with this disease [56]. Myoclonic epilepsy with ragged red fibers (MERRF) has a heterogeneous phenotype that most commonly includes myoclonus, lactic acidosis, cerebellar ataxia, muscle weakness, and ragged red fibers on muscle biopsy [55,57]. Less common symptoms include generalized seizures, short stature, hearing impairment, peripheral neuropathy, headaches, multiple lipomas, vomiting, cognitive dysfunction, and dementia [55,57,58]. Age of onset is typically the second decade of life, and the time of disease progression ranges from 2 to 15 years with a mean time of 8.5 years [58,59]. Reports of the exact incidence of MERRF vary widely, but according to the National Organization for Rare Disorders, the disease occurs in less than 0.9/100,000 patients. Patients often report frequent myoclonic seizures with rare episodes of generalized tonic–clonic seizures, often only partially controlled by anti-epileptic drugs [58]. Reported cardiac abnormalities include Wolff Parkinson White (WPW), supraventricular tachycardia (SVT), right bundle branch block (RBBB), and both dilated and hypertrophic cardiomyopathy (Table 1) [55,59–61].

The A8344G mutation is the most commonly identified mutation in patients with MERRF, occurring in 83–90% of cases [57,58]. One case series found cardiac abnormalities in 53% of MERRF patients with this mutation [61]. T8356C has been reported in one patient to be associated with MERRF

(Table 2) [62]. G8363A was reported in a case series of 9 patients with clinic presentations fitting MERRF and 4/9 patients were found to cardiac abnormalities [60]. This mutation involves coding for the same tRNA gene as other mutations associated with MERRF. Symptomatic treatment of MERRF is focused on symptomatic management of myoclonus and epilepsy with antiepileptic drugs [58].

3.4. Maternally Inherited Diabetes and Deafness (MIDD)

Maternally inherited diabetes and deafness (MIDD), is a mitochondrial disease first characterized in 1992 [63]. Approximately 0.5–2.8% of all diabetic patients have MIDD, with incidences varying by ethnic origin [64,65]. As the name suggests the defining clinical features are diabetes (both type 1 and 2) and bilateral neurosensory hearing loss, each one being equally likely to be the presenting symptom [66]. Typically diabetes develops at a relatively younger age (with half of all patients presenting before age 35), often in a patient with a low or normal BMI [65–68]. Majority of MIDD patients are non-insulin dependent at presentation however approximately half will have relatively rapid progression to inulin dependence within the first several years of diagnosis [65,66,69,70]. Studies have found macular pattern dystrophy in up to 85% of patients [66,71]. Other less frequent findings include myopathy, neuropsychiatric symptoms, short stature and renal disease [66,69]. Brain atrophy, ptosis, constipation, diarrhea, and pseudo-obstruction have also been reported [72–74]. Several case reports have shown a possible association with histories of spontaneous abortion, preterm pregnancy, and placenta accrete (Table 1) [74,75].

Other studies have found left ventricular hypertrophy in up to 55% of patients and cardiomyopathy in up to 15–30% [66,67,76,77]. One study found myocyte hypertrophy and vacuolization, an increased number of mitochondria and evidence of large mitochondria on endomyocardial biopsy [77]. Conduction disorders including WPW, sick sinus syndrome and atrial fibrillation have been found in up to 27% of cases (Table 1) [66–69]. Another study has shown diabetics with the A3243G mutation had more impairment in autonomic nervous function when compared to other diabetics [78]. The mitochondrial mutation A3243G causes a majority of the cases of MIDD, however other mutations have been identified in rare cases, including point mutations at 568 and 8281 (Table 2) [63,64,79].

Treatment of MIDD is primarily symptomatic. MIDD diabetes is managed similarly to other forms with the exception of avoidance of metformin and low threshold for insulin initiation [65,80]. Hearing impairment is closely followed and patients often benefit from cochlear implantation [65,81]. Case reports have shown treatment with Coenzyme Q10 appeared to improve left ventricular function in patients with MIDD [77,82]. One open trial study conducted on 28 patients in Japan found that treatment with CoQ10 reduced progression of insulin secretion defects, exercise intolerance, and hearing loss [83]. Visual symptoms, like acuity loss, are rare in MIDD [71].

3.5. Neuropathy, Ataxia and Retinitis Pigmentosa (NARP)

Classically the syndrome of neuropathy, ataxia, and retinitis pigmentosa (NARP) has been described as a combination of deafness, a myoclonic epilepsy, muscle weakness, retinal pigmentosa, and ataxia [84]. The disease was first described by Fryer et al. in 1994 in a family with seven children who presented with a heterogenous phenotype of Leigh's syndrome [85]. Further investigations however have shown NARP to be phenotypically variable ranging from mild or late-onset symptoms like retinal dystrophy to a more severe multisystemic phenotype that can include developmental delay, dementia, seizures, muscle weakness, sensory neuropathy, ataxia, and retinal pigmentosa and with typical age of onset in the first year of life [84,86]. NARP is estimated to effect about 1/12,000–40,000 according to the National Organization of Rare Disorders and the National Institutes of Health. Several studies have shown a correlation between mutation load and severity of symptoms, especially in the more common mutations at 8993 [87]. Individuals with 80% or more are more likely to have the classic presentation, those below 70% have milder symptoms, and below 50% is often asymptomatic or late onset [86,88–90]. Individuals with >90% mutation load appear to present with Leigh syndrome, indicating clinical presentations are on a NARP/Leigh spectrum (Table 1) [91,92].

Further studies have shown that factors other than mutation load affect a patient's phenotype. Proposed variables for further investigation include mtDNA background, environmental, autosomal, tissue-specific factors, and nuclear modifier genes likely play a role in determining clinical picture and disease severity [93–95]. One case report followed a patient with NARP who developed peripartium dilated cardiomyopathy, ventricular pre-excitation, and non-sustained ventricular tachycardia during 4 years of follow up [96]. However this patient had a A8344G, which has been associated with MERRF and not NARP. Though the 8993 mutation has been linked to cases of hypertrophic cardiomyopathy, cases have been in patients with the more severe Leigh syndrome phenotype [97]. More studies focused on long term follow up to determine late sequelae of NARP are needed to determine cardiac outcomes. NARP is caused by mutations in the MT-ATP6 gene, most commonly T8993G and occasionally T8993C [84,86,88]. Other reported mutations include G8839C, G8989C, 8618insT, T9185C, and a 2-bp microdeletion 9127e9128 del AT [89,91,98–100]. Other mutations in the MT-ATP6 gene have been documented but have been observed to cause the more severe presentations seen in Leigh syndrome [95,101]. A recent study demonstrated the promise of using mitochondrially targeted obligate heterodimeric zinc finger nucleases to target mitochondrial DNA with the NARP T8993G mutation in cell models [102]. Otherwise treatment has primarily been on symptom improvement (Table 2).

3.6. GRACILE

First described in 1998, GRACILE syndrome is a severe mitochondrial disease named after the significant clinical features: growth restriction, aminoaciduria, cholestasis, iron overload, and early death [103]. Incidence is approximated to be at least 1/47,000 based on a study conducted in Finland, however its global prevalence may actually be lower as Finland reports the highest number of cases of GRACILE worldwide [104]. Onset begins with growth restriction at the end of the first trimester, with patient's average birth weight at standard deviations below predicted normal [105]. A study of 29 GRACILE cases found a median lactate of 12.8 mmol/L, pH of 7.00, and all patients had elevated transaminases [106]. The liver develops macrovesicular steatosis, cholestasis with iron accumulation, rapidly progressive fibrosis and cirrhosis [107]. Lactic acidosis is present and often refractory to treatment, further contributing to failure to thrive. Cause of death appears to occur due to energy depletion, with approximately half of all patients dying within the first two weeks of life and the remainder die by 4 months of life [104,106,107]. One patient was found to have prolonged QT [105]. Autopsy-derived myocardial tissue samples showed higher respiratory chain enzyme activity when compared to autopsy controls [104]. Another study on isolated complex III from GRACILE patients found reduced levels and activity of complex III in myocardial tissues, however no cardiac dysfunction or histopathological abnormalities were found (Table 1) [108].

GRACILE is caused by the homozygous point mutation A232G within the BCS1L gene [104]. BCS1L is a mitochondrial chaperone protein that guides the assembly of complex III of the mitochondrial respiratory chain [104]. It is the most common and severe BCS1L disorder, however multiple mutations within the BCS1L gene have been identified and are linked to a variety of phenotypes [109,110]. Identified exclusively in Finland and included as part of the Finnish disease heritage, it is postulated to have accumulated in the Finnish population through founder effect and genetic drift [105,106]. Patients with the homozygous A232G have shown a strong consistency in the resulting phenotype [111]. BCS1L deficiency did not result in decreased complex III activity in tissues from Finnish GRACILE patients, but patients with BCSL1 deficiency did demonstrate reduced Rieske FeS levels [104]. While the pathophysiology is still largely unknown, a recent study showed tissue specific deficiencies in BCS1L and Rieske FeS proteins in the liver, kidney, and heart tissues were associated with decreased levels of assembled complex III (Table 2) [108]. This pathology was identified only in kidney and liver samples, so despite cardiac tissue also having decreased levels/activity of complex III, there appears to still be adequate respiratory chain enzyme activity [107,108]. Given rapid mortality in these patients, treatment is often symptomatic or palliative [112]. Different methods have been implemented to attempt to correct acidosis without clear success [112]. One study in a mouse model of GRACILE syndrome found decreased survival in mice fed a high carbohydrate diet, despite improved levels of several amino acids and urea cycle intermediates [113].

3.7. Mitochondrial Neurogastrointestinal Encephalopathy (MNGIE)

Mitochondrial neurogastrointestinal encephalopathy (MNGIE) is an autosomal recessive disease of multiple organ systems characterized by chronic intestinal dysmotility, leukoencephalopathy, failure to thrive, ptosis, ophthalmoparesis, and peripheral neuropathy [114–116]. Gastrointestinal (GI) symptoms are the most prominent manifestation and include recurrent nausea, vomiting, diarrhea, abdominal pain, gastroparesis, and intestinal pseudo-obstruction with dymotility [117,118]. Brain leukoencephalopathy is present in nearly all cases, but is largely asymptomatic [119]. Brain MRI typically shows symmetric T2 hyperintensities of cerebral white matter [119]. Reported in only ~100 cases, patients classically present between the second and fifth decades of life and die in early adulthood as symptoms progress, with mean age at onset around 18 years of age and mean age at death of about 35 years [117,120,121]. One study found abnormal electrocardiogram (ECG) findings, with 16% of patients in one study demonstrating left ventricular hypertrophy (LVH), and there are single case reports of prolonged QT, cardiac arrest, and SVT (Table 1) [120,121].

MNGIE is caused by loss of function mutations to the thymidine phosphorylase (TP) gene located on chromosome 22q13.32-qter (Table 2) [116]. TP catabolizes thymidine to thymine and loss of enzymatic activity causes accumulation of thymidine and deoxyuridine creating an imbalance in reservoir of cellular nucleosides and nucleotides [117]. This results in impaired mitochondrial DNA replication that can lead to further deletions and mutations [122]. TP is expressed in the GI system, brain, peripheral nerves, spleen and bladder, [120] a distribution pattern that accounts for most clinical findings. Despite low expression in muscles, muscle biopsies show mitochondrial dysfunction with abnormal mtDNA, COX deficiency, and ragged-red fibers [120,121,123]. Given the variability of symptom severity and progression without clear correlation between genotype and phenotype, it is hypothesized that environmental factors and genetic modifiers may play a role in determining a patient's clinical course [121].

Relative to other mitochondrial diseases, significant advancements have been made towards the treatment of MNGIE, but early diagnosis and treatment is crucial to avoid disease progression and accumulation of mutations [124]. Given significant GI manifestations and malnutrition, preventative treatment with nutritional therapy is vital but challenging [125]. Allogeneic hematopoietic stem cell transplant has shown to be a viable treatment option [124,126–128]. Stem cell transplantation can restore TP activity and normalizes the pool of nucleotide and nucleoside [126,127]. Despite these molecular improvements, there remains a high complication rate in transplanted patients, with one study showing only 37.5% of patients alive at time of study follow up [128]. Other treatments that have been studied include platelet infusions, peritoneal dialysis, hemodialysis, and carrier erythrocyte entrapped recombinant TP all of which were shown to partially and temporarily restore TP activity levels to varying degrees [129–132]. Liver transplantation has succeeded in producing lasting restoration of TP activity and symptom improvement in a single case report, though further investigation is needed [133]. Gene therapy-based models for restoration of normal TP enzyme expression has been studied in murine models with promising initial findings [134].

3.8. Barth Syndrome

Barth syndrome, first described in 1983 by Dutch neurologist Dr. Peter Barth, [135] is an X-linked mitochondrial disorder causing congenital dilated cardiomyopathy, skeletal myopathy (predominantly proximal), neutropenia (can be intermittent), and growth retardation in young male infants [135–138]. Prevalence has been estimated to be approximately 1:300,000–400,000 live births, though this is likely an underestimation due to relatively high numbers of spontaneous abortions and still births of male fetuses observed in known Barth syndrome families [139,140]. Disease symptoms typically present within the first year of life with failure to thrive and cardiac abnormalities with or without severe infections, and some studies have even shown cardiac abnormalities in utero [141–143]. Mortality is highest within the first four years of life with most deaths due to either cardiac failure secondary to dilated cardiomyopathy or severe sepsis in the setting of neutropenia [136,137,143]. Reported overall survival rate is 49% at age 5, but this has been steadily increasing in recent years, improving from 20% in patients born before 2000 to 70% in patients born after 2000, likely due to increasing awareness leading to earlier diagnosis and treatment [143]. Despite the high mortality rates in childhood, patients can live into their late 40s (Table 1) [141].

As many as 91–94% of patients develop structural cardiac manifestations including dilated cardiomyopathy, endocardial fibroelastosis, or left-ventricular non-compaction (hypertrabeculation) [137,143–148]. Conduction abnormalities are also common and include prolonged QT, WPW, SVT, and ventricular tachyarrhythmias [143,146,147]. Neutropenia occurs in 70–84% of patients with variable severity and can be persistent or intermittent [148,149]. Elevations in urine 3-methylglutaconic acid and abnormally low cholesterol levels are less common but still present in a significant percentage of patients (Table 1) [143,147,150].

Barth syndrome is an X-lined recessive disorder caused by mutations in the G4.5 gene (TAZ gene) on Xq28, which encodes a highly conserved ascyltransferase (Table 2) [138,151,152]. The TAZ gene encodes an enzyme important in remodeling of cardiolipin [153,154]. Cardiolipin is exclusive to the mitochondrial membrane and plays a key role in proper structure and function of the mitochondria [153,155]. Loss of this enzyme leads to a relative excess of monolysocardiolipin. Measurement of monolysocardilipin/cardiolipin ratio is an important diagnostic test with high sensitivity and specificity for Barth syndrome [156,157]. Though there is currently no curative treatment for Barth syndrome, early recognition and diagnosis can allow for aggressive and prophylactic management [140,158]. Treatment entails typical heart-failure medication regimens and antibiotics during periods of neutropenia or infection [158]. Despite medical management, approximately 12% of patients require cardiac transplantation, with mean age 3.8 years at time of transplant [148].

3.9. Leber's Hereditary Optic Neuropathy (LHON)

This disorder was first described by Dr. Albrecht von Graefe in 1858, but was named after Dr. Theodore Leber who published a case series in 1871 of 15 patients from 4 families afflicted with LHON [159]. LHON classically presents as acute or subacute, painless vision loss typically in young adulthood although symptom onset varies widely and has been reported as early as 2 and as late as 87 years [160–163]. One study showed 11.5% of cases occurring before age 10 [161]. Vision loss typically starts in one eye starting with central vision loss and then progresses to the second eye often days to months later [162,163]. Vision loss is due to degeneration of retinal ganglion cells [164]. Other non-visual, neurologic clinical findings have been reported including: dystonia, peripheral neuropathy, resting tremor, wide spread multiple sclerosis-like white matter lesions and Leigh-like encephalopathy [165–172]. European studies have estimated the prevalence to be between 1:31,000–50,000 with a 80–90% of cases occurring in males [173–175]. Case reports have found left ventricular hypertrabeculation in patients with LHON [176,177]. Another study showed a statistically significant longer QTc in LHON subjects from one American family when compared to controls [178,179]. Other cardiac associations reported include WPW (~9% of LHON subjects) and myocardial thickening (Table 1) [177,179–181].

Approximately 90% cases are caused by one of three mtDNA mutations: G11778A (ND4 gene), G3460A (ND1 gene), and the T14484C (NG6 gene) all of which cause dysfunction in complex I of the mitochondrial respiratory chain (Table 2) [182–185]. Other mutations have been reported in rare cases [186–189]. A majority of mutation carriers do not develop clinical LHON, with 50% of male and 10% of female carriers affected [190]. The reason for this pattern is unclear, but several hypotheses of additional determining factors have emerged including varying levels of oxidative stress, environmental factors, mtDNA haplogroups, and hormones [191–195]. Earlier onset of symptoms and the 14484 mutation have relatively higher rates of spontaneous recovery of vision and are associated with better prognosis [196,197].

Several promising therapies are under investigation. A small, open-label, prospective trial looking at drug EPI-743, which targets glutathione production, showed arrest and reversal of disease progression in 4 of 5 subjects [198]. Some case reports, one double-blinded RCT, and one retrospective study have pointed to beneficial effects on vision with a strong antioxidant, idebenone [199–202]. Given the observed gender bias in disease penetration, studies have begun to investigate the role of estrogen-like molecules on LHON cell-lines with promising preliminary results [203]. A handful of gene-therapy clinical trials are currently underway after promising findings in pre-clinical trials with adeno-associated viral vectors, [204–208] but no studies have evaluated the efficacies of these treatment on cardiac manifestations of this disease.

3.10. Pearson Syndrome

Pearson syndrome (PS), first described by pediatric hematologist-oncologist Dr. Howard Pearson in 1979, is a rare disease affecting the liver, kidney, pancreas, bone marrow and CNS, and more rarely can present with cardiovascular findings. This disease presents initially with transfusion-dependent anemia that may improve, but affected patients develop increasingly severe infections [209]. Incidence was estimated to be roughly 1/1,000,000 in a case series of 11 Italian children, [209] and mortality was high with most infants dying by 3 years of age, [210] although later studies have reported survival of one patient to 6.6 years of age [209]. Multiple cases have been reported of both phenotypic and genetic transformation of the disease from PS to Leigh syndrome (with development of dysphagia, ataxia, peripheral neuropathy and ophthalmoparesis) [211,212] or Kearn's sayre syndrome (with development of progressive external ophtalmoplegia, retinopathy and ataxia) [212–215]. Cardiac abnormalities, while not hallmark symptoms of the disease, have been reported including increased ventricular wall thickness, depolarization abnormalities and prolonged QT. Mortality likely results from failure of other organ symptoms, as most patients die before any severe cardiac abnormalities can result (Table 1) [209].

Genetic deletions of mtDNA in this disorder is widely variable, and may account for why PS can transform into other mitochondrial spectrum disorders like Kearns Sayre Syndrome (KSS), progressive external ophthalmoplegia (PEO) or Leigh Syndrome (LS) [214]. In a study of 15 patients diagnosed with PS, large mitochondrial DNA deletions were typical, with 9 patients having 4.9 kb deletions and 6 having deletions ranging from 9 to 14 kb (Table 2) [210]. Treatment of this disease primarily involves treatment of anemia with transfusions, erythropoietin (EPO) or granulocyte colony stimulating factor (GCSF), and replacement of pancreatic enzymes has been reported in patients with exocrine pancreatic insufficiency [209].

3.11. Kearns–Sayre Syndrome

Kearns–Sayre syndrome (KSS) is a rare mitochondrial disorder that primarily affects the eyes among many other organs including the heart, was first reported by Dr. Kearns with a case series involving nine patients in 1965, and has more recently been described on the spectrum of PEO and PS [212–215]. Most patients with KSS develop the hallmark symptom of progressive external ophthalmoplegia which causes ptosis and weakness or paralysis of the muscles of the eye and some patients may also develop retinopathy [216]. Cardiac conduction defects are common, as are ataxia and abnormally high cerebrospinal fluid (CSF) protein levels (Table 1). This disorder is very rare, effecting only 1–3 per 100,000 individuals and are caused by large deletions in mtDNA ranging from 1000 to 10,000 base pairs that results in loss of genes involved in oxidative phosphorylation (Table 2) [216]. For cardiac manifestations, AV block is a common complication, with case reports of cardiac arrest and conduction abnormalities including complete heart block requiring permanent cardiac pacemaker implantation (Table 1) [217–220]. All patients with KSS or KSS spectrum disorders should be regularly screened with ECGs to monitor for progressive AV block, and there should be low threshold for monitoring in any KSS patient presenting with syncope.

3.12. Chronic Progressive External Ophthalmoplegia

First reported by Zeviani et al. in 1989, [221] chronic progressive external opthalmoplegia (PEO) is an inherited mitochondrial disorder characterized by loss of motor function of the muscles of the eye an eyelid [222–224]. Other associated symptoms include skeletal and cardiac myopathy and dysphagia (Table 1) [223]. Cardiac arrhythmias may also develop. PEO results from large scale mtDNA deletions can occur as part of a spectrum of other large deletion mitochondrial disorders including Kearns–Sayre syndrome [222,223] and Pearson Syndrome, [225–227] as mentioned above. Disease incidence of large mtDNA deletions ranges from 1.2–2.9/100,000 [228,229]. Autosomal dominant PEO [230] has also been reported with mutations reported to 3 nuclear encoded genes mutations have been identified in three nuclear encoded genes: *ANT1*, *C10orf2* and *POLG* (Table 2). As with KSS and other large deletion spectrum disorders, symptomatic supportive care remains the only treatment option [224].

3.13. Friederich's Ataxia

Friederich's ataxia (FA), first described by German physician Dr. Nikolaus Freiderich in 1863, is a neurodegenerative disease that presents with progressive ataxia and areflexia, and progressive life-threatening cardiomyopathy, and both hypertrophic and dilated cardiomyopathies have been reported [231,232]. FA has an incidence of 1–47:1,000,000 [233] that typically presents in childhood, with a mean life expectancy is 40 years of age [234]. About two-thirds of patients will die from cardiac causes (Table 1) [234–236]. FA is an autosomal recessive disease caused by expansion of DNA triplet intron repeat GAA in the frataxin (FXN) gene (Table 2) [233,234,237]. Frataxin is a protein found on the inner mitochondrial membrane and is involved in oxidative phosphorylation, and its deficiency can lead to decreased cellular ATP production and disruption of iron chelation within mitochondria [237]. Treatment relies on antioxidant therapy to reduce buildup of reactive oxygen species and decrease oxidative damage. One novel drug, idebenone, an antioxidant that is similar to coenzyme Q, has been suggested for treatment of FA cardiomyopathy early in disease course based on preclinical studies, [238] and has been shown in randomized blinded trial to reduce measures of cardiac hypertrophy in FA-cardiomyopathy patients [239].

4. Secondary Mitochondrial Myopathies

4.1. Mitochondrial Dysfunction in Ischemia

During myocardial infarction, rupture of an atherosclerotic plaque leads to occlusion of a coronary artery and downstream myocardial ischemia. Endocardial myocytes are the most sensitive to cardiac ischemia, as this segment of the myocardium has the highest imbalance of energy, with cell death starting as early as 20 minutes after occlusion of the infarct related artery [240]. The ischemic insult then moves transmurally from the endocardium to the epicardium. In the era of cardiac catheterization, prompt revascularization has served to rapidly restore blood flow to these damaged tissues, however the consequence of this early restoration of blood flow is reperfusion injury, which produces an additional wave of cell death after the primary insult. The combination of ischemia and reperfusion leaves individual cells in three states of injury: dead cardiomyocytes, reversibly injured cells, and hypoperfused but viable cardiomyocytes [240]. Prompt reperfusion has been successful at saving hypoperfused viable cardiomyocytes, but studies have shown that few reversibly injured cells are rescued after reperfusion [240,241]. Additionally, reperfusion causes a second wave of cell death from altered metabolism of cells damaged by ischemia-reperfusion injury, which results in destruction of mitochondria and release of excessive ROS into damaged cells [240–242]. In animal studies, as many as 38% of cell death results solely from the reperfusion phase of injury, [242] and reperfusion injury accounts for up to 50% of the final infarct size [241].

Damaged mitochondria can continue to propagate myocyte cell death through activation of programmed cell death pathways. Mitochondrial electron transport chains are damaged during the ischemic phase of injury [243]. This results in excessive production and release of ROSs, dysregulation of calcium handling, and abnormal mitochondrial swelling leads to mitochondrial membrane disruption by the mitochondrial permeability transition pore in the inner mitochondrial membrane, [244–246] or via mitochondrial outer membrane permeabilization [246]. Formation of these pore complexes leads to release of toxic mitochondrial ROSs and proteins that activate programmed cell death mechanisms [240,242–244,246,247]. Thus, widespread cell death occurs in several stages following coronary artery occlusion, resulting from the ischemic phase, reperfusion phase, and mitochondrial dysfunction phase resulting in cell death both through necrosis and activation of programmed cell death pathways [240,242,244,247].

4.2. Mitochondrial Dysfunction in Diabetic Cardiomyopathy

There is growing clinical and preclinical evidence that mitochondrial dysfunction is central to cardiomyopathy observed in diabetic patients [248]. The pathogenesis of mitochondrial dysfunction in diabetes may be similar to that of ischemia-reperfusion, but the exact molecular mechanisms of this dysfunction remain poorly understood [248]. Clinically, diabetic cardiomyopathy was first described over 40 years ago in a case series of four patients with heart failure and diabetes, but with normal coronary arteries [249]. Subsequent studies have confirmed these observations [250,251] and more recent studies estimate the prevalence of diastolic heart failure in as many as 60% of type 2 diabetics [252]. While the exact molecular mechanisms of diabetic cardiomyopathy remains unknown, it is likely a multifactorial process involving disruption of normal respiration via the electron transport chain. This leads to increased ROS production and disrupted fatty acid oxidation.

As outlined by the mitochondrial free radial theory of aging, higher levels of ROS lead to hydroxylation and damage of cellular peptides and lipids [248]. These pathologic changes also result in impaired respiration. Normal hearts primarily generate ATP from mitochondrial fatty acid oxidation (60–70% of ATP generated) and less so from glucose, lactate or other substrates (30–40%) [248,253]. However, in the diabetic hearts, mitochondria are more reliant on fatty acid oxidation and suffer from impaired mitophagy, with greater inability to break down oxidative fatty acids, further perpetuating accumulation of oxygen free radical species. This disrupts mitochondrial calcium handling and myocardial E-C coupling, and elevated levels of cellular ROS can lead to disrupted mitochondrial biogenesis, increased mitochondrial permeability and ultimately increased cell death [248].

5. Conclusions

In this review, we seek to improve clinician awareness and recognition of mitochondrial disorders affecting the cardiovascular system. Because of the wide variability of presentations and their relative infrequency in the global population, recognition and diagnosis of these disorders can be challenging. Treatment options for primary mitochondrial diseases are limited and primarily involve support care, although some early studies suggest a role for antioxidant therapy. Future research will be needed to discover novel therapeutic approaches to advance our care of these diseases, including breakthroughs in gene therapy and improved understanding of the genetic expression and penetrance of these mutations. It is our hope that with better recognition of these disorders by clinicians that we can improve diagnosis of these disorders and advance long-term patient care and research into new and more viable treatment options.

Author Contributions: Conceptualization, E.A and J.D.; Writing-original draft preparation, A.M. and J.D.; Writing-review and editing, E.A. and J.D.; Supervision, E.A.

References

1.   Meyers, D.E.; Basha, H.I.; Koenig, M.K. Cardiac manifestations of mitochondrial disorders. *Tex. Heart Inst. J.* **2013**, *40*, 635–636. [PubMed]

2. Meyers, D.E.; Basha, H.I.; Koenig, M.K. Mitochondrial cardiomyopathy: Pathophysiology, diagnosis, and management. *Tex. Heart Inst. J.* **2013**, *40*, 385–394.

3. Chinnery, P.F.; Elliott, H.R.; Hudson, G.; Samuels, D.C.; Relton, C.L. Epigenetics, epidemiology and mitochondrial DNA diseases. *Int. J. Epidemiol.* **2012**, *41*, 177–187. [CrossRef] [PubMed]

4. Elliott, H.R.; Samuels, D.C.; Eden, J.A.; Relton, C.L.; Chinnery, P.F. Pathogenic mitochondrial DNA mutations are common in the general population. *Am. J. Hum. Genet.* **2008**, *83*, 254–260. [CrossRef] [PubMed]

5. Debray, F.G.; Lambert, M.; Chevalier, I.; Robitaille, Y.; Decarie, J.C.; Shoubridge, E.A.; Robinson, B.H.; Mitchell, G.A. Long-term outcome and clinical spectrum of 73 pediatric patients with mitochondrial diseases. *Pediatrics* **2007**, *119*, 722–733. [CrossRef] [PubMed]

6. Anan, R.; Nakagawa, M.; Miyata, M.; Higuchi, I.; Nakao, S.; Suehara, M.; Osame, M.; Tanaka, H. Cardiac involvement in mitochondrial diseases. A study on 17 patients with documented mitochondrial DNA defects. *Circulation* **1995**, *91*, 955–961. [CrossRef] [PubMed]

7. Lane, N. Evolution. The costs of breathing. *Science* **2011**, *334*, 184–185. [CrossRef] [PubMed]

8. Wallace, D.C. Why do we still have a maternally inherited mitochondrial DNA? Insights from evolutionary medicine. *Annu. Rev. Biochem.* **2007**, *76*, 781–821. [CrossRef]

9. Hirano, M.; Davidson, M.; DiMauro, S. Mitochondria and the heart. *Curr. Opin. Cardiol.* **2001**, *16*, 201–210. [CrossRef]

10. Holmgren, D.; Wahlander, H.; Eriksson, B.O.; Oldfors, A.; Holme, E.; Tulinius, M. Cardiomyopathy in children with mitochondrial disease; clinical course and cardiological findings. *Eur. Heart J.* **2003**, *24*, 280–288. [CrossRef]

11. Tocchi, A.; Quarles, E.K.; Basisty, N.; Gitari, L.; Rabinovitch, P.S. Mitochondrial dysfunction in cardiac aging. *Biochim. Biophys. Acta* **2015**, *1847*, 1424–1433. [CrossRef] [PubMed]

12. Bratic, A.; Larsson, N.G. The role of mitochondria in aging. *J. Clin. Investig.* **2013**, *123*, 951–957. [CrossRef]

13. Stadtman, E.R. Protein oxidation and aging. *Science* **1992**, *257*, 1220–1224. [CrossRef] [PubMed]

14. Balaban, R.S.; Nemoto, S.; Finkel, T. Mitochondria, oxidants, and aging. *Cell* **2005**, *120*, 483–495. [CrossRef] [PubMed]

15. Trifunovic, A.; Larsson, N.G. Mitochondrial dysfunction as a cause of ageing. *J. Intern. Med.* **2008**, *263*, 167–178. [CrossRef] [PubMed]

16. Trounce, I.; Byrne, E.; Marzuki, S. Decline in skeletal muscle mitochondrial respiratory chain function: Possible factor in ageing. *Lancet* **1989**, *1*, 637–639. [CrossRef]

17. Kujoth, G.C.; Hiona, A.; Pugh, T.D.; Someya, S.; Panzer, K.; Wohlgemuth, S.E.; Hofer, T.; Seo, A.Y.; Sullivan, R.; Jobling, W.A.; et al. Mitochondrial DNA mutations, oxidative stress, and apoptosis in mammalian aging. *Science* **2005**, *309*, 481–484. [CrossRef]

18. Koga, H.; Kaushik, S.; Cuervo, A.M. Protein homeostasis and aging: The importance of exquisite quality control. *Ageing Res. Rev.* **2011**, *10*, 205–215. [CrossRef]

19. Abbas, A.; Grant, P.J.; Kearney, M.T. Role of IGF-1 in glucose regulation and cardiovascular disease. *Expert Rev. Cardiovasc. Ther.* **2008**, *6*, 1135–1149. [CrossRef]

20. Puglielli, L. Aging of the brain, neurotrophin signaling, and Alzheimer's disease: Is IGF1-R the common culprit? *Neurobiol. Aging* **2008**, *29*, 795–811. [CrossRef]

21. Dai, D.F.; Karunadharma, P.P.; Chiao, Y.A.; Basisty, N.; Crispin, D.; Hsieh, E.J.; Chen, T.; Gu, H.; Djukovic, D.; Raftery, D.; et al. Altered proteome turnover and remodeling by short-term caloric restriction or rapamycin rejuvenate the aging heart. *Aging Cell* **2014**, *13*, 529–539. [CrossRef]

22. Johnson, S.C.; Rabinovitch, P.S.; Kaeberlein, M. mTOR is a key modulator of ageing and age-related disease. *Nature* **2013**, *493*, 338–345. [CrossRef]

23. Pavlakis, S.G.; Phillips, P.C.; DiMauro, S.; De Vivo, D.C.; Rowland, L.P. Mitochondrial myopathy, encephalopathy, lactic acidosis, and strokelike episodes: A distinctive clinical syndrome. *Ann. Neurol.* **1984**, *16*, 481–488. [CrossRef]

24. Yatsuga, S.; Povalko, N.; Nishioka, J.; Katayama, K.; Kakimoto, N.; Matsuishi, T.; Kakuma, T.; Koga, Y.; Taro Matsuoka for, M.S.G.i.J. MELAS: A nationwide prospective cohort study of 96 patients in Japan. *Biochim. Biophys. Acta* **2012**, *1820*, 619–624. [CrossRef]

25. Goto, Y.; Horai, S.; Matsuoka, T.; Koga, Y.; Nihei, K.; Kobayashi, M.; Nonaka, I. Mitochondrial myopathy, encephalopathy, lactic acidosis, and stroke-like episodes (MELAS): A correlative study of the clinical features and mitochondrial DNA mutation. *Neurology* **1992**, *42*, 545–550. [CrossRef]

26. Hirano, M.; Ricci, E.; Koenigsberger, M.R.; Defendini, R.; Pavlakis, S.G.; DeVivo, D.C.; DiMauro, S.; Rowland, L.P. Melas: An original case and clinical criteria for diagnosis. *Neuromuscul. Disord.* **1992**, *2*, 125–135. [CrossRef]

27. Zhang, J.; Guo, J.; Fang, W.; Jun, Q.; Shi, K. Clinical features of MELAS and its relation with A3243G gene point mutation. *Int. J. Clin. Exp. Pathol.* **2015**, *8*, 13411–13415.

28. Mancuso, M.; Orsucci, D.; Angelini, C.; Bertini, E.; Carelli, V.; Comi, G.P.; Donati, A.; Minetti, C.; Moggio, M.; Mongini, T.; et al. The m.3243A>G mitochondrial DNA mutation and related phenotypes. A matter of gender? *J. Neurol.* **2014**, *261*, 504–510. [CrossRef] [PubMed]

29. Okajima, Y.; Tanabe, Y.; Takayanagi, M.; Aotsuka, H. A follow up study of myocardial involvement in patients with mitochondrial encephalomyopathy, lactic acidosis, and stroke-like episodes (MELAS). *Heart* **1998**, *80*, 292–295. [CrossRef] [PubMed]

30. Sproule, D.M.; Kaufmann, P.; Engelstad, K.; Starc, T.J.; Hordof, A.J.; De Vivo, D.C. Wolff-Parkinson-White syndrome in Patients With MELAS. *Arch. Neurol.* **2007**, *64*, 1625–1627. [CrossRef] [PubMed]

31. El-Hattab, A.W.; Adesina, A.M.; Jones, J.; Scaglia, F. MELAS syndrome: Clinical manifestations, pathogenesis, and treatment options. *Mol. Genet. Metab.* **2015**, *116*, 4–12. [CrossRef]

32. Lott, M.T.; Leipzig, J.N.; Derbeneva, O.; Xie, H.M.; Chalkia, D.; Sarmady, M.; Procaccio, V.; Wallace, D.C. mtDNA Variation and Analysis Using Mitomap and Mitomaster. *Curr. Protoc. Bioinformat.* **2013**, *44*, 1–23.

33. El-Hattab, A.W.; Emrick, L.T.; Hsu, J.W.; Chanprasert, S.; Almannai, M.; Craigen, W.J.; Jahoor, F.; Scaglia, F. Impaired nitric oxide production in children with MELAS syndrome and the effect of arginine and citrulline supplementation. *Mol. Genet. Metab.* **2016**, *117*, 407–412. [CrossRef]

34. Ganetzky, R.D.; Falk, M.J. 8-year retrospective analysis of intravenous arginine therapy for acute metabolic strokes in pediatric mitochondrial disease. *Mol. Genet. Metab.* **2018**, *123*, 301–308. [CrossRef]

35. El-Hattab, A.W.; Emrick, L.T.; Williamson, K.C.; Craigen, W.J.; Scaglia, F. The effect of citrulline and arginine supplementation on lactic acidemia in MELAS syndrome. *Meta Gene* **2013**, *1*, 8–14. [CrossRef]

36. El-Hattab, A.W.; Zarante, A.M.; Almannai, M.; Scaglia, F. Therapies for mitochondrial diseases and current clinical trials. *Mol. Genet. Metab.* **2017**, *122*, 1–9. [CrossRef]

37. Steriade, C.; Andrade, D.M.; Faghfoury, H.; Tarnopolsky, M.A.; Tai, P. Mitochondrial encephalopathy with lactic acidosis and stroke-like episodes (MELAS) may respond to adjunctive ketogenic diet. *Pediatr. Neurol.* **2014**, *50*, 498–502. [CrossRef]

38. Rodriguez, M.C.; MacDonald, J.R.; Mahoney, D.J.; Parise, G.; Beal, M.F.; Tarnopolsky, M.A. Beneficial effects of creatine, CoQ10, and lipoic acid in mitochondrial disorders. *Muscle Nerve* **2007**, *35*, 235–242. [CrossRef]

39. Leigh, D. Subacute necrotizing encephalomyelopathy in an infant. *J. Neurol. Neurosurg. Psychiatry* **1951**, *14*, 216–221. [CrossRef]

40. Rahman, S.; Blok, R.B.; Dahl, H.H.; Danks, D.M.; Kirby, D.M.; Chow, C.W.; Christodoulou, J.; Thorburn, D.R. Leigh syndrome: Clinical features and biochemical and DNA abnormalities. *Ann. Neurol.* **1996**, *39*, 343–351. [CrossRef]

41. Darin, N.; Oldfors, A.; Moslemi, A.R.; Holme, E.; Tulinius, M. The incidence of mitochondrial encephalomyopathies in childhood: Clinical features and morphological, biochemical, and DNA abnormalities. *Ann. Neurol.* **2001**, *49*, 377–383. [CrossRef] [PubMed]

42. Lee, H.F.; Tsai, C.R.; Chi, C.S.; Lee, H.J.; Chen, C.C. Leigh syndrome: Clinical and neuroimaging follow-up. *Pediatr. Neurol.* **2009**, *40*, 88–93. [CrossRef] [PubMed]

43. Sofou, K.; De Coo, I.F.; Isohanni, P.; Ostergaard, E.; Naess, K.; De Meirleir, L.; Tzoulis, C.; Uusimaa, J.; De Angst, I.B.; Lonnqvist, T.; et al. A multicenter study on Leigh syndrome: Disease course and predictors of survival. *Orphanet J. Rare Dis.* **2014**, *9*, 52. [CrossRef] [PubMed]

44. Huntsman, R.J.; Sinclair, D.B.; Bhargava, R.; Chan, A. Atypical presentations of leigh syndrome: A case series and review. *Pediatr. Neurol.* **2005**, *32*, 334–340. [CrossRef] [PubMed]

45. Bonfante, E.; Koenig, M.K.; Adejumo, R.B.; Perinjelil, V.; Riascos, R.F. The neuroimaging of Leigh syndrome: Case series and review of the literature. *Pediatr. Radiol.* **2016**, *46*, 443–451. [CrossRef] [PubMed]

46. Sonam, K.; Khan, N.A.; Bindu, P.S.; Taly, A.B.; Gayathri, N.; Bharath, M.M.; Govindaraju, C.; Arvinda, H.R.; Nagappa, M.; Sinha, S.; et al. Clinical and magnetic resonance imaging findings in patients with Leigh syndrome and SURF1 mutations. *Brain Dev.* **2014**, *36*, 807–812. [CrossRef]

47. Hadzsiev, K.; Maasz, A.; Kisfali, P.; Kalman, E.; Gomori, E.; Pal, E.; Berenyi, E.; Komlosi, K.; Melegh, B. Mitochondrial DNA 11777C>A mutation associated Leigh syndrome: Case report with a review of the previously described pedigrees. *Neuromol. Med.* **2010**, *12*, 277–284. [CrossRef]

48. Wang, S.B.; Weng, W.C.; Lee, N.C.; Hwu, W.L.; Fan, P.C.; Lee, W.T. Mutation of mitochondrial DNA G13513A presenting with Leigh syndrome, Wolff-Parkinson-White syndrome and cardiomyopathy. *Pediatr. Neonatol.* **2008**, *49*, 145–149. [CrossRef]

49. Pequignot, M.O.; Dey, R.; Zeviani, M.; Tiranti, V.; Godinot, C.; Poyau, A.; Sue, C.; Di Mauro, S.; Abitbol, M.; Marsac, C. Mutations in the SURF1 gene associated with Leigh syndrome and cytochrome C oxidase deficiency. *Hum. Mutat.* **2001**, *17*, 374–381. [CrossRef]

50. Yang, Y.L.; Sun, F.; Zhang, Y.; Qian, N.; Yuan, Y.; Wang, Z.X.; Qi, Y.; Xiao, J.X.; Wang, X.Y.; Qi, Z.Y.; et al. Clinical and laboratory survey of 65 Chinese patients with Leigh syndrome. *Chin. Med. J.* **2006**, *119*, 373–377. [CrossRef]

51. Tiranti, V.; Hoertnagel, K.; Carrozzo, R.; Galimberti, C.; Munaro, M.; Granatiero, M.; Zelante, L.; Gasparini, P.; Marzella, R.; Rocchi, M.; et al. Mutations of SURF-1 in Leigh disease associated with cytochrome c oxidase deficiency. *Am. J. Hum. Genet.* **1998**, *63*, 1609–1621. [CrossRef]

52. Moslemi, A.R.; Tulinius, M.; Darin, N.; Aman, P.; Holme, E.; Oldfors, A. SURF1 gene mutations in three cases with Leigh syndrome and cytochrome c oxidase deficiency. *Neurology* **2003**, *61*, 991–993. [CrossRef]

53. Poyau, A.; Buchet, K.; Bouzidi, M.F.; Zabot, M.T.; Echenne, B.; Yao, J.; Shoubridge, E.A.; Godinot, C. Missense mutations in SURF1 associated with deficient cytochrome c oxidase assembly in Leigh syndrome patients. *Hum. Genet.* **2000**, *106*, 194–205. [CrossRef]

54. Gerards, M.; Kamps, R.; van Oevelen, J.; Boesten, I.; Jongen, E.; de Koning, B.; Scholte, H.R.; de Angst, I.; Schoonderwoerd, K.; Sefiani, A.; et al. Exome sequencing reveals a novel Moroccan founder mutation in SLC19A3 as a new cause of early-childhood fatal Leigh syndrome. *Brain* **2013**, *136*, 882–890. [CrossRef] [PubMed]

55. Fukuhara, N.; Tokiguchi, S.; Shirakawa, K.; Tsubaki, T. Myoclonus epilepsy associated with ragged-red fibres (mitochondrial abnormalities): Disease entity or a syndrome? Light-and electron-microscopic studies of two cases and review of literature. *J. Neurol. Sci.* **1980**, *47*, 117–133. [CrossRef]

56. Shoffner, J.M.; Lott, M.T.; Lezza, A.M.; Seibel, P.; Ballinger, S.W.; Wallace, D.C. Myoclonic epilepsy and ragged-red fiber disease (MERRF) is associated with a mitochondrial DNA tRNA(Lys) mutation. *Cell* **1990**, *61*, 931–937. [CrossRef]

57. Fang, W.; Huang, C.C.; Chu, N.S.; Lee, C.C.; Chen, R.S.; Pang, C.Y.; Shih, K.D.; Wei, Y.H. Myoclonic epilepsy with ragged-red fibers (MERRF) syndrome: Report of a Chinese family with mitochondrial DNA point mutation in tRNA(Lys) gene. *Muscle Nerve* **1994**, *17*, 52–57. [CrossRef]

58. Lorenzoni, P.J.; Scola, R.H.; Kay, C.S.; Arndt, R.C.; Silvado, C.E.; Werneck, L.C. MERRF: Clinical features, muscle biopsy and molecular genetics in Brazilian patients. *Mitochondrion* **2011**, *11*, 528–532. [CrossRef] [PubMed]

59. Ozawa, M.; Goto, Y.; Sakuta, R.; Tanno, Y.; Tsuji, S.; Nonaka, I. The 8,344 mutation in mitochondrial DNA: A comparison between the proportion of mutant DNA and clinico-pathologic findings. *Neuromuscul. Disord.* **1995**, *5*, 483–488. [CrossRef]

60. Santorelli, F.M.; Mak, S.C.; El-Schahawi, M.; Casali, C.; Shanske, S.; Baram, T.Z.; Madrid, R.E.; DiMauro, S. Maternally inherited cardiomyopathy and hearing loss associated with a novel mutation in the mitochondrial tRNA(Lys) gene (G8363A). *Am. J. Hum. Genet.* **1996**, *58*, 933–939.

61. Catteruccia, M.; Sauchelli, D.; Della Marca, G.; Primiano, G.; Cuccagna, C.; Bernardo, D.; Leo, M.; Camporeale, A.; Sanna, T.; Cianfoni, A.; et al. "Myo-cardiomyopathy" is commonly associated with the A8344G "MERRF" mutation. *J. Neurol.* **2015**, *262*, 701–710. [CrossRef]

62. Silvestri, G.; Moraes, C.T.; Shanske, S.; Oh, S.J.; DiMauro, S. A new mtDNA mutation in the tRNA(Lys) gene associated with myoclonic epilepsy and ragged-red fibers (MERRF). *Am. J. Hum. Genet.* **1992**, *51*, 1213–1217.

63. van den Ouweland, J.M.; Lemkes, H.H.; Ruitenbeek, W.; Sandkuijl, L.A.; de Vijlder, M.F.; Struyvenberg, P.A.; van de Kamp, J.J.; Maassen, J.A. Mutation in mitochondrial tRNA(Leu)(UUR) gene in a large pedigree with maternally transmitted type II diabetes mellitus and deafness. *Nat. Genet.* **1992**, *1*, 368–371. [CrossRef]

64. Maassen, J.A.; Janssen, G.M.; 't Hart, L.M. Molecular mechanisms of mitochondrial diabetes (MIDD). *Ann. Med.* **2005**, *37*, 213–221. [CrossRef] [PubMed]

65. Murphy, R.; Turnbull, D.M.; Walker, M.; Hattersley, A.T. Clinical features, diagnosis and management of maternally inherited diabetes and deafness (MIDD) associated with the 3243A>G mitochondrial point mutation. *Diabet. Med.* **2008**, *25*, 383–399. [CrossRef] [PubMed]

66. Guillausseau, P.J.; Massin, P.; Dubois-LaForgue, D.; Timsit, J.; Virally, M.; Gin, H.; Bertin, E.; Blickle, J.F.; Bouhanick, B.; Cahen, J.; et al. Maternally inherited diabetes and deafness: A multicenter study. *Ann. Intern. Med.* **2001**, *134*, 721–728. [CrossRef]

67. Suzuki, S.; Oka, Y.; Kadowaki, T.; Kanatsuka, A.; Kuzuya, T.; Kobayashi, M.; Sanke, T.; Seino, Y.; Nanjo, K.; Society, R.C.o.S.T.o.D.M.w.G.M.o.t.J.D. Clinical features of diabetes mellitus with the mitochondrial DNA 3243 (A-G) mutation in Japanese: Maternal inheritance and mitochondria-related complications. *Diabetes Res. Clin. Pract.* **2003**, *59*, 207–217. [CrossRef]

68. Zhu, J.; Yang, P.; Liu, X.; Yan, L.; Rampersad, S.; Li, F.; Li, H.; Sheng, C.; Cheng, X.; Zhang, M.; et al. The clinical characteristics of patients with mitochondrial tRNA Leu(UUR)m.3243A > G mutation: Compared with type 1 diabetes and early onset type 2 diabetes. *J. Diabetes Complicat.* **2017**, *31*, 1354–1359. [CrossRef]

69. Guillausseau, P.J.; Dubois-Laforgue, D.; Massin, P.; Laloi-Michelin, M.; Bellanné-Chantelot, C.; Gin, H.; Bertin, E.; Blickle, J.F.; Bauduceau, B.; Bouhanick, B.; et al. Heterogeneity of diabetes phenotype in patients with 3243 bp mutation of mitochondrial DNA (Maternally Inherited Diabetes and Deafness or MIDD). *Diabetes Metab.* **2004**, *30*, 181–186. [CrossRef]

70. Whittaker, R.G.; Schaefer, A.M.; McFarland, R.; Taylor, R.W.; Walker, M.; Turnbull, D.M. Prevalence and progression of diabetes in mitochondrial disease. *Diabetologia* **2007**, *50*, 2085–2089. [CrossRef] [PubMed]

71. Smith, P.R.; Bain, S.C.; Good, P.A.; Hattersley, A.T.; Barnett, A.H.; Gibson, J.M.; Dodson, P.M. Pigmentary retinal dystrophy and the syndrome of maternally inherited diabetes and deafness caused by the mitochondrial DNA 3243 tRNA(Leu) A to G mutation. *Ophthalmology* **1999**, *106*, 1101–1108. [CrossRef]

72. Narbonne, H.; Paquis-Fluckinger, V.; Valero, R.; Heyries, L.; Pellissier, J.F.; Vialettes, B. Gastrointestinal tract symptoms in Maternally Inherited Diabetes and Deafness (MIDD). *Diabetes Metab.* **2004**, *30*, 61–66. [CrossRef]

73. Robberecht, K.; Decock, C.; Stevens, A.; Seneca, S.; De Bleecker, J.; Leroy, B.P. Ptosis as an associated finding in maternally inherited diabetes and deafness. *Ophthalmic Genet.* **2010**, *31*, 240–243. [CrossRef] [PubMed]

74. Lien, L.M.; Lee, H.C.; Wang, K.L.; Chiu, J.C.; Chiu, H.C.; Wei, Y.H. Involvement of nervous system in maternally inherited diabetes and deafness (MIDD) with the A3243G mutation of mitochondrial DNA. *Acta Neurol. Scand.* **2001**, *103*, 159–165. [CrossRef]

75. Aggarwal, P.; Gill-Randall, R.; Wheatley, T.; Buchalter, M.B.; Metcalfe, J.; Alcolado, J.C. Identification of mtDNA mutation in a pedigree with gestational diabetes, deafness, Wolff-Parkinson-White syndrome and placenta accreta. *Hum. Hered.* **2001**, *51*, 114–116. [CrossRef]

76. Majamaa-Voltti, K.; Peuhkurinen, K.; Kortelainen, M.L.; Hassinen, I.E.; Majamaa, K. Cardiac abnormalities in patients with mitochondrial DNA mutation 3243A>G. *BMC Cardiovasc. Disord.* **2002**, *2*, 12. [CrossRef]

77. Azevedo, O.; Vilarinho, L.; Almeida, F.; Ferreira, F.; Guardado, J.; Ferreira, M.; Lourenço, A.; Medeiros, R.; Almeida, J. Cardiomyopathy and kidney disease in a patient with maternally inherited diabetes and deafness caused by the 3243A>G mutation of mitochondrial DNA. *Cardiology* **2010**, *115*, 71–74. [CrossRef] [PubMed]

78. Momiyama, Y.; Suzuki, Y.; Ohtomo, M.; Atsumi, Y.; Matsuoka, K.; Ohsuzu, F.; Kimura, M. Cardiac autonomic nervous dysfunction in diabetic patients with a mitochondrial DNA mutation: Assessment by heart rate variability. *Diabetes Care* **2002**, *25*, 2308–2313. [CrossRef]

79. Tabebi, M.; Charfi, N.; Kallabi, F.; Alila-Fersi, O.; Ben Mahmoud, A.; Tlili, A.; Keskes-Ammar, L.; Kamoun, H.; Abid, M.; Mnif, M.; et al. Whole mitochondrial genome screening of a family with maternally inherited diabetes and deafness (MIDD) associated with retinopathy: A putative haplotype associated to MIDD and a novel MT-CO2 m.8241T>G mutation. *J. Diabetes Complicat.* **2017**, *31*, 253–259. [CrossRef] [PubMed]

80. Maassen, J.A.; 'T Hart, L.M.; Van Essen, E.; Heine, R.J.; Nijpels, G.; Jahangir Tafrechi, R.S.; Raap, A.K.; Janssen, G.M.; Lemkes, H.H. Mitochondrial diabetes: Molecular mechanisms and clinical presentation. *Diabetes* **2004**, *53* (Suppl. 1), S103–S109. [CrossRef]

81. Sinnathuray, A.R.; Raut, V.; Awa, A.; Magee, A.; Toner, J.G. A review of cochlear implantation in mitochondrial sensorineural hearing loss. *Otol. Neurotol.* **2003**, *24*, 418–426. [CrossRef]

82. Salles, J.E.; Moisés, V.A.; Almeida, D.R.; Chacra, A.R.; Moisés, R.S. Myocardial dysfunction in mitochondrial diabetes treated with Coenzyme Q10. *Diabetes Res. Clin. Pract.* **2006**, *72*, 100–103. [CrossRef]

83.   Suzuki, S.; Hinokio, Y.; Ohtomo, M.; Hirai, M.; Hirai, A.; Chiba, M.; Kasuga, S.; Satoh, Y.; Akai, H.; Toyota, T. The effects of coenzyme Q10 treatment on maternally inherited diabetes mellitus and deafness, and mitochondrial DNA 3243 (A to G) mutation. *Diabetologia* **1998**, *41*, 584–588. [CrossRef]

84.   Holt, I.J.; Harding, A.E.; Petty, R.K.; Morgan-Hughes, J.A. A new mitochondrial disease associated with mitochondrial DNA heteroplasmy. *Am. J. Hum. Genet.* **1990**, *46*, 428–433.

85.   Fryer, A.; Appleton, R.; Sweeney, M.G.; Rosenbloom, L.; Harding, A.E. Mitochondrial DNA 8993 (NARP) mutation presenting with a heterogeneous phenotype including 'cerebral palsy'. *Arch. Dis. Child.* **1994**, *71*, 419–422. [CrossRef]

86.   Porto, F.B.; Mack, G.; Sterboul, M.J.; Lewin, P.; Flament, J.; Sahel, J.; Dollfus, H. Isolated late-onset cone-rod dystrophy revealing a familial neurogenic muscle weakness, ataxia, and retinitis pigmentosa syndrome with the T8993G mitochondrial mutation. *Am. J. Ophthalmol.* **2001**, *132*, 935–937. [CrossRef]

87.   Jonckheere, A.I.; Smeitink, J.A.; Rodenburg, R.J. Mitochondrial ATP synthase: Architecture, function and pathology. *J. Inherit. Metab. Dis.* **2012**, *35*, 211–225. [CrossRef]

88.   White, S.L.; Collins, V.R.; Wolfe, R.; Cleary, M.A.; Shanske, S.; DiMauro, S.; Dahl, H.H.; Thorburn, D.R. Genetic counseling and prenatal diagnosis for the mitochondrial DNA mutations at nucleotide 8993. *Am. J. Hum. Genet.* **1999**, *65*, 474–482. [CrossRef]

89.   López-Gallardo, E.; Solano, A.; Herrero-Martín, M.D.; Martínez-Romero, I.; Castaño-Pérez, M.D.; Andreu, A.L.; Herrera, A.; López-Pérez, M.J.; Ruiz-Pesini, E.; Montoya, J. NARP syndrome in a patient harbouring an insertion in the MT-ATP6 gene that results in a truncated protein. *J. Med. Genet.* **2009**, *46*, 64–67. [CrossRef]

90.   Sciacco, M.; Prelle, A.; D'Adda, E.; Lamperti, C.; Bordoni, A.; Rango, M.; Crimi, M.; Comi, G.P.; Bresolin, N.; Moggio, M. Familial mtDNA T8993C transition causing both the NARP and the MILS phenotype in the same generation. A morphological, genetic and spectroscopic study. *J. Neurol.* **2003**, *250*, 1498–1500. [CrossRef]

91.   Childs, A.M.; Hutchin, T.; Pysden, K.; Highet, L.; Bamford, J.; Livingston, J.; Crow, Y.J. Variable phenotype including Leigh syndrome with a 9185T>C mutation in the MTATP6 gene. *Neuropediatrics* **2007**, *38*, 313–316. [CrossRef]

92.   Tatuch, Y.; Christodoulou, J.; Feigenbaum, A.; Clarke, J.T.; Wherret, J.; Smith, C.; Rudd, N.; Petrova-Benedict, R.; Robinson, B.H. Heteroplasmic mtDNA mutation (T——G) at 8993 can cause Leigh disease when the percentage of abnormal mtDNA is high. *Am. J. Hum. Genet.* **1992**, *50*, 852–858.

93.   D'Aurelio, M.; Vives-Bauza, C.; Davidson, M.M.; Manfredi, G. Mitochondrial DNA background modifies the bioenergetics of NARP/MILS ATP6 mutant cells. *Hum. Mol. Genet.* **2010**, *19*, 374–386. [CrossRef]

94.   Claeys, K.G.; Abicht, A.; Häusler, M.; Kleinle, S.; Wiesmann, M.; Schulz, J.B.; Horvath, R.; Weis, J. Novel genetic and neuropathological insights in neurogenic muscle weakness, ataxia, and retinitis pigmentosa (NARP). *Muscle Nerve* **2016**, *54*, 328–333. [CrossRef]

95.   Kara, B.; Arıkan, M.; Maraş, H.; Abacı, N.; Cakırıs, A.; Ustek, D. Whole mitochondrial genome analysis of a family with NARP/MILS caused by m.8993T>C mutation in the MT-ATP6 gene. *Mol. Genet. Metab.* **2012**, *107*, 389–393. [CrossRef]

96.   Limongelli, G.; Tome-Esteban, M.; Dejthevaporn, C.; Rahman, S.; Hanna, M.G.; Elliott, P.M. Prevalence and natural history of heart disease in adults with primary mitochondrial respiratory chain disease. *Eur. J. Heart Fail.* **2010**, *12*, 114–121. [CrossRef]

97.   Pastores, G.M.; Santorelli, F.M.; Shanske, S.; Gelb, B.D.; Fyfe, B.; Wolfe, D.; Willner, J.P. Leigh syndrome and hypertrophic cardiomyopathy in an infant with a mitochondrial DNA point mutation (T8993G). *Am. J. Med. Genet.* **1994**, *50*, 265–271. [CrossRef]

98.   Duno, M.; Wibrand, F.; Baggesen, K.; Rosenberg, T.; Kjaer, N.; Frederiksen, A.L. A novel mitochondrial mutation m.8989G>C associated with neuropathy, ataxia, retinitis pigmentosa—The NARP syndrome. *Gene* **2013**, *515*, 372–375. [CrossRef]

99.   Mordel, P.; Schaeffer, S.; Dupas, Q.; Laville, M.A.; Gérard, M.; Chapon, F.; Allouche, S. A 2 bp deletion in the mitochondrial ATP 6 gene responsible for the NARP (neuropathy, ataxia, and retinitis pigmentosa) syndrome. *Biochem. Biophys. Res. Commun.* **2017**, *494*, 133–137. [CrossRef]

100. Blanco-Grau, A.; Bonaventura-Ibars, I.; Coll-Cantí, J.; Melià, M.J.; Martinez, R.; Martínez-Gallo, M.; Andreu, A.L.; Pinós, T.; García-Arumí, E. Identification and biochemical characterization of the novel mutation m.8839G>C in the mitochondrial ATP6 gene associated with NARP syndrome. *Genes Brain Behav.* **2013**, *12*, 812–820. [CrossRef]

101. Moslemi, A.R.; Darin, N.; Tulinius, M.; Oldfors, A.; Holme, E. Two new mutations in the MTATP6 gene associated with Leigh syndrome. *Neuropediatrics* **2005**, *36*, 314–318. [CrossRef]

102. Gammage, P.A.; Rorbach, J.; Vincent, A.I.; Rebar, E.J.; Minczuk, M. Mitochondrially targeted ZFNs for selective degradation of pathogenic mitochondrial genomes bearing large-scale deletions or point mutations. *EMBO Mol. Med.* **2014**, *6*, 458–466. [CrossRef]

103. Fellman, V.; Rapola, J.; Pihko, H.; Varilo, T.; Raivio, K.O. Iron-overload disease in infants involving fetal growth retardation, lactic acidosis, liver haemosiderosis, and aminoaciduria. *Lancet* **1998**, *351*, 490–493. [CrossRef]

104. Visapää, I.; Fellman, V.; Vesa, J.; Dasvarma, A.; Hutton, J.L.; Kumar, V.; Payne, G.S.; Makarow, M.; Van Coster, R.; Taylor, R.W.; et al. GRACILE syndrome, a lethal metabolic disorder with iron overload, is caused by a point mutation in BCS1L. *Am. J. Hum. Genet.* **2002**, *71*, 863–876. [CrossRef]

105. Fellman, V. The GRACILE syndrome, a neonatal lethal metabolic disorder with iron overload. *Blood Cells Mol. Dis.* **2002**, *29*, 444–450. [CrossRef]

106. Fellman, V.; Kotarsky, H. Mitochondrial hepatopathies in the newborn period. *Semin. Fetal Neonatal Med.* **2011**, *16*, 222–228. [CrossRef]

107. Rapola, J.; Heikkilä, P.; Fellman, V. Pathology of lethal fetal growth retardation syndrome with aminoaciduria, iron overload, and lactic acidosis (GRACILE). *Pediatr. Pathol. Mol. Med.* **2002**, *21*, 183–193. [CrossRef]

108. Kotarsky, H.; Karikoski, R.; Mörgelin, M.; Marjavaara, S.; Bergman, P.; Zhang, D.L.; Smet, J.; van Coster, R.; Fellman, V. Characterization of complex III deficiency and liver dysfunction in GRACILE syndrome caused by a BCS1L mutation. *Mitochondrion* **2010**, *10*, 497–509. [CrossRef]

109. de Lonlay, P.; Valnot, I.; Barrientos, A.; Gorbatyuk, M.; Tzagoloff, A.; Taanman, J.W.; Benayoun, E.; Chrétien, D.; Kadhom, N.; Lombès, A.; et al. A mutant mitochondrial respiratory chain assembly protein causes complex III deficiency in patients with tubulopathy, encephalopathy and liver failure. *Nat. Genet.* **2001**, *29*, 57–60. [CrossRef]

110. Serdaroğlu, E.; Takcı, Ş.; Kotarsky, H.; Çil, O.; Utine, E.; Yiğit, Ş.; Fellman, V. A Turkish BCS1L mutation causes GRACILE-like disorder. *Turk. J. Pediatr.* **2016**, *58*, 658–661. [CrossRef]

111. Fellman, V.; Lemmelä, S.; Sajantila, A.; Pihko, H.; Järvelä, I. Screening of BCS1L mutations in severe neonatal disorders suspicious for mitochondrial cause. *J. Hum. Genet.* **2008**, *53*, 554–558. [CrossRef]

112. Lee, W.S.; Sokol, R.J. Mitochondrial hepatopathies: Advances in genetics, therapeutic approaches, and outcomes. *J. Pediatr.* **2013**, *163*, 942–948. [CrossRef]

113. Rajendran, J.; Tomašić, N.; Kotarsky, H.; Hansson, E.; Velagapudi, V.; Kallijärvi, J.; Fellman, V. Effect of High-Carbohydrate Diet on Plasma Metabolome in Mice with Mitochondrial Respiratory Chain Complex III Deficiency. *Int. J. Mol. Sci.* **2016**, *17*, 1824. [CrossRef] [PubMed]

114. Bardosi, A.; Creutzfeldt, W.; DiMauro, S.; Felgenhauer, K.; Friede, R.L.; Goebel, H.H.; Kohlschütter, A.; Mayer, G.; Rahlf, G.; Servidei, S. Myo-, neuro-, gastrointestinal encephalopathy (MNGIE syndrome) due to partial deficiency of cytochrome-c-oxidase. A new mitochondrial multisystem disorder. *Acta Neuropathol.* **1987**, *74*, 248–258. [CrossRef] [PubMed]

115. Hirano, M.; Silvestri, G.; Blake, D.M.; Lombes, A.; Minetti, C.; Bonilla, E.; Hays, A.P.; Lovelace, R.E.; Butler, I.; Bertorini, T.E. Mitochondrial neurogastrointestinal encephalomyopathy (MNGIE): Clinical, biochemical, and genetic features of an autosomal recessive mitochondrial disorder. *Neurology* **1994**, *44*, 721–727. [CrossRef] [PubMed]

116. Nishino, I.; Spinazzola, A.; Hirano, M. Thymidine phosphorylase gene mutations in MNGIE, a human mitochondrial disorder. *Science* **1999**, *283*, 689–692. [CrossRef] [PubMed]

117. Nishino, I.; Spinazzola, A.; Papadimitriou, A.; Hammans, S.; Steiner, I.; Hahn, C.D.; Connolly, A.M.; Verloes, A.; Guimarães, J.; Maillard, I.; et al. Mitochondrial neurogastrointestinal encephalomyopathy: An autosomal recessive disorder due to thymidine phosphorylase mutations. *Ann. Neurol.* **2000**, *47*, 792–800. [CrossRef]

118. Blondon, H.; Polivka, M.; Joly, F.; Flourie, B.; Mikol, J.; Messing, B. Digestive smooth muscle mitochondrial myopathy in patients with mitochondrial-neuro-gastro-intestinal encephalomyopathy (MNGIE). *Gastroenterol. Clin. Biol.* **2005**, *29*, 773–778. [CrossRef]

119. Scarpelli, M.; Ricciardi, G.K.; Beltramello, A.; Zocca, I.; Calabria, F.; Russignan, A.; Zappini, F.; Cotelli, M.S.; Padovani, A.; Tomelleri, G.; et al. The role of brain MRI in mitochondrial neurogastrointestinal encephalomyopathy. *Neuroradiol. J.* **2013**, *26*, 520–530. [CrossRef]

120. Hirano, M.; Nishigaki, Y.; Martí, R. Mitochondrial neurogastrointestinal encephalomyopathy (MNGIE): A disease of two genomes. *Neurologist* **2004**, *10*, 8–17. [CrossRef]

121. Garone, C.; Tadesse, S.; Hirano, M. Clinical and genetic spectrum of mitochondrial neurogastrointestinal encephalomyopathy. *Brain* **2011**, *134*, 3326–3332. [CrossRef]

122. Viscomi, C.; Zeviani, M. MtDNA-maintenance defects: Syndromes and genes. *J. Inherit. Metab. Dis.* **2017**, *40*, 587–599. [CrossRef] [PubMed]

123. Filosto, M.; Tomelleri, G.; Tonin, P.; Scarpelli, M.; Vattemi, G.; Rizzuto, N.; Padovani, A.; Simonati, A. Neuropathology of mitochondrial diseases. *Biosci. Rep.* **2007**, *27*, 23–30. [CrossRef]

124. Halter, J.; Schüpbach, W.; Casali, C.; Elhasid, R.; Fay, K.; Hammans, S.; Illa, I.; Kappeler, L.; Krähenbühl, S.; Lehmann, T.; et al. Allogeneic hematopoietic SCT as treatment option for patients with mitochondrial neurogastrointestinal encephalomyopathy (MNGIE): A consensus conference proposal for a standardized approach. *Bone Marrow Transplant.* **2011**, *46*, 330–337. [CrossRef] [PubMed]

125. Wang, J.; Chen, W.; Wang, F.; Wu, D.; Qian, J.; Kang, J.; Li, H.; Ma, E. Nutrition Therapy for Mitochondrial Neurogastrointestinal Encephalopathy with Homozygous Mutation of the TYMP Gene. *Clin. Nutr. Res.* **2015**, *4*, 132–136. [CrossRef] [PubMed]

126. Hirano, M.; Martí, R.; Casali, C.; Tadesse, S.; Uldrick, T.; Fine, B.; Escolar, D.M.; Valentino, M.L.; Nishino, I.; Hesdorffer, C.; et al. Allogeneic stem cell transplantation corrects biochemical derangements in MNGIE. *Neurology* **2006**, *67*, 1458–1460. [CrossRef] [PubMed]

127. Filosto, M.; Scarpelli, M.; Tonin, P.; Lucchini, G.; Pavan, F.; Santus, F.; Parini, R.; Donati, M.A.; Cotelli, M.S.; Vielmi, V.; et al. Course and management of allogeneic stem cell transplantation in patients with mitochondrial neurogastrointestinal encephalomyopathy. *J. Neurol.* **2012**, *259*, 2699–2706. [CrossRef] [PubMed]

128. Halter, J.P.; Michael, W.; Schüpbach, M.; Mandel, H.; Casali, C.; Orchard, K.; Collin, M.; Valcarcel, D.; Rovelli, A.; Filosto, M.; et al. Allogeneic haematopoietic stem cell transplantation for mitochondrial neurogastrointestinal encephalomyopathy. *Brain* **2015**, *138*, 2847–2858. [CrossRef] [PubMed]

129. Lara, M.C.; Weiss, B.; Illa, I.; Madoz, P.; Massuet, L.; Andreu, A.L.; Valentino, M.L.; Anikster, Y.; Hirano, M.; Martí, R. Infusion of platelets transiently reduces nucleoside overload in MNGIE. *Neurology* **2006**, *67*, 1461–1463. [CrossRef]

130. Yavuz, H.; Ozel, A.; Christensen, M.; Christensen, E.; Schwartz, M.; Elmaci, M.; Vissing, J. Treatment of mitochondrial neurogastrointestinal encephalomyopathy with dialysis. *Arch. Neurol.* **2007**, *64*, 435–438. [CrossRef]

131. Bax, B.E.; Bain, M.D.; Scarpelli, M.; Filosto, M.; Tonin, P.; Moran, N. Clinical and biochemical improvements in a patient with MNGIE following enzyme replacement. *Neurology* **2013**, *81*, 1269–1271. [CrossRef]

132. Röeben, B.; Marquetand, J.; Bender, B.; Billing, H.; Haack, T.B.; Sanchez-Albisua, I.; Schöls, L.; Blom, H.J.; Synofzik, M. Hemodialysis in MNGIE transiently reduces serum and urine levels of thymidine and deoxyuridine, but not CSF levels and neurological function. *Orphanet J. Rare Dis.* **2017**, *12*, 135. [CrossRef] [PubMed]

133. De Giorgio, R.; Pironi, L.; Rinaldi, R.; Boschetti, E.; Caporali, L.; Capristo, M.; Casali, C.; Cenacchi, G.; Contin, M.; D'Angelo, R.; et al. Liver transplantation for mitochondrial neurogastrointestinal encephalomyopathy. *Ann. Neurol.* **2016**, *80*, 448–455. [CrossRef] [PubMed]

134. Torres-Torronteras, J.; Cabrera-Pérez, R.; Barba, I.; Costa, C.; de Luna, N.; Andreu, A.L.; Barquinero, J.; Hirano, M.; Cámara, Y.; Martí, R. Long-Term Restoration of Thymidine Phosphorylase Function and Nucleoside Homeostasis Using Hematopoietic Gene Therapy in a Murine Model of Mitochondrial Neurogastrointestinal Encephalomyopathy. *Hum. Gene Ther.* **2016**, *27*, 656–667. [CrossRef] [PubMed]

135. Barth, P.G.; Scholte, H.R.; Berden, J.A.; Van der Klei-Van Moorsel, J.M.; Luyt-Houwen, I.E.; Van 't Veer-Korthof, E.T.; Van der Harten, J.J.; Sobotka-Plojhar, M.A. An X-linked mitochondrial disease affecting cardiac muscle, skeletal muscle and neutrophil leucocytes. *J. Neurol. Sci* **1983**, *62*, 327–355. [CrossRef]

136. Lev, D.; Nissenkorn, A.; Leshinsky-Silver, E.; Sadeh, M.; Zeharia, A.; Garty, B.Z.; Blieden, L.; Barash, V.; Lerman-Sagie, T. Clinical presentations of mitochondrial cardiomyopathies. *Pediatr. Cardiol.* **2004**, *25*, 443–450. [CrossRef] [PubMed]

137. Adès, L.C.; Gedeon, A.K.; Wilson, M.J.; Latham, M.; Partington, M.W.; Mulley, J.C.; Nelson, J.; Lui, K.; Sillence, D.O. Barth syndrome: Clinical features and confirmation of gene localisation to distal Xq28. *Am. J. Med. Genet.* **1993**, *45*, 327–334. [CrossRef]

138. D'Adamo, P.; Fassone, L.; Gedeon, A.; Janssen, E.A.; Bione, S.; Bolhuis, P.A.; Barth, P.G.; Wilson, M.; Haan, E.; Orstavik, K.H.; et al. The X-linked gene G4.5 is responsible for different infantile dilated cardiomyopathies. *Am. J. Hum. Genet.* **1997**, *61*, 862–867. [CrossRef] [PubMed]

139. Steward, C.G.; Newbury-Ecob, R.A.; Hastings, R.; Smithson, S.F.; Tsai-Goodman, B.; Quarrell, O.W.; Kulik, W.; Wanders, R.; Pennock, M.; Williams, M.; et al. Barth syndrome: An X-linked cause of fetal cardiomyopathy and stillbirth. *Prenat. Diagn.* **2010**, *30*, 970–976. [CrossRef]

140. Clarke, S.L.; Bowron, A.; Gonzalez, I.L.; Groves, S.J.; Newbury-Ecob, R.; Clayton, N.; Martin, R.P.; Tsai-Goodman, B.; Garratt, V.; Ashworth, M.; et al. Barth syndrome. *Orphanet J. Rare Dis.* **2013**, *8*, 23. [CrossRef]

141. Barth, P.G.; Valianpour, F.; Bowen, V.M.; Lam, J.; Duran, M.; Vaz, F.M.; Wanders, R.J. X-linked cardioskeletal myopathy and neutropenia (Barth syndrome): An update. *Am. J. Med. Genet. A* **2004**, *126A*, 349–354. [CrossRef] [PubMed]

142. Brady, A.N.; Shehata, B.M.; Fernhoff, P.M. X-linked fetal cardiomyopathy caused by a novel mutation in the TAZ gene. *Prenat. Diagn.* **2006**, *26*, 462–465. [CrossRef] [PubMed]

143. Rigaud, C.; Lebre, A.S.; Touraine, R.; Beaupain, B.; Ottolenghi, C.; Chabli, A.; Ansquer, H.; Ozsahin, H.; Di Filippo, S.; De Lonlay, P.; et al. Natural history of Barth syndrome: A national cohort study of 22 patients. *Orphanet J. Rare Dis.* **2013**, *8*, 70. [CrossRef] [PubMed]

144. Bleyl, S.B.; Mumford, B.R.; Thompson, V.; Carey, J.C.; Pysher, T.J.; Chin, T.K.; Ward, K. Neonatal, lethal noncompaction of the left ventricular myocardium is allelic with Barth syndrome. *Am. J. Hum. Genet.* **1997**, *61*, 868–872. [CrossRef] [PubMed]

145. Chin, T.K.; Perloff, J.K.; Williams, R.G.; Jue, K.; Mohrmann, R. Isolated noncompaction of left ventricular myocardium. A study of eight cases. *Circulation* **1990**, *82*, 507–513. [CrossRef]

146. Pignatelli, R.H.; McMahon, C.J.; Dreyer, W.J.; Denfield, S.W.; Price, J.; Belmont, J.W.; Craigen, W.J.; Wu, J.; El Said, H.; Bezold, L.I.; et al. Clinical characterization of left ventricular noncompaction in children: A relatively common form of cardiomyopathy. *Circulation* **2003**, *108*, 2672–2678. [CrossRef]

147. Spencer, C.T.; Bryant, R.M.; Day, J.; Gonzalez, I.L.; Colan, S.D.; Thompson, W.R.; Berthy, J.; Redfearn, S.P.; Byrne, B.J. Cardiac and clinical phenotype in Barth syndrome. *Pediatrics* **2006**, *118*, e337–e346. [CrossRef]

148. Roberts, A.E.; Nixon, C.; Steward, C.G.; Gauvreau, K.; Maisenbacher, M.; Fletcher, M.; Geva, J.; Byrne, B.J.; Spencer, C.T. The Barth Syndrome Registry: Distinguishing disease characteristics and growth data from a longitudinal study. *Am. J. Med. Genet. A* **2012**, *158A*, 2726–2732. [CrossRef]

149. Steward, C.G.; Groves, S.J.; Taylor, C.T.; Maisenbacher, M.K.; Versluys, B.; Newbury-Ecob, R.A.; Ozsahin, H.; Damin, M.K.; Bowen, V.M.; McCurdy, K.R.; et al. Neutropenia in Barth syndrome: Characteristics, risks, and management. *Curr. Opin. Hematol.* **2019**, *26*, 6–15. [CrossRef]

150. Kelley, R.I.; Cheatham, J.P.; Clark, B.J.; Nigro, M.A.; Powell, B.R.; Sherwood, G.W.; Sladky, J.T.; Swisher, W.P. X-linked dilated cardiomyopathy with neutropenia, growth retardation, and 3-methylglutaconic aciduria. *J. Pediatr.* **1991**, *119*, 738–747. [CrossRef]

151. Bolhuis, P.A.; Hensels, G.W.; Hulsebos, T.J.; Baas, F.; Barth, P.G. Mapping of the locus for X-linked cardioskeletal myopathy with neutropenia and abnormal mitochondria (Barth syndrome) to Xq28. *Am. J. Hum. Genet.* **1991**, *48*, 481–485. [PubMed]

152. Bione, S.; D'Adamo, P.; Maestrini, E.; Gedeon, A.K.; Bolhuis, P.A.; Toniolo, D. A novel X-linked gene, G4.5. is responsible for Barth syndrome. *Nat. Genet.* **1996**, *12*, 385–389. [CrossRef] [PubMed]

153. Vreken, P.; Valianpour, F.; Nijtmans, L.G.; Grivell, L.A.; Plecko, B.; Wanders, R.J.; Barth, P.G. Defective remodeling of cardiolipin and phosphatidylglycerol in Barth syndrome. *Biochem. Biophys. Res. Commun.* **2000**, *279*, 378–382. [CrossRef] [PubMed]

154. Gaspard, G.J.; McMaster, C.R. Cardiolipin metabolism and its causal role in the etiology of the inherited cardiomyopathy Barth syndrome. *Chem. Phys. Lipids* **2015**, *193*, 1–10. [CrossRef] [PubMed]

155. Houtkooper, R.H.; Turkenburg, M.; Poll-The, B.T.; Karall, D.; Pérez-Cerdá, C.; Morrone, A.; Malvagia, S.; Wanders, R.J.; Kulik, W.; Vaz, F.M. The enigmatic role of tafazzin in cardiolipin metabolism. *Biochim. Biophys. Acta* **2009**, *1788*, 2003–2014. [CrossRef] [PubMed]

156. Valianpour, F.; Mitsakos, V.; Schlemmer, D.; Towbin, J.A.; Taylor, J.M.; Ekert, P.G.; Thorburn, D.R.; Munnich, A.; Wanders, R.J.; Barth, P.G.; et al. Monolysocardiolipins accumulate in Barth syndrome but do not lead to enhanced apoptosis. *J. Lipid Res.* **2005**, *46*, 1182–1195. [CrossRef] [PubMed]

157. Kulik, W.; van Lenthe, H.; Stet, F.S.; Houtkooper, R.H.; Kemp, H.; Stone, J.E.; Steward, C.G.; Wanders, R.J.; Vaz, F.M. Bloodspot assay using HPLC-tandem mass spectrometry for detection of Barth syndrome. *Clin. Chem* **2008**, *54*, 371–378. [CrossRef] [PubMed]

158. Jefferies, J.L. Barth syndrome. *Am. J. Med. Genet. C Semin. Med. Genet.* **2013**, *163C*, 198–205. [CrossRef]

159. Meyerson, C.; Van Stavern, G.; McClelland, C. Leber hereditary optic neuropathy: Current perspectives. *Clin. Ophthalmol* **2015**, *9*, 1165–1176.

160. Giraudet, S.; Lamirel, C.; Amati-Bonneau, P.; Reynier, P.; Bonneau, D.; Miléa, D.; Cochereau, I. Never too old to harbour a young man's disease? *Br. J. Ophthalmol.* **2011**, *95*, 887–896. [CrossRef]

161. Barboni, P.; Savini, G.; Valentino, M.L.; La Morgia, C.; Bellusci, C.; De Negri, A.M.; Sadun, F.; Carta, A.; Carbonelli, M.; Sadun, A.A.; et al. Leber's hereditary optic neuropathy with childhood onset. *Invest. Ophthalmol. Vis. Sci.* **2006**, *47*, 5303–5309. [CrossRef]

162. Carelli, V.; Ross-Cisneros, F.N.; Sadun, A.A. Mitochondrial dysfunction as a cause of optic neuropathies. *Prog. Retin. Eye Res.* **2004**, *23*, 53–89. [CrossRef]

163. Newman, N.J. Leber's hereditary optic neuropathy. New genetic considerations. *Arch. Neurol.* **1993**, *50*, 540–548. [CrossRef] [PubMed]

164. Chao de la Barca, J.M.; Simard, G.; Amati-Bonneau, P.; Safiedeen, Z.; Prunier-Mirebeau, D.; Chupin, S.; Gadras, C.; Tessier, L.; Gueguen, N.; Chevrollier, A.; et al. The metabolomic signature of Leber's hereditary optic neuropathy reveals endoplasmic reticulum stress. *Brain* **2016**, *139*, 2864–2876. [CrossRef]

165. Jun, A.S.; Brown, M.D.; Wallace, D.C. A mitochondrial DNA mutation at nucleotide pair 14459 of the NADH dehydrogenase subunit 6 gene associated with maternally inherited Leber hereditary optic neuropathy and dystonia. *Proc. Natl. Acad. Sci. USA* **1994**, *91*, 6206–6210. [CrossRef]

166. Harding, A.E.; Sweeney, M.G.; Miller, D.H.; Mumford, C.J.; Kellar-Wood, H.; Menard, D.; McDonald, W.I.; Compston, D.A. Occurrence of a multiple sclerosis-like illness in women who have a Leber's hereditary optic neuropathy mitochondrial DNA mutation. *Brain* **1992**, *115 (Pt. 4)*, 979–989. [CrossRef]

167. Funalot, B.; Reynier, P.; Vighetto, A.; Ranoux, D.; Bonnefont, J.P.; Godinot, C.; Malthièry, Y.; Mas, J.L. Leigh-like encephalopathy complicating Leber's hereditary optic neuropathy. *Ann. Neurol.* **2002**, *52*, 374–377. [CrossRef] [PubMed]

168. Nikoskelainen, E.K.; Marttila, R.J.; Huoponen, K.; Juvonen, V.; Lamminen, T.; Sonninen, P.; Savontaus, M.L. Leber's "plus": Neurological abnormalities in patients with Leber's hereditary optic neuropathy. *J. Neurol. Neurosurg. Psychiatry* **1995**, *59*, 160–164. [CrossRef] [PubMed]

169. Perez, F.; Anne, O.; Debruxelles, S.; Menegon, P.; Lambrecq, V.; Lacombe, D.; Martin-Negrier, M.L.; Brochet, B.; Goizet, C. Leber's optic neuropathy associated with disseminated white matter disease: A case report and review. *Clin. Neurol. Neurosurg.* **2009**, *111*, 83–86. [CrossRef]

170. Kellar-Wood, H.; Robertson, N.; Govan, G.G.; Compston, D.A.; Harding, A.E. Leber's hereditary optic neuropathy mitochondrial DNA mutations in multiple sclerosis. *Ann. Neurol.* **1994**, *36*, 109–112. [CrossRef]

171. Meire, F.M.; Van Coster, R.; Cochaux, P.; Obermaier-Kusser, B.; Candaele, C.; Martin, J.J. Neurological disorders in members of families with Leber's hereditary optic neuropathy (LHON) caused by different mitochondrial mutations. *Ophthalmic Genet.* **1995**, *16*, 119–126. [CrossRef] [PubMed]

172. Pfeffer, G.; Burke, A.; Yu-Wai-Man, P.; Compston, D.A.; Chinnery, P.F. Clinical features of MS associated with Leber hereditary optic neuropathy mtDNA mutations. *Neurology* **2013**, *81*, 2073–2081. [CrossRef] [PubMed]

173. Yu-Wai-Man, P.; Griffiths, P.G.; Brown, D.T.; Howell, N.; Turnbull, D.M.; Chinnery, P.F. The epidemiology of Leber hereditary optic neuropathy in the North East of England. *Am. J. Hum. Genet.* **2003**, *72*, 333–339. [CrossRef]

174. Puomila, A.; Hämäläinen, P.; Kivioja, S.; Savontaus, M.L.; Koivumäki, S.; Huoponen, K.; Nikoskelainen, E. Epidemiology and penetrance of Leber hereditary optic neuropathy in Finland. *Eur. J. Hum. Genet.* **2007**, *15*, 1079–1089. [CrossRef] [PubMed]

175. Mascialino, B.; Leinonen, M.; Meier, T. Meta-analysis of the prevalence of Leber hereditary optic neuropathy mtDNA mutations in Europe. *Eur. J. Ophthalmol.* **2012**, *22*, 461–465. [CrossRef] [PubMed]

176. Finsterer, J.; Stöllberger, C.; Prainer, C.; Hochwarter, A. Lone noncompaction in Leber's hereditary optic neuropathy. *Acta Cardiol.* **2004**, *59*, 187–190. [CrossRef]

177. Finsterer, J.; Stöllberger, C.; Michaela, J. Familial left ventricular hypertrabeculation in two blind brothers. *Cardiovasc. Pathol.* **2002**, *11*, 146–148. [CrossRef]

178. Ortiz, R.G.; Newman, N.J.; Manoukian, S.V.; Diesenhouse, M.C.; Lott, M.T.; Wallace, D.C. Optic disk cupping and electrocardiographic abnormalities in an American pedigree with Leber's hereditary optic neuropathy. *Am. J. Ophthalmol.* **1992**, *113*, 561–566. [CrossRef]

179. Finsterer, J.; Stollberger, C.; Gatterer, E. Wolff-Parkinson-White syndrome and noncompaction in Leber's hereditary optic neuropathy due to the variant m.3460G>A. *J. Int. Med. Res.* **2018**, *46*, 2054–2060. [CrossRef]

180. Nikoskelainen, E.K.; Savontaus, M.L.; Huoponen, K.; Antila, K.; Hartiala, J. Pre-excitation syndrome in Leber's hereditary optic neuropathy. *Lancet* **1994**, *344*, 857–858. [CrossRef]

181. Mashima, Y.; Kigasawa, K.; Hasegawa, H.; Tani, M.; Oguchi, Y. High incidence of pre-excitation syndrome in Japanese families with Leber's hereditary optic neuropathy. *Clin. Genet.* **1996**, *50*, 535–537. [CrossRef] [PubMed]

182. Wallace, D.C.; Singh, G.; Lott, M.T.; Hodge, J.A.; Schurr, T.G.; Lezza, A.M.; Elsas, L.J.; Nikoskelainen, E.K. Mitochondrial DNA mutation associated with Leber's hereditary optic neuropathy. *Science* **1988**, *242*, 1427–1430. [CrossRef] [PubMed]

183. Huoponen, K.; Vilkki, J.; Aula, P.; Nikoskelainen, E.K.; Savontaus, M.L. A new mtDNA mutation associated with Leber hereditary optic neuroretinopathy. *Am. J. Hum. Genet.* **1991**, *48*, 1147–1153.

184. Johns, D.R.; Neufeld, M.J.; Park, R.D. An ND-6 mitochondrial DNA mutation associated with Leber hereditary optic neuropathy. *Biochem. Biophys. Res. Commun.* **1992**, *187*, 1551–1557. [CrossRef]

185. Riordan-Eva, P.; Harding, A.E. Leber's hereditary optic neuropathy: The clinical relevance of different mitochondrial DNA mutations. *J. Med. Genet.* **1995**, *32*, 81–87. [CrossRef]

186. Valentino, M.L.; Barboni, P.; Ghelli, A.; Bucchi, L.; Rengo, C.; Achilli, A.; Torroni, A.; Lugaresi, A.; Lodi, R.; Barbiroli, B.; et al. The ND1 gene of complex I is a mutational hot spot for Leber's hereditary optic neuropathy. *Ann. Neurol.* **2004**, *56*, 631–641. [CrossRef]

187. Valentino, M.L.; Avoni, P.; Barboni, P.; Pallotti, F.; Rengo, C.; Torroni, A.; Bellan, M.; Baruzzi, A.; Carelli, V. Mitochondrial DNA nucleotide changes C14482G and C14482A in the ND6 gene are pathogenic for Leber's hereditary optic neuropathy. *Ann. Neurol.* **2002**, *51*, 774–778. [CrossRef]

188. Chinnery, P.F.; Brown, D.T.; Andrews, R.M.; Singh-Kler, R.; Riordan-Eva, P.; Lindley, J.; Applegarth, D.A.; Turnbull, D.M.; Howell, N. The mitochondrial ND6 gene is a hot spot for mutations that cause Leber's hereditary optic neuropathy. *Brain* **2001**, *124*, 209–218. [CrossRef] [PubMed]

189. Achilli, A.; Iommarini, L.; Olivieri, A.; Pala, M.; Hooshiar Kashani, B.; Reynier, P.; La Morgia, C.; Valentino, M.L.; Liguori, R.; Pizza, F.; et al. Rare primary mitochondrial DNA mutations and probable synergistic variants in Leber's hereditary optic neuropathy. *PLoS ONE* **2012**, *7*, e42242. [CrossRef]

190. Yu-Wai-Man, P.; Turnbull, D.M.; Chinnery, P.F. Leber hereditary optic neuropathy. *J. Med. Genet.* **2002**, *39*, 162–169.

191. Battisti, C.; Formichi, P.; Cardaioli, E.; Bianchi, S.; Mangiavacchi, P.; Tripodi, S.A.; Tosi, P.; Federico, A. Cell response to oxidative stress induced apoptosis in patients with Leber's hereditary optic neuropathy. *J. Neurol. Neurosurg. Psychiatry* **2004**, *75*, 1731–1736. [CrossRef] [PubMed]

192. Giordano, C.; Montopoli, M.; Perli, E.; Orlandi, M.; Fantin, M.; Ross-Cisneros, F.N.; Caparrotta, L.; Martinuzzi, A.; Ragazzi, E.; Ghelli, A.; et al. Oestrogens ameliorate mitochondrial dysfunction in Leber's hereditary optic neuropathy. *Brain* **2011**, *134*, 220–234. [CrossRef] [PubMed]

193. Sadun, A.A.; Carelli, V.; Salomao, S.R.; Berezovsky, A.; Quiros, P.A.; Sadun, F.; DeNegri, A.M.; Andrade, R.; Moraes, M.; Passos, A.; et al. Extensive investigation of a large Brazilian pedigree of 11778/haplogroup J Leber hereditary optic neuropathy. *Am. J. Ophthalmol.* **2003**, *136*, 231–238. [CrossRef]

194. Kirkman, M.A.; Yu-Wai-Man, P.; Korsten, A.; Leonhardt, M.; Dimitriadis, K.; De Coo, I.F.; Klopstock, T.; Chinnery, P.F. Gene-environment interactions in Leber hereditary optic neuropathy. *Brain* **2009**, *132*, 2317–2326. [CrossRef]

195. Khan, N.A.; Govindaraj, P.; Soumittra, N.; Sharma, S.; Srilekha, S.; Ambika, S.; Vanniarajan, A.; Meena, A.K.; Uppin, M.S.; Sundaram, C.; et al. Leber's Hereditary Optic Neuropathy-Specific Mutation m.11778G>A

196. Mascialino, B.; Leinonen, M.; Meier, T. Meta-analysis of the prevalence of Leber hereditary optic mtDNA mutations in Europe. *Eur. J. Ophthalmol.* **2012**, *22*, 461–465. [CrossRef] [PubMed]

197. Johns, D.R.; Heher, K.L.; Miller, N.R.; Smith, K.H. Leber's hereditary optic neuropathy. Clinical manifestations of the 14484 mutation. *Arch. Ophthalmol.* **1993**, *111*, 495–498. [CrossRef]

198. Sadun, A.A.; Chicani, C.F.; Ross-Cisneros, F.N.; Barboni, P.; Thoolen, M.; Shrader, W.D.; Kubis, K.; Carelli, V.; Miller, G. Effect of EPI-743 on the clinical course of the mitochondrial disease Leber hereditary optic neuropathy. *Arch. Neurol.* **2012**, *69*, 331–338. [CrossRef]

199. Klopstock, T.; Yu-Wai-Man, P.; Dimitriadis, K.; Rouleau, J.; Heck, S.; Bailie, M.; Atawan, A.; Chattopadhyay, S.; Schubert, M.; Garip, A.; et al. A randomized placebo-controlled trial of idebenone in Leber's hereditary optic neuropathy. *Brain* **2011**, *134*, 2677–2686. [CrossRef]

200. Mashima, Y.; Hiida, Y.; Oguchi, Y. Remission of Leber's hereditary optic neuropathy with idebenone. *Lancet* **1992**, *340*, 368–369. [CrossRef]

201. Mashima, Y.; Kigasawa, K.; Wakakura, M.; Oguchi, Y. Do idebenone and vitamin therapy shorten the time to achieve visual recovery in Leber hereditary optic neuropathy? *J. Neuroophthalmol.* **2000**, *20*, 166–170. [CrossRef]

202. Carelli, V.; La Morgia, C.; Valentino, M.L.; Rizzo, G.; Carbonelli, M.; De Negri, A.M.; Sadun, F.; Carta, A.; Guerriero, S.; Simonelli, F.; et al. Idebenone treatment in Leber's hereditary optic neuropathy. *Brain* **2011**, *134*, e188. [CrossRef]

203. Pisano, A.; Preziuso, C.; Iommarini, L.; Perli, E.; Grazioli, P.; Campese, A.F.; Maresca, A.; Montopoli, M.; Masuelli, L.; Sadun, A.A.; et al. Targeting estrogen receptor β as preventive therapeutic strategy for Leber's hereditary optic neuropathy. *Hum. Mol. Genet.* **2015**, *24*, 6921–6931. [CrossRef] [PubMed]

204. Guy, J.; Qi, X.; Koilkonda, R.D.; Arguello, T.; Chou, T.H.; Ruggeri, M.; Porciatti, V.; Lewin, A.S.; Hauswirth, W.W. Efficiency and safety of AAV-mediated gene delivery of the human ND4 complex I subunit in the mouse visual system. *Invest. Ophthalmol. Vis. Sci.* **2009**, *50*, 4205–4214. [CrossRef]

205. Ellouze, S.; Augustin, S.; Bouaita, A.; Bonnet, C.; Simonutti, M.; Forster, V.; Picaud, S.; Sahel, J.A.; Corral-Debrinski, M. Optimized allotopic expression of the human mitochondrial ND4 prevents blindness in a rat model of mitochondrial dysfunction. *Am. J. Hum. Genet.* **2008**, *83*, 373–387. [CrossRef] [PubMed]

206. Yang, S.; Ma, S.Q.; Wan, X.; He, H.; Pei, H.; Zhao, M.J.; Chen, C.; Wang, D.W.; Dong, X.Y.; Yuan, J.J.; et al. Long-term outcomes of gene therapy for the treatment of Leber's hereditary optic neuropathy. *EBioMedicine* **2016**, *10*, 258–268. [CrossRef] [PubMed]

207. Koilkonda, R.D.; Yu, H.; Chou, T.H.; Feuer, W.J.; Ruggeri, M.; Porciatti, V.; Tse, D.; Hauswirth, W.W.; Chiodo, V.; Boye, S.L.; et al. Safety and effects of the vector for the Leber hereditary optic neuropathy gene therapy clinical trial. *JAMA Ophthalmol.* **2014**, *132*, 409–420. [CrossRef] [PubMed]

208. Guy, J.; Feuer, W.J.; Davis, J.L.; Porciatti, V.; Gonzalez, P.J.; Koilkonda, R.D.; Yuan, H.; Hauswirth, W.W.; Lam, B.L. Gene Therapy for Leber Hereditary Optic Neuropathy: Low- and Medium-Dose Visual Results. *Ophthalmology* **2017**, *124*, 1621–1634. [CrossRef]

209. Farruggia, P.; Di Cataldo, A.; Pinto, R.M.; Palmisani, E.; Macaluso, A.; Valvo, L.L.; Cantarini, M.E.; Tornesello, A.; Corti, P.; Fioredda, F.; et al. Pearson Syndrome: A Retrospective Cohort Study from the Marrow Failure Study Group of A.I.E.O.P. (Associazione Italiana Emato-Oncologia Pediatrica). *JIMD Rep.* **2016**, *26*, 37–43. [PubMed]

210. Rotig, A.; Bourgeron, T.; Chretien, D.; Rustin, P.; Munnich, A. Spectrum of mitochondrial DNA rearrangements in the Pearson marrow-pancreas syndrome. *Hum. Mol. Genet.* **1995**, *4*, 1327–1330. [CrossRef] [PubMed]

211. Santorelli, F.M.; Barmada, M.A.; Pons, R.; Zhang, L.L.; DiMauro, S. Leigh-type neuropathology in Pearson syndrome associated with impaired ATP production and a novel mtDNA deletion. *Neurology* **1996**, *47*, 1320–1323. [CrossRef]

212. Lee, H.F.; Lee, H.J.; Chi, C.S.; Tsai, C.R.; Chang, T.K.; Wang, C.J. The neurological evolution of Pearson syndrome: Case report and literature review. *Eur. J. Paediatr. Neurol.* **2007**, *11*, 208–214. [CrossRef] [PubMed]

213. McShane, M.A.; Hammans, S.R.; Sweeney, M.; Holt, I.J.; Beattie, T.J.; Brett, E.M.; Harding, A.E. Pearson syndrome and mitochondrial encephalomyopathy in a patient with a deletion of mtDNA. *Am. J. Hum. Genet.* **1991**, *48*, 39–42. [PubMed]

214. Mancuso, M.; Orsucci, D.; Angelini, C.; Bertini, E.; Carelli, V.; Comi, G.P.; Donati, M.A.; Federico, A.; Minetti, C.; Moggio, M.; et al. Redefining phenotypes associated with mitochondrial DNA single deletion. *J. Neurol.* **2015**, *262*, 1301–1309. [CrossRef] [PubMed]

215. Crippa, B.L.; Leon, E.; Calhoun, A.; Lowichik, A.; Pasquali, M.; Longo, N. Biochemical abnormalities in Pearson syndrome. *Am. J. Med. Genet. A* **2015**, *167A*, 621–628. [CrossRef] [PubMed]

216. Yamashita, S.; Nishino, I.; Nonaka, I.; Goto, Y. Genotype and phenotype analyses in 136 patients with single large-scale mitochondrial DNA deletions. *J. Hum. Genet.* **2008**, *53*, 598–606. [CrossRef] [PubMed]

217. Puri, A.; Pradhan, A.; Chaudhary, G.; Singh, V.; Sethi, R.; Narain, V.S. Symptomatic complete heart block leading to a diagnosis of Kearns-Sayre syndrome. *Indian Heart J.* **2012**, *64*, 515–517. [CrossRef]

218. Gobu, P.; Karthikeyan, B.; Prasath, A.; Santhosh, S.; Balachander, J. Kearns Sayre Syndrome (KSS) - A Rare Cause For Cardiac Pacing. *Indian Pacing Electrophysiol. J.* **2011**, *10*, 547–550.

219. van Beynum, I.; Morava, E.; Taher, M.; Rodenburg, R.J.; Karteszi, J.; Toth, K.; Szabados, E. Cardiac arrest in kearns-sayre syndrome. *JIMD Rep.* **2012**, *2*, 7–10.

220. Kabunga, P.; Lau, A.K.; Phan, K.; Puranik, R.; Liang, C.; Davis, R.L.; Sue, C.M.; Sy, R.W. Systematic review of cardiac electrical disease in Kearns-Sayre syndrome and mitochondrial cytopathy. *Int. J. Cardiol.* **2015**, *181*, 303–310. [CrossRef]

221. Zeviani, M.; Servidei, S.; Gellera, C.; Bertini, E.; DiMauro, S.; DiDonato, S. An autosomal dominant disorder with multiple deletions of mitochondrial DNA starting at the D-loop region. *Nature* **1989**, *339*, 309–311. [CrossRef]

222. Kearns, T.P.; Sayre, G.P. Retinitis pigmentosa, external ophthalmophegia, and complete heart block: Unusual syndrome with histologic study in one of two cases. *AMA Arch. Ophthalmol.* **1958**, *60*, 280–289. [CrossRef]

223. Akaike, M.; Kawai, H.; Yokoi, K.; Kunishige, M.; Mine, H.; Nishida, Y.; Saito, S. Cardiac dysfunction in patients with chronic progressive external ophthalmoplegia. *Clin. Cardiol.* **1997**, *20*, 239–243. [CrossRef]

224. Aure, K.; Ogier de Baulny, H.; Laforet, P.; Jardel, C.; Eymard, B.; Lombes, A. Chronic progressive ophthalmoplegia with large-scale mtDNA rearrangement: Can we predict progression? *Brain* **2007**, *130*, 1516–1524. [CrossRef]

225. Poulton, J.; Deadman, M.E.; Ramacharan, S.; Gardiner, R.M. Germ-line deletions of mtDNA in mitochondrial myopathy. *Am. J. Hum. Genet.* **1991**, *48*, 649–653.

226. Bernes, S.M.; Bacino, C.; Prezant, T.R.; Pearson, M.A.; Wood, T.S.; Fournier, P.; Fischel-Ghodsian, N. Identical mitochondrial DNA deletion in mother with progressive external ophthalmoplegia and son with Pearson marrow-pancreas syndrome. *J. Pediatr.* **1993**, *123*, 598–602. [CrossRef]

227. Shanske, S.; Tang, Y.; Hirano, M.; Nishigaki, Y.; Tanji, K.; Bonilla, E.; Sue, C.; Krishna, S.; Carlo, J.R.; Willner, J.; et al. Identical mitochondrial DNA deletion in a woman with ocular myopathy and in her son with pearson syndrome. *Am. J. Hum. Genet.* **2002**, *71*, 679–683. [CrossRef]

228. Remes, A.M.; Majamaa-Voltti, K.; Karppa, M.; Moilanen, J.S.; Uimonen, S.; Helander, H.; Rusanen, H.; Salmela, P.I.; Sorri, M.; Hassinen, I.E.; et al. Prevalence of large-scale mitochondrial DNA deletions in an adult Finnish population. *Neurology* **2005**, *64*, 976–981. [CrossRef]

229. Chinnery, P.F.; Johnson, M.A.; Wardell, T.M.; Singh-Kler, R.; Hayes, C.; Brown, D.T.; Taylor, R.W.; Bindoff, L.A.; Turnbull, D.M. The epidemiology of pathogenic mitochondrial DNA mutations. *Ann. Neurol.* **2000**, *48*, 188–193. [CrossRef]

230. Kiechl, S.; Horvath, R.; Luoma, P.; Kiechl-Kohlendorfer, U.; Wallacher-Scholz, B.; Stucka, R.; Thaler, C.; Wanschitz, J.; Suomalainen, A.; Jaksch, M.; et al. Two families with autosomal dominant progressive external ophthalmoplegia. *J. Neurol. Neurosurg. Psychiatry* **2004**, *75*, 1125–1128. [CrossRef]

231. Harding, A.E. Friedreich's ataxia: A clinical and genetic study of 90 families with an analysis of early diagnostic criteria and intrafamilial clustering of clinical features. *Brain* **1981**, *104*, 589–620. [CrossRef]

232. Durr, A.; Cossee, M.; Agid, Y.; Campuzano, V.; Mignard, C.; Penet, C.; Mandel, J.L.; Brice, A.; Koenig, M. Clinical and genetic abnormalities in patients with Friedreich's ataxia. *N. Engl. J. Med.* **1996**, *335*, 1169–1175. [CrossRef] [PubMed]

233. Koeppen, A.H. Friedreich's ataxia: Pathology, pathogenesis, and molecular genetics. *J. Neurol. Sci.* **2011**, *303*, 1–12. [CrossRef] [PubMed]

234. Jensen, M.K.; Bundgaard, H. Cardiomyopathy in Friedreich ataxia: Exemplifying the challenges faced by cardiologists in the management of rare diseases. *Circulation* **2012**, *125*, 1591–1593. [CrossRef]

235. Tsou, A.Y.; Paulsen, E.K.; Lagedrost, S.J.; Perlman, S.L.; Mathews, K.D.; Wilmot, G.R.; Ravina, B.; Koeppen, A.H.; Lynch, D.R. Mortality in Friedreich ataxia. *J. Neurol. Sci.* **2011**, *307*, 46–49. [CrossRef]

236. Schultz, J.C.; Hilliard, A.A.; Cooper, L.T., Jr.; Rihal, C.S. Diagnosis and treatment of viral myocarditis. *Mayo Clin. Proc.* **2009**, *84*, 1001–1009. [CrossRef]

237. Drinkard, B.E.; Keyser, R.E.; Paul, S.M.; Arena, R.; Plehn, J.F.; Yanovski, J.A.; Di Prospero, N.A. Exercise capacity and idebenone intervention in children and adolescents with Friedreich ataxia. *Arch. Phys. Med. Rehabil.* **2010**, *91*, 1044–1050. [CrossRef]

238. Rustin, P.; von Kleist-Retzow, J.C.; Chantrel-Groussard, K.; Sidi, D.; Munnich, A.; Rotig, A. Effect of idebenone on cardiomyopathy in Friedreich's ataxia: A preliminary study. *Lancet* **1999**, *354*, 477–479. [CrossRef]

239. Mariotti, C.; Solari, A.; Torta, D.; Marano, L.; Fiorentini, C.; Di Donato, S. Idebenone treatment in Friedreich patients: One-year-long randomized placebo-controlled trial. *Neurology* **2003**, *60*, 1676–1679. [CrossRef]

240. Lesnefsky, E.J.; Chen, Q.; Tandler, B.; Hoppel, C.L. Mitochondrial Dysfunction and Myocardial Ischemia-Reperfusion: Implications for Novel Therapies. *Annu. Rev. Pharmacol. Toxicol.* **2017**, *57*, 535–565. [CrossRef]

241. Yellon, D.M.; Hausenloy, D.J. Myocardial reperfusion injury. *N. Engl. J. Med.* **2007**, *357*, 1121–1135. [CrossRef]

242. Murphy, E.; Steenbergen, C. Mechanisms underlying acute protection from cardiac ischemia-reperfusion injury. *Physiol. Rev.* **2008**, *88*, 581–609. [CrossRef] [PubMed]

243. Chen, Q.; Camara, A.K.; Stowe, D.F.; Hoppel, C.L.; Lesnefsky, E.J. Modulation of electron transport protects cardiac mitochondria and decreases myocardial injury during ischemia and reperfusion. *Am. J. Physiol. Cell Physiol.* **2007**, *292*, C137–C147. [CrossRef] [PubMed]

244. Lesnefsky, E.J.; Chen, Q.; Hoppel, C.L. Mitochondrial Metabolism in Aging Heart. *Circ. Res.* **2016**, *118*, 1593–1611. [CrossRef] [PubMed]

245. Halestrap, A.P.; Clarke, S.J.; Javadov, S.A. Mitochondrial permeability transition pore opening during myocardial reperfusion–a target for cardioprotection. *Cardiovasc. Res.* **2004**, *61*, 372–385. [CrossRef]

246. Kubli, D.A.; Gustafsson, A.B. Mitochondria and mitophagy: The yin and yang of cell death control. *Circ. Res.* **2012**, *111*, 1208–1221. [CrossRef]

247. Kung, G.; Konstantinidis, K.; Kitsis, R.N. Programmed necrosis, not apoptosis, in the heart. *Circ. Res.* **2011**, *108*, 1017–1036. [CrossRef]

248. Bugger, H.; Abel, E.D. Mitochondria in the diabetic heart. *Cardiovasc. Res.* **2010**, *88*, 229–240. [CrossRef] [PubMed]

249. Rubler, S.; Dlugash, J.; Yuceoglu, Y.Z.; Kumral, T.; Branwood, A.W.; Grishman, A. New type of cardiomyopathy associated with diabetic glomerulosclerosis. *Am. J. Cardiol.* **1972**, *30*, 595–602. [CrossRef]

250. Hamby, R.I.; Zoneraich, S.; Sherman, L. Diabetic cardiomyopathy. *JAMA* **1974**, *229*, 1749–1754. [CrossRef]

251. Regan, T.J.; Lyons, M.M.; Ahmed, S.S.; Levinson, G.E.; Oldewurtel, H.A.; Ahmad, M.R.; Haider, B. Evidence for cardiomyopathy in familial diabetes mellitus. *J. Clin. Investig.* **1977**, *60*, 884–899. [CrossRef] [PubMed]

252. Bell, D.S. Diabetic cardiomyopathy. *Diabetes Care* **2003**, *26*, 2949–2951. [CrossRef] [PubMed]

253. Duncan, J.G. Mitochondrial dysfunction in diabetic cardiomyopathy. *Biochim. Biophys. Acta* **2011**, *1813*, 1351–1359. [CrossRef] [PubMed]

11

Mitochondria's Role in Skin Ageing

Roisin Stout and Mark Birch-Machin *

Dermatological Sciences, Institute of Cellular Medicine, Medical School, Newcastle University, Newcastle upon Tyne NE2 4HH, UK; r.stout2@newcastle.ac.uk
* Correspondence: mark.birch-machin@newcastle.ac.uk

Abstract: Skin ageing is the result of a loss of cellular function, which can be further accelerated by external factors. Mitochondria have important roles in skin function, and mitochondrial damage has been found to accumulate with age in skin cells, but also in response to solar light and pollution. There is increasing evidence that mitochondrial dysfunction and oxidative stress are key features in all ageing tissues, including skin. This is directly linked to skin ageing phenotypes: wrinkle formation, hair greying and loss, uneven pigmentation and decreased wound healing. The loss of barrier function during skin ageing increases susceptibility to infection and affects wound healing. Therefore, an understanding of the mechanisms involved is important clinically and also for the development of antiageing skin care products.

Keywords: mitochondria; skin; ageing; reactive oxygen species; photoageing

1. Skin Structure

Skin is the largest organ of the human body and made up of three distinct layers: the epidermis, the dermis and subcutaneous fat. It functions as a barrier against the environment, providing protection against microbes as well as fluid and temperature homeostasis. The epidermis is a thin layer of densely packed keratinised epithelial cells (keratinocytes) which contains no nerves or blood vessels and relies on the thick dermal layer underneath for metabolism. The dermis is the main living tissue in the skin, consisting of fibroblast cells in an extracellular matrix interspersed with sweat glands, hair follicles, muscle, capillaries and nerve endings. The epidermal basal layer is the innermost layer of the epidermis dispersed with melanocytes [1]. It separates the outer layers of the epidermis from the nutrient-providing papillary dermis and the thick supporting reticular dermis layer below, all of which rest on a layer of subcutaneous fat. With skin taking a large environmental insult, the keratinocytes undergo constant turnover by epidermal stem cells to replace damaged cells [2]. Melanocytes produce melanin, which is transported to keratinocytes to produce skin pigmentation and provide some solar protection. Structural integrity, repair and strength within the dermal layer of the skin are provided by type I collagen fibres, produced from procollagen bodies. Collagen regulation occurs through synthesis promotion by cytokine TGF-β, inhibition by transcription factor AP-1 and active degradation by the collagenase enzymes matrix metalloproteinases (MMPs) [3].

2. Mitochondria's Role in Skin

Mitochondria play a vital role in the skin. While the energy requirement may not be as great as other organs, such as skeletal muscle, it is still integral for processes like cell signalling, wound healing, pigmentation, vasculature homeostasis and hair growth. They are critical in microbial defence; glycolysis and ATP production have been found to rapidly increase in response to *Staphylococcus aureus* infection on the skin, in response to hypoxia induced metabolic stress [4]. This implements mitochondrial reactive oxygen species (ROS) signalling in the defence against skin infection through hypoxia-inducible factor 1-alpha (HIF1α) activation and immune cell recruitment [5]. Mitochondrial function and ROS production aid the regulation of stem cell differentiation, and have further been specifically linked to epidermal homeostasis and hair follicle development [6]. Reactive oxygen species signalling via mitochondria is therefore specifically involved in skin structure and function.

In patients with genetic mitochondrial disease, skin manifestations are often neglected as the disease predominantly affects the neuromuscular system, due to its high energy requirements. Various abnormalities in mitochondrial function, such as mutations of mitochondrial repair genes and haem synthesis, have been directly linked to a multitude of skin aberrations [7]. Lipomas and pigmentation disorders are the most commonly recorded skin complaints in mitochondrial disease patients [7,8]. This is likely due to mitochondrial defects in brown fat [9] and the direct effect of mitochondrial function in pigment production, respectively. Skin complaints can therefore be directly linked to genetic mitochondrial dysfunction and through complex ROS signalling. However, the correlation between the skin and mitochondria should be approached with caution, many other skin disorders are a result of secondary factors in diseases which do not primarily affect the mitochondrion itself, such as skin blistering in epidermolysis bullosa simplex [10].

3. Hallmarks of Skin Ageing

Wrinkles are one of the first features thought of when considering facial appearance and ageing. Intrinsic ageing is the result of chronological, inevitable senescence of the skin cells which varies depending on ethnicity, hormones and the anatomical region of affected skin. Extrinsic skin ageing is a result of all the external factors that can induce skin ageing, such as lifestyle, smoking, UV exposure and the environment, which have a cumulative effect over time [11]. Fine lines, breakdown of the skin structure, reddening due to increased visible vasculature and a reduction of elasticity are the main clinical features of intrinsic ageing; extrinsic ageing produces much deeper wrinkles, dryer skin, spider veins and uneven pigmentation [12].

As skin is constantly defending against environmental insult, it is important to maintain its integrity: ageing skin has reduced wound healing capacity and increased water loss. This increases susceptibility to cuts and infection, and makes it more prone to irritation and dermatoses [13]. It is essential to maintain an adequate skin barrier and understand the mechanisms involved in its loss to protect against age related dysregulation.

4. Mitochondria and Ageing

The "Free Radical Theory of Ageing" was first proposed by Harman in the 1950s [14]. It states that mutations acquired in mitochondrial DNA (mtDNA) during life, both spontaneously and through stress, can disrupt cellular metabolism like oxidative phosphorylation in the mitochondria and ultimately increase ROS. This, in turn, results in the oxidation of cellular components including proteins, lipids, DNA and RNA, which creates a cycle of altered metabolism and further damage. Ultimately, this results in the subsequent decline of cellular function seen in ageing and degenerative diseases.

Since it was first proposed, there have been a multitude of studies attempting to corroborate this theory by analysing mtDNA damage in ageing. As of yet there is no consensus, but there is a correlation between mtDNA damage, increasing oxidative stress and ageing. In skin samples, an accumulation of mtDNA deletions has been found to not only increase with age, but also in sun exposed areas compared to protected areas [15]. In this study by Ray et al., epidermal skin had a significantly greater increase in mtDNA deletions with chronic sun exposure compared to dermal skin, which had no significant change in mtDNA deletion quantity to protected skin. This was higher than those found in normal ageing. Additionally, an increase in point mutations has been observed in aged human fibroblasts which suggest that there are different types of mtDNA damage that could contribute to skin ageing [16]. Mitochondrial mutations and deletions have also been found to increase with ageing in other tissues. An accumulation of somatic mtDNA point mutations has been observed in the noncoding region of muscle tissue [17,18], and an increase in the frequency of a common 4977 bp deletion has been observed with increasing age in both breast and brain tissue [19,20]. This specific deletion has been found to increase in an age dependent manner in whole human skin [21], however more recent studies suggests that this increase only correlates with sun exposure [22] and particularly in the dermis [23]. The T414G transversion mutation in the mtDNA promoter region has a strong correlation with dermal fibroblast ageing, which is significantly increased in UV exposed regions [24]. This mutation has been found in tissues affected by age-related conditions such as in the brain of Alzheimer's patients [25], precancerous cells in the colon [26] and an age-dependent increase in this mutation has also been found in muscle tissue [27]. This demonstrates that mtDNA damage increases with age in a variety of tissues and UV stress can accelerate this damage in the skin. However, it has been difficult to determine whether these mutations are generated by or induce ROS production, which is the centre of many debates surrounding this theory [28,29].

UV-induced oxidative stress and its role in signalling during extrinsic ageing have been well documented in the skin [30], but oxidative stress can also have ageing effects elsewhere. Reducing calorie intake by 10 to 50% is believed to decrease metabolic stress and scavenge ROS. It has been shown to increase lifespan in many organisms, including yeast [31] and mice [32], and decrease ageing biomarkers in nonhuman primates [33], making it a good candidate as a model to test Harman's theory. Altogether, tissue-specific increase in mitochondrial efficiency and the oxidative stress response [34] and consequential reduction in ROS and oxidative stress have been shown following CR; and while not all CR study models increased in lifespan, there is evidence to suggest improved ageing health [35]. The focus of these studies is primarily lifespan and effects on organs other than the skin. However, a report on CR in Rhesus monkeys presented with subjective increase in hair loss in the ad libitum control compared to the CR monkey [36], therefore CR and the resulting metabolic changes could also have an impact on the skin.

Skin changes with CR were further investigated by Forni et al. [37] in mice. Caloric restriction resulted in increased mitochondrial function in the dermis, but not the epidermis, and fur remodelling and impaired vasoconstriction relating to thermoregulation. This implicates mitochondria as energy providers for cold adaptation in the skin, which agrees with previous observations of mitochondrial uncoupling as a preventative mechanism to cold stress [38]. In terms of skin ageing, CR promotes epidermal thickening and increases hair follicle stem cell pool which could indicate a rejuvenation of the skin by preventing skin thinning and hair loss indicative of skin ageing. This is coupled by evidence that mice without mitochondrial matrix antioxidant superoxide dismutase SOD2, which converts superoxide anon to hydrogen peroxide for further metabolism, exhibit normal ageing phenotypes at a younger age, particularly cellular senescence in the skin [39]. Therefore, the reduced capacity to break down superoxide anion results in higher oxidative stress and accelerated skin ageing in this model.

Another important discovery in mice looked at the induction of mtDNA depletion by an amino acid substitution in POLG1. Mice with this mutation showed a significant reduction in all OXPHOS complex activities in the skin and phenotypical ageing symptoms such as hair greying and loss, curvature of the spine, reduced movement and wrinkling of the skin [40]. The skin and hair changes are attributed to deformities of the hair follicle, increased epidermal cell proliferation causing deep wrinkles and epidermal thickening. Skin is not often commented on when addressing symptoms of POLG mutations in humans, so a satisfactory comparison cannot yet be made.

So far, research has demonstrated an increase of mtDNA mutations in ageing and a link between lower metabolic stress and increased ageing health, but does not show cause and effect. The problem with these models is two-fold. Firstly, is the amount of mutant mtDNA present in the cell enough to cause a pathogenic effect and secondly, do the observed age-related mutations dysregulate the respiratory chain? This can be partially answered with an observed decrease in mitochondrial function and metabolism in ageing muscle tissue in parallel with an increasing mutation load with ageing [41,42]. This does not rule out other mechanisms of mitochondrial dysfunction unrelated to the observed mutations [43], nor does it prove that ROS is a confounding factor in the pathogenesis.

5. Pigmentation

Melanin pigment is formed in response to oxidation reactions in melanocytes. Pheomelanin is the yellow-red pigment associated with red head and freckles and eumelanin which is more prevalent in dark haired individuals, the ratio of these is regulated by the melanocortin 1 receptor (MCR1) gene which has been previously reviewed [44]. Pheomelanin has been shown to have higher prooxidant effects on the cell as it sequesters cysteine and glutathione antioxidant during synthesis, and the loss-of-function in MCR1 results in the inability to produce eumelanin in response to α-melanocyte-stimulating-hormone (α-MSH), the process of which produces some antioxidant properties [45]. In terms of skin ageing, loss of MCR1 function has been linked to increased perceived age by an average of two years and heterozygous variants without complete loss-of-function had an increased perceived age of one year on average [46]. It has been suggested that this could be the effect of oxidative effects of pheomelanin production or changes to fibroblast function in the absence of MCR1 activity. In relation to mitochondrial function, melanocytes pretreated with α-MSH have been shown to have a protective effect on mtDNA copy number in response to UVB light. This could infer that stimulation of eumelanin rather than pheomelanin could have photoprotective properties; however, no quantification pheomelanin/eumelanin was performed [47]. Links between mitochondrial function, mtDNA and pheomelanin/eumelanin ratio have not yet been formally researched, which could provide an insight into the mechanisms involved in skin ageing though oxidative stress.

Uneven pigmentation is one of the hallmarks of skin ageing. Mitochondria have even been implicated in the biosynthesis of melanin in melanocytes, required to create pigmentation in response to UV light. Prohibitin proteins found localised in the inner mitochondrial membrane were found to bind directly to melanogenin, a synthetic pigmentation promotor. Prohibitin silencing directly interfered with melanogenin activity and is thought to be involved in the regulation of rate limiting melanin enzyme tyrosinase [48]. In addition to this, mitochondria in melanocytes have been shown to interact with melanosomes, suggesting a functional role in melanosome biogenesis and therefore melanin production [49].

Melatonin is a hormone predominantly produced in the brain to regulate sleep, and its metabolism relies heavily on mitochondria and ROS signalling [50]. It exhibits antioxidant effects and can inhibit melanogenesis in animal models at high concentrations, which can help modulate coat colour [51]. Studies observing changes in human skin pigmentation with intake of oral melatonin found no effects over a 30-day period in patients with hyperpigmentation of varying causes [52], melanoma patients or a control group [53]. However, melatonin and its metabolites have been detected in human skin in vivo, and all were found to inhibit melanocyte proliferation and tyrosinase activity in vitro [54]. All of the above suggests that mitochondrial function is a modulator of skin pigmentation, and also that dysfunction could interfere with melanin production both directly and indirectly through excessive ROS signalling and melatonin production.

These findings correspond with the observation from individuals with vitiligo—a condition which results in areas of the skin with inactive melanocytes—of reduced energy production in cultured melanocytes with depleted skin pigmentation, compared to healthy melanocytes [55], and the increased presence of vitiligo in patients with genetic mitochondrial dysfunction [56].

6. Photoageing

Sun damage is a well-known cause of skin cancer and ageing, and photoageing is the process of chronic sun exposure leading to extrinsic skin ageing. Solar light is composed of ultraviolet radiation (UVR) (10–380 nm), visible light (380–780 nm) and infrared radiation (IR) (above 780 nm). UVR is the most notorious for causing skin damage, so protection against both UVA and UVB is found in most sunscreens. UVB radiation was once believed to be the only contributor to photoageing due to higher energy levels than UVA, but it is now proven that UVA is the key player, though each can affect skin in different ways. UVA makes up the majority of solar UVR but only affects DNA indirectly, whereas UVB radiation represents a small portion but causes direct DNA damage [57].

The epidermis is the first line of defence against UVB damage and absorbs the majority of the radiation. The level of which depends on ethnicity, site of skin, hydration and many other factors [58]. Pigmentation from melanin plays a large part in the initial protection against UVR [59], and higher melanin has an inverse correlation with DNA lesions in humans [60] and this is also seen in other species, such as whales [61]. UVA, visible and infrared light can penetrate deeper into the skin than UVB (Figure 1), and it has been shown that dermal fibroblasts are in fact more susceptible to DNA damage from longer wavelengths of light (>300 nm) [62]. There is also evidence of visible and infrared light induced skin damage, and even a synergistic effect of all wavelengths [63].

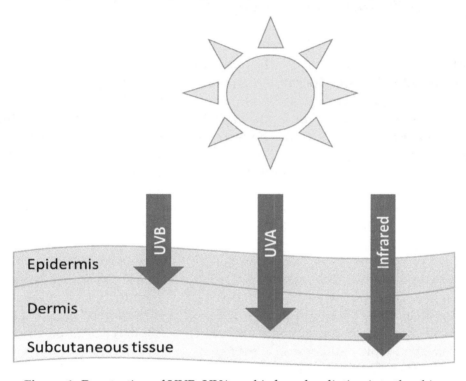

Figure 1. Penetration of UVB, UVA and infrared radiation into the skin.

Ageing is a natural process, and even without UV insult would occur over time due to the gradual shortening of telomere caps in nuclear DNA, loss-of-functionality in ageing and consequent cellular senescence [64]. This ageing damage profile has been found in a number of age related diseases including dementia and atherosclerosis [65,66]. It can also be induced in vitro in skin fibroblasts using UVA radiation [67] and in keratinocytes using UVB exposure [68], which further demonstrates a role for UVR in ageing. In addition to this, mtDNA damage is repeatedly seen in higher levels in photoexposed skin leading to an accumulation of cellular damage and a decrease in mitochondrial activity in the skin [24,69–71].

Although the precise mechanisms of photoageing are still being researched, collagen, mtDNA damage and increased ROS production are all key features. Inflammation induces the breakdown of matrix proteins to help the recruitment and migration of immune cells, therefore chronic inflammation can result in detrimental breakdown of tissues [72]. Inflammation due to UVA and UVB exposure has been shown to induce the enzymatic activity of MMPs in the dermis and epidermis, respectively, through ROS signalling and the activation of transcription factor AP-1 and NFκB [73–76]. AP-1 production reduces synthesis of procollagen type I and III, thereby disrupting the formation of new collagen at the same time as degrading it [77]. This is supported by the presence of ultrastructural changes and degradation of collagen fibre bundles from the dermis in photoexposed areas of human skin and UV irradiated mouse models [78]. Infrared radiation can also induce MMPs in dermal fibroblasts [79]. Therefore, sun exposure is directly linked to the active breakdown of collagen and the reduction of collagen synthesis through ROS signalling, leading to the formation of deep wrinkles and extrinsic skin ageing. Hypothetically, the mtDNA damage observed in photoexposed areas could cause dysregulation of OXPHOS and an increase in ROS production, as theorised in the 'Free Radical Theory of Ageing', and this could then lead to accelerated skin ageing.

The process of photodegradation of melanin results in singlet oxygen production, which has been shown in synthetic models [80], and UVA irradiation of pheomelanin exhibited conformational changes in catalase antioxidant which was attenuated with a singlet oxygen quencher [81]. In humans, a six-fold increase in photoageing was observed in those with homozygous loss of MC1R gene variants compared to those with wild type gene [82]. This all suggests that photodegradation of melanin could also be an important mechanism in the oxidative stress and mtDNA damage exhibited in photoexposed skin.

7. Pollution

With climate change a major danger to human health, research into the effects of air pollution has received growing attention. Outdoor pollutants predominantly originate from vehicle emissions, combustion of fossil fuels and industrial processes. Small particulate matter ($PM_{2.5}$) and ozone has been shown to increase DNA and protein damage through ROS and oxidative stress in vitro and in mouse models [83,84], and have a positive association with skin ageing though pigmentation spots and skin wrinkling in Chinese [85] and German populations [86]. Activation of the aryl hydrocarbon receptor (AhR) is key in modulating the effects of pollution. Its activation by ligands, including ozone and $PM_{2.5}$ [87,88], increases the expression of cytochrome P450, which can metabolise polycyclic aromatic hydrocarbons into carcinogenic substances capable of inducing DNA damage. These mechanisms have been further reviewed elsewhere [12,89,90].

Lentigines are hyperpigmented lesions in the skin as a consequence of excess melanocytes, which often become more abundant during ageing. Solar lentigines are associated with the level of sun exposure of the skin [91], and are the product of excess melanin production. Traffic-associated particles and soot have also been associated with the formation of these pigment spots on the forehead and cheeks [86,92], suggesting a common mechanism between UVR and pollution stressors. It has been suggested that one factor in this could be due to the age-dependent decline of mitochondrial complex II: succinate dehydrogenase [93]. Complex II is entirely transcribed by nuclear DNA and has been shown to decrease it's activity in comparison to complex I and IV in an age dependent manner in senescent cells, predominantly in the epidermis [69]. Inducing hyperpigmentation in melanoma cells results in the inhibition of complex II activity and an initial increase in superoxide ROS formation, and increasing melanin concentration was capable of attenuating further formation [94]. Therefore, lentigine formation could be a protective mechanism against the increase ROS production from senescent skin cells, due to a decline in complex II function.

8. Hair Follicles

Hair loss and greying is another key observable ageing phenotype. Unfortunately, this is one ageing phenotype which is poorly understood and as yet cannot be prevented. Hair follicles are situated within the dermis, and melanocytes and keratinocytes are responsible for the colour and growth of hair; it is therefore important to mention hair within the context of skin and ageing.

One theory of hair greying involves the acquisition of mitochondrial DNA damage with increased oxidative stress; the 'common' 4977 bp deletion has been discovered in higher levels in greying and unpigmented hair follicles (40% and 20%, respectively) than in pigmented (5%) [95]. Greying hair can be characterised by the gradual loss of melanocytes in the pigmentary units by apoptosis, until the hair follicle is unpigmented [96]. This pigmentary unit in greying hair was found to have the highest level of oxidative stress in melanocytes and a loss of ROS scavenging Bcl-2 activity. Bcl-2 is an inhibitor of the mitochondrial pathway of apoptosis, so the diminished expression can explain the increased apoptosis of melanocytes in response to cell stressors. These findings are in line with the grey hair phenotype of Bcl2−/− mice [97]. This details the mechanisms associated with mitochondrial function;

but all of three theorised mechanisms, as reviewed by SK Jo et al. (2018) [98], point to a role of oxidative or genotoxic stress induced damage, which supports mitochondrial involvement.

Hair loss can occur though ageing, nutrient deficiency and temporary or permanent alopecia, all of which present differently. Like hair greying, hair loss is little understood. Mice with PolgA mutations leading to a faulty mtDNA repair mechanism, have an increased mtDNA mutation abundance and an accelerated ageing phenotype which exhibits a reduction in hair density [99]. Age-related hair loss in humans is predominantly androgenic with a higher prevalence in men [100]. Dermal papilla cells from balding regions have been found to express higher levels of senescence markers and have antioxidant superoxide dismutase expression localised in the nuclear region. This is in contrast to the cytoplasmic or mitochondrial localisation found in nonbalding counterparts [101]. This translocation of superoxide dismutase in response to oxidative stress in the cell is a protective mechanism as it is suggested to promote oxidative resistance and repair and function as a transcription factor [22].

Mice with mitochondrial transcription factor A (TFAM) knockdown, which causes mtDNA depletion and loss of electron transport chain (ETC) complexes, in the epidermis and hair follicle epithelium show a reduction in proliferation, increase in apoptosis and exhibit abnormalities in melanin production and function in the hair follicles [102]. ROS signalling from mitochondrial function is required for hair growth, as shown by high mitochondrial membrane potential and a burst of ROS production at the matrix epidermal cell and hair shaft interface in growing cultured bovine and human hair follicles [103]. These epithelial cells subsequently underwent mitochondrial de-polarisation as they converted to hair shaft matrix. Both these studies demonstrate critical mitochondrial function and ROS signalling in the morphogenesis of hair follicles and hair shaft elongation, and the importance of functional ETC in these processes.

Although there is a limited understanding of hair ageing, there is evidence to support mitochondrial involvement in both, predominantly through the increase of oxidative stress and a reduced capacity to cope.

9. Summary

Mitochondria are important for skin function and mtDNA mutations; functional decline is linked to skin ageing through stress-induced wrinkle formation, pigmentation and hair greying and loss. Many of the mechanisms contributing to skin ageing are not fully understood, and it is likely that mitochondrial function is part of a complex set of processes that lead to tissue functional decline and ageing. It is important scientifically to understand the mechanisms behind skin ageing to clinically develop prevention strategies, but it is also useful in industry to improve antiageing formulas and those targeted to mature skin.

Abbreviations

UVA	Ultraviolet A
UVB	Ultraviolet B
IR	Infrared
MMPs	Matrix metalloproteinases
ROS	Reactive oxygen species
AP-1	activator protein-1
NFκB	Nuclear factor kappa-light-chain-enhancer of activated B cells
TGF-β	Transforming growth factor beta
PM$_{2.5}$	Small particulate matter
AhR	Aryl hydrocarbon receptor
Bcl-2	B-cell lymphoma 2
ETC	Electron transport chain

References

1.   Thingnes, J.; Lavelle, T.J.; Hovig, E.; Omholt, S.W. Understanding the Melanocyte Distribution in Human Epidermis: An Agent-Based Computational Model Approach. *PLoS ONE* **2012**, *7*, e40377. [CrossRef]
2.   Koster, M.I. Making an epidermis. *Ann. N. Y. Acad. Sci.* **2009**, *1170*, 7–10. [CrossRef] [PubMed]
3.   Poon, F.; Kang, S.; Chien, A.L. Mechanisms and treatments of photoaging. *Photodermatol. Photoimmunol. Photomed.* **2015**, *31*, 65–74. [CrossRef]
4.   Wickersham, M.; Wachtel, S.; Wong Fok Lung, T.; Soong, G.; Jacquet, R.; Richardson, A.; Parker, D.; Prince, A. Metabolic Stress Drives Keratinocyte Defenses against Staphylococcus aureus Infection. *Cell Rep.* **2017**, *18*, 2742–2751. [CrossRef] [PubMed]
5.   Hamanaka, R.B.; Chandel, N.S. Mitochondrial reactive oxygen species regulate hypoxic signaling. *Curr. Opin. Cell Biol.* **2009**, *21*, 894–899. [CrossRef]
6.   Hamanaka, R.B.; Chandel, N.S. Mitochondrial metabolism as a regulator of keratinocyte differentiation. *Cell. Logist.* **2013**, *3*, e25456. [CrossRef]
7.   Feichtinger, R.G.; Sperl, W.; Bauer, J.W.; Kofler, B. Mitochondrial dysfunction: A neglected component of skin diseases. *Exp. Dermatol.* **2014**, *23*, 607–614. [CrossRef] [PubMed]
8.   Birch-Machin, M.A. Mitochondria and skin disease. *Clin. Exp. Dermatol.* **2000**, *25*, 141–146. [CrossRef]
9.   Plummer, C.; Spring, P.J.; Marotta, R.; Chin, J.; Taylor, G.; Sharpe, D.; Athanasou, N.A.; Thyagarajan, D.; Berkovic, S.F. Multiple Symmetrical Lipomatosis—A mitochondrial disorder of brown fat. *Mitochondrion* **2013**, *13*, 269–276. [CrossRef]
10. Boulton, S.J.; Bowman, A.; Koohgoli, R.; Birch-Machin, M.A. Skin manifestations of mitochondrial dysfunction: More important than previously thought. *Exp. Dermatol.* **2015**, *24*, 12–13. [CrossRef]
11. Farage, M.A.; Miller, K.W.; Elsner, P.; Maibach, H.I. Intrinsic and extrinsic factors in skin ageing: A review. *Int. J. Cosmet. Sci.* **2008**, *30*, 87–95. [CrossRef]
12. Naidoo, K.; Birch-Machin, M. Oxidative Stress and Ageing: The Influence of Environmental Pollution, Sunlight and Diet on Skin. *Cosmetics* **2017**, *4*, 4. [CrossRef]
13. Wey, S.-J.; Chen, D.-Y. Common cutaneous disorders in the elderly. *J. Clin. Gerontol. Geriatr.* **2010**, *1*, 36–41. [CrossRef]
14. Harman, D. Aging: A Theory Based on Free Radical and Radiation Chemistry. *J. Gerontol.* **1956**, *11*, 298–300. [CrossRef] [PubMed]
15. Ray, A.J.; Turner, R.; Nikaido, O.; Rees, J.L.; Birch-Machin, M.A. The Spectrum of Mitochondrial DNA Deletions is a Ubiquitous Marker of Ultraviolet Radiation Exposure in Human Skin. *J. Investig. Dermatol.* **2000**, *115*, 674–679. [CrossRef] [PubMed]
16. Michikawa, Y.; Mazzucchelli, F.; Bresolin, N.; Scarlato, G.; Attardi, G. Aging-Dependent Large Accumulation of Point Mutations in the Human mtDNA Control Region for Replication. *Science (New York N. Y.)* **1999**, *286*, 774–779. [CrossRef]
17. Wang, Y.; Michikawa, Y.; Mallidis, C.; Bai, Y.; Woodhouse, L.; Yarasheski, K.E.; Miller, C.A.; Askanas, V.; Engel, W.K.; Bhasin, S.; et al. Muscle-specific mutations accumulate with aging in critical human mtDNA control sites for replication. *Proc. Natl. Acad. Sci. USA* **2001**, *98*, 4022–4027. [CrossRef] [PubMed]
18. Del Bo, R.; Crimi, M.; Sciacco, M.; Malferrari, G.; Bordoni, A.; Napoli, L.; Prelle, A.; Biunno, I.; Moggio, M.; Bresolin, N.; et al. High mutational burden in the mtDNA control region from aged muscles: A single-fiber study. *Neurobiol. Aging* **2003**, *24*, 829–838. [CrossRef]
19. Pavicic, W.H.; Richard, S.M. Correlation analysis between mtDNA 4977-bp deletion and ageing. *Mutat. Res./Fundam. Mol. Mech. Mutagen.* **2009**, *670*, 99–102. [CrossRef] [PubMed]
20. Corral-Debrinski, M.; Horton, T.; Lott, M.T.; Shoffner, J.M.; Flint Beal, M.; Wallace, D.C. Mitochondrial DNA deletions in human brain: Regional variability and increase with advanced age. *Nat. Genet.* **1992**, *2*, 324. [CrossRef]
21. Yang, J.H.; Lee, H.C.; Lin, K.J.; Wei, Y.H. A specific 4977-bp deletion of mitochondrial DNA in human ageing skin. *Arch. Dermatol. Res.* **1994**, *286*, 386–390. [CrossRef] [PubMed]
22. Powers, J.M.; Murphy, G.; Ralph, N.; O'Gorman, S.M.; Murphy, J.E.J. Mitochondrial DNA deletion percentage in sun exposed and non sun exposed skin. *J. Photochem. Photobiol. B Biol.* **2016**, *165*, 277–282. [CrossRef] [PubMed]

23. Eshaghian, A.; Vleugels, R.A.; Canter, J.A.; McDonald, M.A.; Stasko, T.; Sligh, J.E. Mitochondrial DNA Deletions Serve as Biomarkers of Aging in the Skin, but Are Typically Absent in Nonmelanoma Skin Cancers. *J. Investig. Dermatol.* **2006**, *126*, 336–344. [CrossRef] [PubMed]

24. Birket, M.J.; Birch-Machin, M.A. Ultraviolet radiation exposure accelerates the accumulation of the aging-dependent T414G mitochondrial DNA mutation in human skin. *Aging Cell* **2007**, *6*, 557–564. [CrossRef]

25. Coskun, P.E.; Beal, M.F.; Wallace, D.C. Alzheimer's brains harbor somatic mtDNA control-region mutations that suppress mitochondrial transcription and replication. *Proc. Natl. Acad. Sci. USA* **2004**, *101*, 10726–10731. [CrossRef] [PubMed]

26. Kassem, A.M.; El-Guendy, N.; Tantawy, M.; Abdelhady, H.; El-Ghor, A.; Wahab, A.H.A. Mutational Hotspots in the Mitochondrial D-Loop Region of Cancerous and Precancerous Colorectal Lesions in Egyptian Patients. *DNA Cell Biol.* **2011**, *30*, 899–906. [CrossRef]

27. Murdock, D.G.; Christacos, N.C.; Wallace, D.C. The age-related accumulation of a mitochondrial DNA control region mutation in muscle, but not brain, detected by a sensitive PNA-directed PCR clamping based method. *Nucleic Acids Res.* **2000**, *28*, 4350–4355. [CrossRef]

28. Zhang, R.; Wang, Y.; Ye, K.; Picard, M.; Gu, Z. Independent impacts of aging on mitochondrial DNA quantity and quality in humans. *BMC Genom.* **2017**, *18*, 890. [CrossRef]

29. Payne, B.A.I.; Chinnery, P.F. Mitochondrial dysfunction in aging: Much progress but many unresolved questions. *Biochim. Biophys. Acta* **2015**, *1847*, 1347–1353. [CrossRef]

30. Rinnerthaler, M.; Bischof, J.; Streubel, M.K.; Trost, A.; Richter, K. Oxidative stress in aging human skin. *Biomolecules* **2015**, *5*, 545–589. [CrossRef]

31. Lin, S.-J.; Kaeberlein, M.; Andalis, A.A.; Sturtz, L.A.; Defossez, P.-A.; Culotta, V.C.; Fink, G.R.; Guarente, L. Calorie restriction extends Saccharomyces cerevisiae lifespan by increasing respiration. *Nature* **2002**, *418*, 344. [CrossRef]

32. Bartke, A.; Wright, J.C.; Mattison, J.A.; Ingram, D.K.; Miller, R.A.; Roth, G.S. Extending the lifespan of long-lived mice. *Nature* **2001**, *414*, 412. [CrossRef]

33. Lane, M.A.; Ingram, D.K.; Ball, S.S.; Roth, G.S. Dehydroepiandrosterone Sulfate: A Biomarker of Primate Aging Slowed by Calorie Restriction. *J. Clin. Endocrinol. Metab.* **1997**, *82*, 2093–2096. [CrossRef]

34. Lanza, I.R.; Zabielski, P.; Klaus, K.A.; Morse, D.M.; Heppelmann, C.J.; Bergen, H.R., 3rd; Dasari, S.; Walrand, S.; Short, K.R.; Johnson, M.L.; et al. Chronic caloric restriction preserves mitochondrial function in senescence without increasing mitochondrial biogenesis. *Cell Metab.* **2012**, *16*, 777–788. [CrossRef]

35. Mattison, J.A.; Roth, G.S.; Beasley, T.M.; Tilmont, E.M.; Handy, A.M.; Herbert, R.L.; Longo, D.L.; Allison, D.B.; Young, J.E.; Bryant, M.; et al. Impact of caloric restriction on health and survival in rhesus monkeys from the NIA study. *Nature* **2012**, *489*, 318. [CrossRef]

36. Colman, R.J.; Anderson, R.M.; Johnson, S.C.; Kastman, E.K.; Kosmatka, K.J.; Beasley, T.M.; Allison, D.B.; Cruzen, C.; Simmons, H.A.; Kemnitz, J.W.; et al. Caloric Restriction Delays Disease Onset and Mortality in Rhesus Monkeys. *Science (New York N. Y.)* **2009**, *325*, 201–204. [CrossRef]

37. Forni, M.F.; Peloggia, J.; Braga, T.T.; Chinchilla, J.E.O.; Shinohara, J.; Navas, C.A.; Camara, N.O.S.; Kowaltowski, A.J. Caloric Restriction Promotes Structural and Metabolic Changes in the Skin. *Cell Rep.* **2017**, *20*, 2678–2692. [CrossRef]

38. Stier, A.; Bize, P.; Habold, C.; Bouillaud, F.; Massemin, S.; Criscuolo, F. Mitochondrial uncoupling prevents cold-induced oxidative stress: A case study using UCP1 knockout mice. *J. Exp. Biol.* **2014**, *217*, 624–630. [CrossRef]

39. Weyemi, U.; Parekh, P.R.; Redon, C.E.; Bonner, W.M. SOD2 deficiency promotes aging phenotypes in mouse skin. *Aging* **2012**, *4*, 116–118. [CrossRef]

40. Singh, B.; Schoeb, T.R.; Bajpai, P.; Slominski, A.; Singh, K.K. Reversing wrinkled skin and hair loss in mice by restoring mitochondrial function. *Cell Death Dis.* **2018**, *9*, 735. [CrossRef]

41. McCully, K.K.; Fielding, R.A.; Evans, W.J.; Leigh, J.S., Jr.; Posner, J.D. Relationships between in vivo and in vitro measurements of metabolism in young and old human calf muscles. *J. Appl. Physiol. (Bethesda Md. 1985)* **1993**, *75*, 813–819. [CrossRef]

42. Short, K.R.; Bigelow, M.L.; Kahl, J.; Singh, R.; Coenen-Schimke, J.; Raghavakaimal, S.; Nair, K.S. Decline in skeletal muscle mitochondrial function with aging in humans. *Proc. Natl. Acad. Sci. USA* **2005**, *102*, 5618–5623. [CrossRef]

43. Niyazov, D.M.; Kahler, S.G.; Frye, R.E. Primary Mitochondrial Disease and Secondary Mitochondrial Dysfunction: Importance of Distinction for Diagnosis and Treatment. *Mol. Syndromol.* **2016**, *7*, 122–137. [CrossRef]

44. Denat, L.; Kadekaro, A.L.; Marrot, L.; Leachman, S.A.; Abdel-Malek, Z.A. Melanocytes as instigators and victims of oxidative stress. *J. Investig. Dermatol.* **2014**, *134*, 1512–1518. [CrossRef]

45. Song, X.; Mosby, N.; Yang, J.; Xu, A.; Abdel-Malek, Z.; Kadekaro, A.L. alpha-MSH activates immediate defense responses to UV-induced oxidative stress in human melanocytes. *Pigment Cell Melanoma Res.* **2009**, *22*, 809–818. [CrossRef]

46. Liu, F.; Hamer, M.A.; Deelen, J.; Lall, J.S.; Jacobs, L.; van Heemst, D.; Murray, P.G.; Wollstein, A.; de Craen, A.J.; Uh, H.W.; et al. The MC1R Gene and Youthful Looks. *Curr. Biol. CB* **2016**, *26*, 1213–1220. [CrossRef]

47. Böhm, M.; Hill, H.Z. Ultraviolet B, melanin and mitochondrial DNA: Photo-damage in human epidermal keratinocytes and melanocytes modulated by alpha-melanocyte-stimulating hormone. *F1000 Res.* **2016**, *5*, 881. [CrossRef]

48. Snyder, J.R.; Hall, A.; Ni-Komatsu, L.; Khersonsky, S.M.; Chang, Y.-T.; Orlow, S.J. Dissection of Melanogenesis with Small Molecules Identifies Prohibitin as a Regulator. *Chem. Biol.* **2005**, *12*, 477–484. [CrossRef]

49. Daniele, T.; Hurbain, I.; Vago, R.; Casari, G.; Raposo, G.; Tacchetti, C.; Schiaffino, M.V. Mitochondria and melanosomes establish physical contacts modulated by Mfn2 and involved in organelle biogenesis. *Curr. Biol. CB* **2014**, *24*, 393–403. [CrossRef]

50. Slominski, A.T.; Semak, I.; Fischer, T.W.; Kim, T.-K.; Kleszczyński, K.; Hardeland, R.; Reiter, R.J. Metabolism of melatonin in the skin: Why is it important? *Exp. Dermatol.* **2017**, *26*, 563–568. [CrossRef]

51. Slominski, A.; Pruski, D. Melatonin inhibits proliferation and melanogenesis in rodent melanoma cells. *Exp. Cell Res.* **1993**, *206*, 189–194. [CrossRef]

52. Lerner, A.B.; Nordlund, J.J. The Effects of Oral Melatonin on Skin Color and on the Release of Pituitary Hormones. *J. Clin. Endocrinol. Metab.* **1977**, *45*, 768–774. [CrossRef]

53. McElhinney, D.B.; Hoffman, S.J.; Robinson, W.A.; Ferguson, J.A.N. Effect of Melatonin on Human Skin Color. *J. Investig. Dermatol.* **1994**, *102*, 258–259. [CrossRef]

54. Kim, T.-K.; Lin, Z.; Tidwell, W.J.; Li, W.; Slominski, A.T. Melatonin and its metabolites accumulate in the human epidermis in vivo and inhibit proliferation and tyrosinase activity in epidermal melanocytes in vitro. *Mol. Cell. Endocrinol.* **2015**, *404*, 1–8. [CrossRef]

55. Dell'Anna, M.L.; Ottaviani, M.; Kovacs, D.; Mirabilii, S.; Brown, D.A.; Cota, C.; Migliano, E.; Bastonini, E.; Bellei, B.; Cardinali, G.; et al. Energetic mitochondrial failing in vitiligo and possible rescue by cardiolipin. *Sci. Rep.* **2017**, *7*, 13663. [CrossRef]

56. Karvonen, S.L.; Haapasaari, K.M.; Kallioinen, M.; Oikarinen, A.; Hassinen, I.E.; Majamaa, K. Increased prevalence of vitiligo, but no evidence of premature ageing, in the skin of patients with bp 3243 mutation in mitochondrial DNA in the mitochondrial encephalomyopathy, lactic acidosis and stroke-like episodes syndrome (MELAS). *Br. J. Dermatol.* **1999**, *140*, 634–639. [CrossRef]

57. Rünger, T.M.; Epe, B.; Möller, K. Processing of Directly and Indirectly Ultraviolet-Induced DNA Damage in Human Cells. *Recent Results Cancer Res.* **1995**, *139*, 31–42.

58. Sklar, L.R.; Almutawa, F.; Lim, H.W.; Hamzavi, I. Effects of ultraviolet radiation, visible light, and infrared radiation on erythema and pigmentation: A review. *Photochem. Photobiol. Sci.* **2013**, *12*, 54–64. [CrossRef]

59. Swalwell, H.; Latimer, J.; Haywood, R.M.; Birch-Machin, M.A. Investigating the role of melanin in UVA/UVB- and hydrogen peroxide-induced cellular and mitochondrial ROS production and mitochondrial DNA damage in human melanoma cells. *Free Radic. Biol. Med.* **2012**, *52*, 626–634. [CrossRef]

60. Wenczl, E.; van der Schans, G.P.; Roza, L.; Kolb, R.; Smit, N.; Schothorst, A.A. UVA-induced oxidative DNA damage in human melanocytes is related to their (pheo)melanin content. *J. Dermatol. Sci.* **1998**, *16*, S221. [CrossRef]

61. Martinez-Levasseur, L.M.; Birch-Machin, M.A.; Bowman, A.; Gendron, D.; Weatherhead, E.; Knell, R.J.; Acevedo-Whitehouse, K. Whales use distinct strategies to counteract solar ultraviolet radiation. *Sci. Rep.* **2013**, *3*, 2386. [CrossRef]

62. Latimer, J.A.; Lloyd, J.J.; Diffey, B.L.; Matts, P.J.; Birch-Machin, M.A. Determination of the Action Spectrum of UVR-Induced Mitochondrial DNA Damage in Human Skin Cells. *J. Investig. Dermatol.* **2015**, *135*, 2512–2518. [CrossRef]

63. Rashdan, E.; Wilkinson, S.; Birch-Machin, M. British Society for Investigative Dermatology Annual Meeting 2018 26–28 March 2018 Blizard Institute, Barts and The London School of Medicine and Dentistry. *Br. J. Dermatol.* **2018**. [CrossRef]

64. Harley, C.B.; Futcher, A.B.; Greider, C.W. Telomeres shorten during ageing of human fibroblasts. *Nature* **1990**, *345*, 458. [CrossRef]

65. Saretzki, G.; Zglinicki, T. Replicative Aging, Telomeres, and Oxidative Stress. *Ann. N. Y. Acad. Sci.* **2006**, *959*, 24–29. [CrossRef]

66. Samani, N.J.; Boultby, R.; Butler, R.; Thompson, J.R.; Goodall, A.H. Telomere shortening in atherosclerosis. *Lancet* **2001**, *358*, 472–473. [CrossRef]

67. Ma, H.M.; Liu, W.; Zhang, P.; Yuan, X.Y. Human skin fibroblast telomeres are shortened after ultraviolet irradiation. *J. Int. Med. Res.* **2012**, *40*, 1871–1877. [CrossRef]

68. Nistico, S.; Ehrlich, J.; Gliozzi, M.; Maiuolo, J.; Del Duca, E.; Muscoli, C.; Mollace, V. Telomere and telomerase modulation by bergamot polyphenolic fraction in experimental photoageing in human keratinocytes. *J. Biol. Regul. Homeost. Agents* **2015**, *29*, 723–728.

69. Bowman, A.; Birch-Machin, M.A. Age-Dependent Decrease of Mitochondrial Complex II Activity in Human Skin Fibroblasts. *J. Investig. Dermatol.* **2016**, *136*, 912–919. [CrossRef]

70. Krishnan, K.J.; Harbottle, A.; Birch-Machin, M.A. The Use of a 3895 bp Mitochondrial DNA Deletion as a Marker for Sunlight Exposure in Human Skin. *J. Investig. Dermatol.* **2004**, *123*, 1020–1024. [CrossRef]

71. Berneburg, M.; Gattermann, N.; Stege, H.; Grewe, M.; Vogelsang, K.; Ruzicka, T.; Krutmann, J. Chronically Ultraviolet-exposed Human Skin Shows a Higher Mutation Frequency of Mitochondrial DNA as Compared to Unexposed Skin and the Hematopoietic System. *Photochem. Photobiol.* **1997**, *66*, 271–275. [CrossRef]

72. Manicone, A.M.; McGuire, J.K. Matrix metalloproteinases as modulators of inflammation. *Semin. Cell Dev. Biol.* **2008**, *19*, 34–41. [CrossRef]

73. Vicentini, F.T.; He, T.; Shao, Y.; Fonseca, M.J.; Verri, W.A., Jr.; Fisher, G.J.; Xu, Y. Quercetin inhibits UV irradiation-induced inflammatory cytokine production in primary human keratinocytes by suppressing NF-kappaB pathway. *J. Dermatol. Sci.* **2011**, *61*, 162–168. [CrossRef]

74. Kang, S.; Chung, J.H.; Lee, J.H.; Fisher, G.J.; Wan, Y.S.; Duell, E.A.; Voorhees, J.J. Topical N-Acetyl Cysteine and Genistein Prevent Ultraviolet-Light-Induced Signaling That Leads to Photoaging in Human Skin in vivo. *J. Investig. Dermatol.* **2003**, *120*, 835–841. [CrossRef]

75. Tewari, A.; Grys, K.; Kollet, J.; Sarkany, R.; Young, A.R. Upregulation of MMP12 and its activity by UVA1 in human skin: Potential implications for photoaging. *J. Investig. Dermatol.* **2014**, *134*, 2598–2609. [CrossRef]

76. Chiang, H.M.; Chen, H.C.; Lin, T.J.; Shih, I.C.; Wen, K.C. Michelia alba extract attenuates UVB-induced expression of matrix metalloproteinases via MAP kinase pathway in human dermal fibroblasts. *Food Chem. Toxicol.* **2012**, *50*, 4260–4269. [CrossRef]

77. Fisher, G.J.; Datta, S.; Wang, Z.; Li, X.Y.; Quan, T.; Chung, J.H.; Kang, S.; Voorhees, J.J. c-Jun-dependent inhibition of cutaneous procollagen transcription following ultraviolet irradiation is reversed by all-trans retinoic acid. *J. Clin. Investig.* **2000**, *106*, 663–670. [CrossRef]

78. Edwards, C.; Pearse, A.; Marks, R.; Nishimori, Y.; Matsumoto, K.; Kawai, M. Degenerative Alterations of Dermal Collagen Fiber Bundles in Photodamaged Human Skin and UV-Irradiated Hairless Mouse Skin: Possible Effect on Decreasing Skin Mechanical Properties and Appearance of Wrinkles. *J. Investig. Dermatol.* **2001**, *117*, 1458–1463. [CrossRef]

79. Schieke, S.M.; Stege, H.; Kürten, V.; Grether-Beck, S.; Sies, H.; Krutmann, J. Infrared-A Radiation-Induced Matrix Metalloproteinase 1 Expression is Mediated Through Extracellular Signal-regulated Kinase 1/2 Activation in Human Dermal Fibroblasts. *J. Investig. Dermatol.* **2002**, *119*, 1323–1329. [CrossRef]

80. Szewczyk, G.; Zadlo, A.; Sarna, M.; Ito, S.; Wakamatsu, K.; Sarna, T. Aerobic photoreactivity of synthetic eumelanins and pheomelanins: Generation of singlet oxygen and superoxide anion. *Pigment Cell Melanoma Res.* **2016**, *29*, 669–678. [CrossRef]

81. Maresca, V.; Flori, E.; Briganti, S.; Camera, E.; Cario-André, M.; Taïeb, A.; Picardo, M. UVA-Induced Modification of Catalase Charge Properties in the Epidermis Is Correlated with the Skin Phototype. *J. Investig. Dermatol.* **2006**, *126*, 182–190. [CrossRef]

82. Elfakir, A.; Ezzedine, K.; Latreille, J.; Ambroisine, L.; Jdid, R.; Galan, P.; Hercberg, S.; Gruber, F.; Malvy, D.; Tschachler, E.; et al. Functional MC1R-Gene Variants Are Associated with Increased Risk for Severe Photoaging of Facial Skin. *J. Investig. Dermatol.* **2010**, *130*, 1107–1115. [CrossRef]

83. Piao, M.J.; Ahn, M.J.; Kang, K.A.; Ryu, Y.S.; Hyun, Y.J.; Shilnikova, K.; Zhen, A.X.; Jeong, J.W.; Choi, Y.H.; Kang, H.K.; et al. Particulate matter 2.5 damages skin cells by inducing oxidative stress, subcellular organelle dysfunction, and apoptosis. *Arch. Toxicol.* **2018**, *92*, 2077–2091. [CrossRef]

84. Valacchi, G.; van der Vliet, A.; Schock, B.C.; Okamoto, T.; Obermuller-Jevic, U.; Cross, C.E.; Packer, L. Ozone exposure activates oxidative stress responses in murine skin. *Toxicology* **2002**, *179*, 163–170. [CrossRef]

85. Ding, A.; Yang, Y.; Zhao, Z.; Hüls, A.; Vierkötter, A.; Yuan, Z.; Cai, J.; Zhang, J.; Gao, W.; Li, J.; et al. Indoor PM2.5 exposure affects skin aging manifestation in a Chinese population. *Sci. Rep.* **2017**, *7*, 15329. [CrossRef]

86. Vierkötter, A.; Schikowski, T.; Ranft, U.; Sugiri, D.; Matsui, M.; Krämer, U.; Krutmann, J. Airborne Particle Exposure and Extrinsic Skin Aging. *J. Investig. Dermatol.* **2010**, *130*, 2719–2726. [CrossRef]

87. Gualtieri, M.; Øvrevik, J.; Mollerup, S.; Asare, N.; Longhin, E.; Dahlman, H.-J.; Camatini, M.; Holme, J.A. Airborne urban particles (Milan winter-PM2.5) cause mitotic arrest and cell death: Effects on DNA, mitochondria, AhR binding and spindle organization. *Mutat. Res./Fundam. Mol. Mech. Mutagen.* **2011**, *713*, 18–31. [CrossRef]

88. Afaq, F.; Zaid, M.A.; Pelle, E.; Khan, N.; Syed, D.N.; Matsui, M.S.; Maes, D.; Mukhtar, H. Aryl Hydrocarbon Receptor Is an Ozone Sensor in Human Skin. *J. Investig. Dermatol.* **2009**, *129*, 2396–2403. [CrossRef]

89. Koohgoli, R.; Hudson, L.; Naidoo, K.; Wilkinson, S.; Chavan, B.; Birch-Machin, M.A. Bad air gets under your skin. *Exp. Dermatol.* **2017**, *26*, 384–387. [CrossRef]

90. Shimada, T.; Fujii-Kuriyama, Y. Metabolic activation of polycyclic aromatic hydrocarbons to carcinogens by cytochromes P450 1A1 and 1B1. *Cancer Sci.* **2004**, *95*, 1–6. [CrossRef]

91. Bastiaens, M.; Hoefnagel, J.; Westendorp, R.; Vermeer, B.-J.; Bouwes Bavinck, J.N. Solar Lentigines are Strongly Related to Sun Exposure in Contrast to Ephelides. *Pigment Cell Res.* **2004**, *17*, 225–229. [CrossRef]

92. Hüls, A.; Vierkötter, A.; Gao, W.; Krämer, U.; Yang, Y.; Ding, A.; Stolz, S.; Matsui, M.; Kan, H.; Wang, S.; et al. Traffic-Related Air Pollution Contributes to Development of Facial Lentigines: Further Epidemiological Evidence from Caucasians and Asians. *J. Investig. Dermatol.* **2016**, *136*, 1053–1056. [CrossRef]

93. Chang, A.L.S. Expanding Our Understanding of Human Skin Aging. *J. Investig. Dermatol.* **2016**, *136*, 897–899. [CrossRef] [PubMed]

94. Boulton, S.J.; Birch-Machin, M.A. Impact of hyperpigmentation on superoxide flux and melanoma cell metabolism at mitochondrial complex II. *FASEB J.* **2015**, *29*, 346–353. [CrossRef] [PubMed]

95. Arck, P.C.; Overall, R.; Spatz, K.; Liezman, C.; Handjiski, B.; Klapp, B.F.; Birch-Machin, M.A.; Peters, E.M.J. Towards a "free radical theory of graying": Melanocyte apoptosis in the aging human hair follicle is an indicator of oxidative stress induced tissue damage. *FASEB J.* **2006**, *20*, 1567–1569. [CrossRef]

96. Commo, S.; Gallard, O.; Bernard, B.A. Human hair greying is linked to a specific depletion of hair follicle melanocytes affecting both the bulb and the outer root sheath. *Br. J. Dermatol.* **2004**, *150*, 435–443.

97. Veis, D.J.; Sorenson, C.M.; Shutter, J.R.; Korsmeyer, S.J. Bcl-2-deficient mice demonstrate fulminant lymphoid apoptosis, polycystic kidneys, and hypopigmented hair. *Cell* **1993**, *75*, 229–240. [CrossRef]

98. Jo, S.K.; Lee, J.Y.; Lee, Y.; Kim, C.D.; Lee, J.-H.; Lee, Y.H. Three Streams for the Mechanism of Hair Graying. *Ann. Dermatol.* **2018**, *30*, 397–401. [CrossRef]

99. Trifunovic, A.; Wredenberg, A.; Falkenberg, M.; Spelbrink, J.N.; Rovio, A.T.; Bruder, C.E.; Bohlooly, -Y.M.; Gidlöf, S.; Oldfors, A.; Wibom, R.; et al. Premature ageing in mice expressing defective mitochondrial DNA polymerase. *Nature* **2004**, *429*, 417. [CrossRef]

100. Trüeb, R.M. Oxidative stress in ageing of hair. *Int. J. Trichol.* **2009**, *1*, 6–14. [CrossRef]

101. Bahta, A.W.; Farjo, N.; Farjo, B.; Philpott, M.P. Premature Senescence of Balding Dermal Papilla Cells In Vitro Is Associated with p16INK4a Expression. *J. Investig. Dermatol.* **2008**, *128*, 1088–1094. [CrossRef]

102. Kloepper, J.E.; Baris, O.R.; Reuter, K.; Kobayashi, K.; Weiland, D.; Vidali, S.; Tobin, D.J.; Niemann, C.; Wiesner, R.J.; Paus, R. Mitochondrial Function in Murine Skin Epithelium Is Crucial for Hair Follicle Morphogenesis and Epithelial–Mesenchymal Interactions. *J. Investig. Dermatol.* **2015**, *135*, 679–689. [CrossRef]

103. Lemasters, J.J.; Ramshesh, V.K.; Lovelace, G.L.; Lim, J.; Wright, G.D.; Harland, D.; Dawson, T.L. Compartmentation of Mitochondrial and Oxidative Metabolism in Growing Hair Follicles: A Ring of Fire. *J. Investig. Dermatol.* **2017**, *137*, 1434–1444. [CrossRef]

12

Mitochondrial Dysfunction in Parkinson's Disease—Cause or Consequence?

Chun Chen [1,2], **Doug M. Turnbull** [1,2] **and Amy K. Reeve** [1,2,*]

[1] Wellcome Centre for Mitochondrial Research, Institute for Neuroscience, Newcastle University Institute for Ageing, Newcastle University, Newcastle upon Tyne, NE2 4HH, UK; c.chen20@ncl.ac.uk (C.C.); doug.turnbull@newcastle.ac.uk (D.M.T.)

[2] Newcastle University LLHW Centre for Ageing and Vitality, Newcastle University, Newcastle upon Tyne, NE2 4HH, UK

[*] Correspondence: amy.reeve@newcastle.ac.uk

Abstract: James Parkinson first described the motor symptoms of the disease that took his name over 200 years ago. While our knowledge of many of the changes that occur in this condition has increased, it is still unknown what causes this neurodegeneration and why it only affects some individuals with advancing age. Here we review current literature to discuss whether the mitochondrial dysfunction we have detected in Parkinson's disease is a pathogenic cause of neuronal loss or whether it is itself a consequence of dysfunction in other pathways. We examine research data from cases of idiopathic Parkinson's with that from model systems and individuals with familial forms of the disease. Furthermore, we include data from healthy aged individuals to highlight that many of the changes described are also present with advancing age, though not normally in the presence of severe neurodegeneration. While a definitive answer to this question may still be just out of reach, it is clear that mitochondrial dysfunction sits prominently at the centre of the disease pathway that leads to catastrophic neuronal loss in those affected by this disease.

Keywords: Parkinson's disease; mitochondria; ageing; neurodegenerative disease

---

1. Introduction

Mitochondrial dysfunction was proposed to be an integral player in the development of Parkinson's disease (PD) nearly 40 years ago, and since those initial discoveries, evidence of the role it may play in this neurodegeneration continues to increase. There is now evidence to suggest a role not only for a loss of mitochondrial function in terms of ATP provision and calcium buffering capacity, but also the degradation of these organelles through mitophagy and the interaction of mitochondria with other organelles and proteins in this disease. Furthermore, over the last 30 years, our understanding of the molecular pathways involved in the development of PD has grown immensely. These developments have been driven in part by improved genetic techniques allowing large-scale screens to be performed, but also by the speed with which disease-causing genes can be identified within affected families. In light of this, the number of genes associated with both early onset familial PD and the sporadic form of the disease continues to increase. This growing body of work continues to highlight pathways likely to be important for the development of PD, many of which centre around the function of mitochondria.

2. Mitochondrial Function

2.1. Mitochondrial Respiratory Chain

The first link between mitochondrial dysfunction and PD became evident in 1983, when 1-methyl-4-phenyl-1,2,3,6-tetrahydropyridine (MPTP) was found to cause parkinsonian-like symptoms in intravenous drug users [1,2]. Once MPTP penetrates the blood-brain barrier, this lipophilic compound is bio-transformed into its toxic form 1-methyl-4-phenylpyridinium (MPP+) by glial monoamine oxidase (MAO) [3]. MPP+ specifically interferes with the activity of respiratory chain (RC) complex I (NADH: Ubiquinone oxidoreductase) in dopaminergic (DA) neurons, causing selective neurodegeneration in both human and mouse substantia nigra (SN) [2,4,5]. Since this original study, several environmental toxins which also are capable of potent inhibition of mitochondrial complex I have been implicated in the epidemiology of sporadic PD. This raised awareness of the association of environmental exposure with the risk of developing PD later in life, via damage of RC function and increased oxidative stress (reviewed in [6,7]). These neurotoxins include rotenone, a wide spectrum insecticide [8]; organochlorine pesticides, such as chloripyrifos and permethrin, and macromolecular solvents such as 1-trichloromethyl-1,2,3,4-tetrahydro-β-carboline (TaClo) and trichloroethylene (TCE) (reviewed in [6]). However, the toxicity of these molecules may not simply lie in their inhibition of Complex I, but may also be related to exposure level, and their effect on other cellular processes, for example intracellular dopamine oxidation [9–12].

In post-mortem studies, varying degrees of Complex I (Figure 1) and complex II (succinate dehydrogenase, SDH) deficiency have been found in individual SN neurons from PD patients (~60% Complex I and ~65% Complex II deficiency [13]). A widespread decrease in complex I expression has also been observed in multiple brain regions in PD, including hippocampus, putamen, and pedunculopontine nucleus [14,15]. While immunofluorescent (protein expression) [13] and COX (Complex IV, cytochrome c oxidase)/SDH (enzyme activity) [16,17] assays have identified that 25–30% of SN neurons show a deficiency for Complex IV (Figure 1). This deficiency commonly presents alongside the aforementioned Complex I or Complex II deficiency in both PD and normal ageing [13,18]. It is possible that the predisposition for Complex I deficiency in SN neurons is due to a low reserve for Complex I function [19]. Furthermore, the high number of mitochondrial DNA (mtDNA) encoded subunits required for Complex I assembly confers that this complex is more likely to be affected by pathogenic mtDNA mutations in the susceptible neuronal populations. However, the causal role of Complex I deficiency in SN neuronal loss remains unclear. The loss of Complex I seems to be better tolerated than that of other RC subunits, given that defects in the expression of this complex are commonly detected in surviving SN neurons in PD cases and aged matched individuals, as well as in neurons from multiple other regions [13,14,18]. Mutations in the gene encoding the mitochondrial polymerase, *POLG*, in mitochondrial disease patients cause accumulated mitochondrial dysfunction similar to that detected in PD and ageing [20]. Complex I-negative neurons are found in infant *POLG* patients, before the prominent loss of neurons, which could further support a less detrimental effect of Complex I deficiency on neuronal survival, compared to the loss of other RC complexes [21].

Single neuron studies have attempted to interrogate the relationship between mitochondrial dysfunction and the formation of alpha-synuclein pathology [14,22]. Significantly higher expression of Complex I and Complex IV was found in SN neurons with alpha-synuclein pathology [22], whilst the presence of alpha-synuclein aggregation was less frequent in Complex I deficient SN neurons [14,22]. Both post-mortem studies suggested that alpha-synuclein pathology and abnormal RC function may be two independent factors in PD pathogenesis.

Figure 1. Mitochondrial respiratory chain (RC) deficiency in substantia nigra (SN) neurons of an individual with Parkinson's disease (PD). Immunofluorescent images demonstrating SN neurons with normal Complex I (CI) and Complex IV (CIV) expression, Complex I deficiency and normal Complex IV expression, and deficiency of both Complex I and Complex IV. Scale bar, 20 μm.

2.2. Mitochondrial DNA Defects

The potential consequences of clonally expanded mtDNA deletions and related biochemical defects on the survival of SN neurons have been investigated in several studies. Indeed, somatic mtDNA deletions reaching 50% have been described at the single SN neuron level in both PD and healthy ageing, with much higher levels in COX-deficient cells [16,17]. These deletions were found to be of various sizes (~2000 to ~9500bp), located within the major arc of mtDNA, and involve both tRNA and mitochondrial RC protein genes [20]. It is therefore evident that these multiple mtDNA deletions are somatically acquired, with the clonal expansion of different-sized deletions within each individual SN neuron, thus yielding a wide spectrum of mtDNA deletion breakpoints within an individual [20]. A recent post-mortem study revealed an accumulation of mtDNA deletions with advancing age in individual SN neurons, whilst such a trend did not occur in cortical or cerebellar neurons and the deletion load was much lower in these neuronal populations [23].

Although the mechanism for the formation of mtDNA deletions is still under debate, the necessity of mtDNA replication activity in deletion formation [24] was challenged by the absence of 3'-repeat retention in some of the detected mtDNA deletion species in SN neurons [20]. According to the "slipped-replication" theory, a single stranded loop occurs between 3'5' direct repeats which is then exposed and degraded during mtDNA replication, leading to the occurrence of deletions that are often located within the major arc of mtDNA [24]. Krishnan et al. proposed another possibility that mtDNA deletion formation may initiate from 3'–5' exonuclease activity during the repair of damage to mtDNA in the SN neuronal population [25]. MtDNA damage leads to the formation of double strand breaks (DSB), and misrepair of such breaks could cause the loss of several kilobases of mtDNA on both strands. Single strand mtDNA generated from this process would then anneal with homologous sequences, resulting in the double-stranded deleted molecule with both a 5' and 3' repeat [25]. The relationship between DSB repair and the generation of mtDNA deletions has been supported by several studies using inducible mitochondrial-targeted restriction endonuclease, *Pst*I, to trigger mtDNA DSB. Multiple mtDNA deletions were found in cultured *Pst*I neurons [26] and in DA neurons of a *Pst*I mouse model [27]. These mice also developed nigrostriatal degeneration and PD-related behavioral phenotypes [27]. Later, Moraes' team reported an acceleration effect of mtDNA DSB on neuronal ageing through reactive oxygen species (ROS) induced damage [28]. The nature of deletion formation through repair could therefore be regarded as an inevitable cost of mtDNA self-rescue/regulation against oxidative damage. This fits well with the strikingly high deletion load of mtDNA detected in aged SN neurons of both healthy individuals and PD patients [20,23], as ROS-induced mtDNA damage advances with ageing.

In addition to the higher mtDNA deletion load in the SN than other aged brain regions, such as the basal ganglia, cortical areas and cerebellum [23,29,30], Dolle et al. also revealed a age-related increase of mtDNA copy number within individual SN neurons [23]. More importantly, the upregulation of mtDNA copy number also correlates with the increase in mtDNA deletion load within the SN neuronal population. The corresponding increase of mtDNA copy number with mtDNA deletion level, together with an enhancement of mitochondrial function, were mirrored in a study of DA neurons from a premature ageing model (POLG[D257A] mice) [31]. These findings suggested an ability of age SN neurons to adapt to mitochondrial dysfunction via the maintenance of their mtDNA population. Failure of such regulatory mechanisms of mtDNA copy number is described in PD patients in several studies. Grunewald et al. suggested depletion of mtDNA copy number and low expression of an essential mtDNA nucleoid protein, mitochondrial transcription factor A (TFAM) in the SN neurons of PD patients [13]. However, another study showed a decrease in mtDNA wildtype copy number but not in total copy number, alongside a decreased correlation between mtDNA copy number and deletion level in PD neurons compared to healthy aged neurons [23]. Reduction of mtDNA copy number in the peripheral blood [32] and cerebrospinal fluid [33,34] has also been detected in patients with PD and neurodegenerative disease.

These studies all suggest that the formation and accumulation of high levels of mtDNA deletions leads to mitochondrial dysfunction that will have an impact on the health and survival of SN neurons. However, many of the reported findings are also found in normal ageing in the SN. Therefore, mtDNA alterations are certainly one cause of the mitochondrial deficiency detected within these neurons and will undoubtedly increase the vulnerability of these neurons to loss in PD, but the question still remains whether these defects are causative of PD itself.

2.3. ROS Production and Oxidative Stress

The accumulation of somatic mtDNA deletions and the subsequent development of RC deficiency within aged SN neurons may lead to impaired mitochondrial membrane potential ($\Delta\Psi$m), reduced synthesis of ATP, and an increase in release of ROS leading to oxidative stress [35]. A higher rate of electron flux due to an increase in respiratory capacity to adapt to high metabolic demands in SN neurons has also been thought to cause increased ROS generation. The increase in numbers of electrons being transferred would increase the probability of electron capture by O_2 to generate superoxide before they reach COX [36]. In addition to the production and release of ROS from mitochondria, the process of dopamine metabolism by monoamine oxidase could also account for the accumulation of toxic oxidative species such as hydroxyl radicals [37]. Oxidative damage to mtDNA results in further deficiency in RC expression and creates a vicious circle of oxidative stress and bioenergetics failure. This "mitochondrial theory of ageing" has long been regarded as a rationale for mitochondrial changes with advancing age [38], which could contribute to the increase in SN neuronal vulnerability. However, this theory was challenged by more recent studies which manipulated the antioxidant capacity of several mouse models, finding impaired integrity of the mitochondrial genome which was not necessarily associated with an age-related phenotype or shortened lifespan (reviewed in [39]). Evidence from a premature ageing mouse model (POLG[D257A] mutant) found that the generation of mitochondrial ROS or mtDNA damage did not increase with a high heteroplasmic level of mtDNA point mutation, and that there seems to be a threshold for mtDNA deletions to cause accelerated ageing [40].

In addition to mitochondrial ROS, other factors that may contribute to increased oxidative damage include iron accumulation and an increase in lipid peroxidation burden [41,42], while accumulation of hydroxyl and superoxide radicals due to a decline in glutathione content [43] have also been reported in the brain of PD patients. Recent studies also highlighted a direct toxicity of alpha-synuclein oligomers on mitochondria via induction of mitochondrial lipid peroxidation and oxidation of ATP synthase [44,45]. It was shown that alpha-synuclein leads to increased permeability of mitochondrial membranes and ROS production, ultimately leading to neuronal death [45].

2.4. Calcium Handling

Emerging evidence has suggested the importance of cytosolic calcium ions (Ca^{2+}) in the regionally selective nature of neuronal loss in PD pathogenesis. Dopaminergic neurons in the SN exhibit autonomous pacemaking activity in order to maintain regular release of dopamine to the striatum, facilitated by CaV1.3 L-type calcium channels. Action potentials generated from this process are broad, with a relatively slow rate (2–10 Hz), promoting a slow rhythmic activity accompanied with a slow oscillation in cytosolic Ca^{2+}. A relationship between Ca^{2+} oscillations and PD neuronal loss was initially proposed by experiments showing a decline in the number of calbindin (a Ca^{2+} binding protein), positive neurons in PD patients [46,47]. These slow Ca^{2+} oscillations promote the import of Ca^{2+} into the mitochondrial intermembrane space and matrix. Intramitochondrial Ca^{2+} is required for the activation of pyruvate dehydrogenase, isocitrate dehydrogenase and α-ketoglutarate (important enzymes in the tricarboxylic acid (TCA) cycle) and promotes RC function and ATP production. Mitochondrial sequestration of Ca^{2+} benefits synaptic neurotransmission in terms of assisting in the stabilization of the cytosolic Ca^{2+} concentration during vesicle exocytosis [48] and promoting the recovery of synaptic excitation after exocytosis [48,49]. The unique feature of CaV1.3 channels is that they open at relatively hyperpolarized $\Delta\Psi m$. Even so, the lack of powerful intracellular buffering of Ca^{2+} from the endoplasmic reticulum (ER) in DA neurons drives a sustained Ca^{2+} flux to enter mitochondria. This is able to promote ATP synthesis in the absence of a strong energy demand [50,51]. Ca^{2+} overload may force the opening of mitochondrial permeability transition pore (mPTP), leading to retrograde electron flux through the electron transport chain, resulting in increased ROS production, release of cytochrome c, and activation of apoptosis [52,53]. The increase in mitochondrial oxidative stress has also been identified in other neuronal populations, including the dorsal motor nucleus of the vagus (DMV) and the locus coeruleus (LC), which also express CaV1.3 channels. DA neurons in the ventral tegmental area (VTA) which have modest CaV1.3 channel currents however, demonstrate low mitochondrial oxidative stress and an improved ability to buffer cytosolic Ca^{2+} with ageing [54,55]. All of these indicate that CaV1.3 channels cause extra oxidative burden on mitochondria that may contribute to the selectively vulnerability of SN neurons (reviewed in Reference [56]). A recent report showed depletion of alpha-synuclein prevents the elevation of cytosolic Ca^{2+} concentration induced by MPP+ in mouse SN neurons, suggesting synergistic detrimental effects of these two pathological aspects in PD neurodegeneration [57].

2.5. Two Novel Familial PD Genes Associated with Mitochondrial Function

2.5.1. VPS35

A novel autosomal dominant PD related pathogenic mutation was identified in the vascular protein sorting associated protein 35 (*VPS35*, PARK17, OMIM 614203) gene [58,59], and has been linked to impaired RC complex I and II subunit assembly and activity [60]. The VPS35 protein is a core subunit of the cargo recognition subcomplex that mediates the sorting, trafficking, and endocytosis of synaptic vesicles [35]. The *VPS35* mutation-induced mitochondrial dysfunction has been suggested to be a consequence of impaired mitochondrial fusion, tipping the balance of the fission and fusion cycle toward excessive fission. VPS35 promotes the degradation of mitochondrial E3 ubiquitin ligase1 (MUL1), and stabilizes mitofusin 2 (MFN2) preventing its degradation by MUL1 [61]. VPS35 deficiency impairs the regulatory machinery of mitochondrial dynamics via degradation of MFN2 by MUL1 in DA neurons, leading to mitochondrial dysfunction and fragmentation, which may underlie related PD pathogenesis [61]. Furthermore, a recent report has shown prominent changes in dopaminergic synaptic function, including increased dopamine turnover, loss of the dopamine transporter (DAT) and increased vesicular monoamine transporter 2 (VMAT2) expression in a *VPS35* knock-in mouse model [62].

2.5.2. CHCHD2

Mutations in the coiled-coil-helix-coiled-coil-helix domain containing 2 (*CHCHD2*, PARK22, OMIM 616244) gene have recently been associated with autosomal dominant PD in Japanese families [63]. The role of *CHCHD2* as a PD-related gene was confirmed by genetic screening of affected Chinese families [64], however, studies in Caucasians, south Italians [65,66], and Brazilians [67] did not support its causative role in PD. It has been proposed that the localization of the CHCHD2 protein in the mitochondrial intermembrane space is beneficial to the maintenance of mitochondrial cristae structure and integrity of the mitochondrial RC [68,69]. Inhibition of CHCHD2 was found to impair mitochondrial Complex III (cytochrome bc_1 complex) and Complex IV activity, leading to decreases in OXPHOS activity and increased oxidative damage [69,70]. These mitochondrial structural and biochemical defects have also been shown in fibroblasts generated from a PD patient who carried a homozygous variant in *CHCHD2* [71]. In addition to the mitochondrial structural and biochemical defects, *Drosophila* carrying the *CHCHD2* mutations identified in patients also manifest motor symptoms and DA neurodegeneration [69].

2.6. Does Mitochondrial Dysfunction Drive the Development of Neurodegeneration in PD?

It is evident from other conditions, for example, mitochondrial disorders associated with mutations in the polymerase gamma gene, *POLG*, that a primary mitochondrial defect is sufficient to cause loss of SN neurons (and other neuronal populations) [18,72]. Furthermore, such mutations are often associated with the development of PD-like symptoms (reviewed in Reference [73]). However, attempting to disentangle "cause and effect" in the contribution of mitochondrial dysfunction to the pathogenesis of PD is difficult, since many of the changes we detect in those with PD are also present in healthy aged individuals. The mitochondrial defects present in these individuals often exist in the absence of cell loss or parkinsonian symptoms. For example, equivalent levels of mtDNA deletions are detected in SN neurons from individuals with PD and healthy controls [16,17] and neurons showing deficiencies for both Complex I and Complex IV are also detected in both instances [18]. Many of the processes described above initiate changes in other pathways and thus activate well defined responses which exist to mitigate to these changes, for example, ROS and antioxidants. Therefore, it might be suggested that in PD it is the ability of neurons to respond to mitochondrial functional changes that is impaired. Thus, neurons become more sensitive to changes in other pathways, which ultimately leads to their degeneration and loss.

3. Mitochondrial Turnover

3.1. Mitophagy

Mitophagy contributes to mitochondrial quality control by the selective clearance of damaged mitochondria, targeting an entire mitochondrion or fission fragmented mitochondria for autophagy. As a specialized form of autophagy, mitophagy comprises three necessary stages: the recognition of impaired mitochondria, the formation of autophagic membranes around the target, and the fusion of the mitoautophagosome with a lysosome (reviewed in Reference [74] and Reference [75]). Two familial PD-associated proteins, phosphatase and tensin homolog (PTEN)-induced putative kinase 1 (PINK1, PARK6, OMIM 608309) and E3 ubiquitin ligase, Parkin (PARK2, OMIM 602544), have been strongly implicated in the identification of damaged mitochondria for degradation via mitophagy [76]. PINK1 is a serine/threonine kinase localized to both mitochondria and the cytosol [77]. It accumulates on the outer membrane of damaged mitochondria, following a reduction in $\Delta\Psi m$, and recruits Parkin to trigger the engulfment of mitochondria by autophagosomes [78]. The recruitment of Parkin requires PINK1-mediated phosphorylation of both Parkin and ubiquitin, which activates a ubiquitin phosphorylation cascade for mitophagy adapters. This feed-forward amplification loop leads to further recruitment and ubiquitylation-activation of Parkin so that the engulfment can proceed [79]. However, several studies have described a Parkin-independent mitophagy pathway associated with other E3 ubiquitin ligases including Glycoprotein 78 (Gp78) [80] and Ariadne RBR Ubiquitin E3 ligase 1 (ARIH1) [81].

3.2. Mitochondrial Biogenesis

The constant generation of new mitochondria is a key process for the maintenance of a healthy mitochondrial population with advancing age. The fact that the mitochondrial genome has limited protein coding capacity determines the dependence of mitochondrial biogenesis on synchronized transcription activity from both the mitochondrial and nuclear genomes. This provides building blocks which aid the replacement of mitochondria or can be inserted into remaining functional mitochondria [82]. Central to the regulation of mitochondrial biogenesis is the nuclear transcription cascade, mediated by peroxisome proliferator-activated receptor γ (PPARγ) coactivator 1α (PGC-1α) [83,84]. PGC-1α and its downstream cofactors nuclear respiratory factors (NRF1, 2) largely contribute to the regulation of transcription initiation of all nuclear-encoded RC proteins that are expressed by the nuclear genome. TFAM and dimethyladenosine transferase 2 (TFB2M) can then act in response to intracellular oxidative stress [85,86]. Reduction in the mRNA level of nuclear-encoded RC genes that are responsive to PGC-1α has been identified in individual DA neurons of PD patients, and in neurons in regions with subclinical PD-related Lewy body neuropathology [87]. The transcriptional decline in genes that control mitochondrial biogenesis and oxidative energy metabolism, including RC related genes and some cytosolic ribosomal genes (related to protein synthesis), are altered with advancing age [88,89]. This is supported by the discovery of downregulated AMP- activated protein kinase (AMPK) signalling, a key player in the control of PGC-1α expression, alongside decreased mitochondrial biogenesis in aged individuals [90]. These data strongly indicate the contribution of impaired biogenesis to the accumulation of mitochondrial dysfunction during ageing and the neurodegenerative process.

PGC-1α and its transcriptional control is critical for maintaining neuron function. Loss of dopaminergic neurons and striatal degeneration have been demonstrated in animal models where the PGC-1α gene is silenced or knockout [57,91,92]. Several ex vivo and in vivo studies have demonstrated the beneficial effects of PGC-1α overexpression and the corresponding increase in transcription activities in the rescue of dopaminergic neuronal loss induced by MPTP [93], rotenone, or alpha-synuclein mediated toxicity [94–96]. In addition to enhancing mitochondrial biogenesis, PGC-1α is also capable of activating the expression of antioxidant enzymes in response to oxidative stress [97,98] and protecting DA neurons against neuroinflammation [99]. However, there is still a lack of consensus on the value of upregulating PGC-1α expression as a PD therapeutic intervention. An increase in PGC-1α expression is not necessarily associated with an activation of its target cofactors that facilitate mitochondrial biogenesis [40]. Major alterations in energy metabolism that impair normal neuronal function have been found in a study of long term overexpression of PGC-1α in an alpha-synuclein mutant mouse, carrying the A53T mutation [33]. However, mitochondrial hyperactivity and increased ROS production were also described in this model, and may also contribute to the severe DA neuronal loss.

Shin et al. first identified a link between Parkin and PGC-1α in the regulation of PGC-1α expression via a Parkin interacting substrate, PARIS (also known as zinc finger protein 746, ZNF746). Parkin mediates the proteasomal degradation of PARIS. In the absence of Parkin, PARIS is bound to the promoter of PGC-1α gene and suppresses its expression [100]. This causes declines in mitochondrial respiratory capacity and mitochondrial mass, ultimately leading to dopaminergic neuronal death [33,34,101]. The parkin-mediated PARIS-dependent control of mitochondrial biogenesis, adds further evidence that impaired mitochondrial turnover contributes to the neuronal loss in PD.

It is hypothesized that mitochondrial turnover is slowed in aged and PD neurons due to defective nuclear transcriptional control of mitochondrial proteins. Alongside this, there is a decline in the clearance of dysfunctional mitochondria that occurs in coordination with a decrease in biogenic activity and, as a result, mutant mitochondria accumulate in the neurodegenerative process. Evidence for a decline in mitophagy during ageing has been highlighted in several recent reviews [102–105]. The abnormal accumulation of alpha-synuclein in PD neurons may put an additional burden on protein degradation pathways, increasing the vulnerability of SN neurons to mitochondrial dysfunction and pushing these neurons toward early cell death (reviewed in [106]).

3.3. Familial PD Associated Genes Related to Mitochondrial Turnover

3.3.1. PINK1 and Parkin

Among many genes that are associated with familiar PD, *PINK1* and *Parkin* are highlighted due to their substantial involvement in mitochondrial maintenance. Although the PINK1/Parkin pathway is the key mediator of the process of mitophagy, recently more attention has been given to their regulatory roles in neuronal mitochondrial dynamics via their interactions with the Mitochondrial Rho GTPase1 (MIRO)/Milton complex (see below). In addition, the association of PINK1 and Parkin with the removal of mitochondrial proteins and impaired mitochondrial biogenesis has been suggested (reviewed in Reference [107]).

PINK1 has been suggested to also be important for the mitochondrial unfolded protein response (UPR^{mt}). The UPR^{mt} was first reported in cell lines with a mutant form of ornithine transcarbamylase (OTC) [108], which led to accumulation of a misfolded form of the protein which subsequently drove expression of mitochondrial quality control genes. Believed to be a stress response to damaged mitochondrial proteins and hence dysfunction, alterations in the UPR^{mt} pathway may be of pathogenic importance in PD. For example, PINK1 has been proposed to be involved in this pathway through its interaction with HTRA serine peptidase 2 (HTRA2, PARK13, OMIM 606441) [109] and tumor necrosis factor receptor-associated protein 1 (TRAP1) [110]. Importantly, mutations in the genes encoding both these proteins have been associated with the development of PD [111,112]. In addition, the brains of those individuals carrying *PINK1* mutations show decreased levels of HTRA2 phosphorylation [109], while the brains of mice with a knockout of *HTRA2* show an accumulation of misfolded proteins within the mitochondria leading to reduced respiratory function and neurodegeneration [113]. TRAP1 is a mitochondrial chaperone protein, whose knockout in *Drosophila* causes an age-related decrease in climbing ability and dopamine levels in the brain, increased sensitivity to mitochondrial toxins including rotenone and a decrease in ATP levels [114]. It is also a PINK1 effector whose expression in PINK1 deficient *Drosophila* rescues morphological and mitochondrial defects and is capable of reducing dopamine deficits [114,115]. Given the importance of the UPR^{mt} for the maintenance of mitochondrial function, this pathway may prove to be an important therapeutic target. Upregulation of the UPR^{mt} for example, may allow mitochondrial function to be improved through either degradation of unfolded mitochondrial proteins or increases in the upstream signalling cascade.

3.3.2. DJ-1 and LRRK2

The functions of DJ-1 (PARK7, OMIM 606324) and leucine-rich repeat kinase 2 (LRRK2, PARK8, OMIM 609007) are less well characterized in terms of mitochondrial health. Downregulation of DJ-1 causes multiple mitochondrial abnormalities, including increased mitochondrial fragmentation and reduced ΔΨm and connectivity [116,117]. Interestingly, this effect can be blocked by overexpression of Parkin and PINK1 [118]. A recent study using induced pluripotent stem cells (iPSC)-derived neurons reports the beneficial effect of LRRK2 in the removal of MIRO, and thus enhanced arrest of damaged mitochondria. Pathogenic *LRRK2* mutations disrupt this function, speeding up mitochondrial mobility and consequentially slowing the initiation of mitophagy [119].

3.3.3. ATP13A2 and GBA

Novel mutations in *ATP13A2* (ATPase type 13A2, PARK9, OMIM 610513) have been identified as a genetic cause of a rare juvenile-onset form of PD, named Kufor–Rakeb syndrome [120,121]. *ATP13A2* encodes an isoform of type P5B ATPase, which functions as a lysosomal ATPase transporter. It is believed to play critical roles in the regulation of vesicular transportation [122], endolysosomal activity [123,124], and glycolysis [125]. Deficiency of ATP13A2 causes lysosomal defects, and thus affects cation homeostasis, for example Zn^{2+}, leading to impaired mitochondrial respiratory function and defective mitophagy [89,122]. A recent study also found gliosis in multiple brain regions of heterozygous *ATP13A2* knockout mice, suggestive of the neuroinflammation which occurs in the early stages of PD development [123]. Another heterozygous mutation in the gene that encodes the lysosomal enzyme glucocerebrosidase (*GBA*, OMIM 606463) has also been identified as a powerful genetic risk factor for PD [126,127]. Those PD patients who carried a *GBA* mutation tended to have an earlier age of onset and an increased risk of developing dementia compared to idiopathic PD patients [128]. Together, this evidence highlights that lysosomal alterations may be crucial to the pathogenesis PD, exacerbating the accumulation of mitochondrial damage and abnormal protein aggregation [129].

3.4. Does Mitochondrial Turnover Drive the Development of Neurodegeneration in PD?

Although the process is still not clearly defined in neurons, data suggests that the degradation of dysfunctional mitochondria occurs through the autophagy related pathway, mitophagy. A number of studies have suggested that there is a decline in mitophagy with age (reviewed in References [102,103]). Furthermore, many of the genes that control the degradation of mitochondria through this pathway have been linked to ageing and lifespan in model organisms (reviewed in [130]). A decline in lysosome function has also been shown to occur with advancing age, mainly through the accumulation of lipofuscin within these organelles [131]. However, the fact that many of the genes responsible for familial PD have been shown to have important roles in autophagy or lysosomal pathways suggests that this is an important driver of the pathogenesis of PD. Alterations in the efficiency of such pathways will clearly exacerbate mitochondrial dysfunction, allowing defective mitochondria to accumulate. Mitochondrial dysfunction itself may also increase oxidative damage to proteins and organelles which may overwhelm these systems in PD, leading to neuronal loss. Again, we are faced with a vicious circle of damage, whereby mitochondrial dysfunction may be caused by defects in genes such as *ATP13A2*. However, lysosomal dysfunction may increase oxidative stress, which would then cause further mitochondrial and cellular damage.

4. Mitochondrial Dynamics, Transport, and Distribution

The precise distribution of mitochondria within neurons is a fundamental aspect of the correct function of these cells. Neuronal communication through electrical impulse and chemical synapses is fundamental for brain function, and, in PD, a loss of synapses has been shown to precede the loss of cell bodies from the substantia nigra. This decline in synaptic terminal density may begin decades before the first symptoms appear in affected individuals (reviewed in Reference [132]). Therefore, understanding the causes of this synaptic loss may be key to unlocking new therapies for PD.

As described above, mitochondrial production relies on signalling between the nucleus and the mitochondria, while the degradation of dysfunctional mitochondria requires the interaction of a number of proteins and signalling pathways that we are only just beginning to understand. Mitochondrial biogenesis generally occurs at the soma, in close proximity to the nucleus, although evidence has suggested that mtDNA replication may occur within axons at sites distant from the cell body [133–135]. The degradation of damaged mitochondria has generally been thought to occur within the cell body, since this was thought to be the only location of lysosomes, though recently this convention has also been challenged [136]. Data has also suggested that mitochondria may be donated to and removed from neurons by astrocytes, with such processes occurring in response to cellular stress [137,138]. Therefore, neurons require processes which allow mitochondrial movements to be responsive to changes within the local and intracellular environments.

Mitochondria perform a variety of roles within neurons to support their function. They provide localized ATP to regions of the neuron which are particularly energy demanding (including the nodes of Ranvier and pre-synaptic terminals) and buffer cytosolic calcium. These two functions of mitochondria support the release and recycling of synaptic vesicles and the maintenance of electrochemical gradients, which are intimately dependent on each other since they both rely on calcium signalling. Therefore, as the main organelles which support these processes, there is a need for mitochondria to be dynamic and responsive in their distribution. The movement and localization of mitochondria can be affected by their function. A loss of mitochondrial membrane potential, for example, has been proposed to drive directional mitochondrial movement. Vice versa, incorrect positioning of mitochondria within neurons may have a detrimental effect on the health and function of neurons (reviewed in [139,140]).

4.1. Fission and Fusion

The processes of fission and fusion control the network connectivity of mitochondria within neurons. These processes allow the creation or destruction of a mitochondrial syncytium, in which mitochondrial contents may be shared, or dysfunctional mitochondria partitioned for destruction. The degradation of dysfunctional mitochondria through mitophagy and the manipulation of this process has been suggested to be an important therapeutic avenue for many degenerative diseases [141]. While many of the specifics of exactly how mitochondria are detected as being targets for degradation remain unclear, it is likely that the fission of such organelles from the network will be a key process [142]. Fragmentation of the mitochondrial network occurs rapidly following the loss of mitochondrial membrane potential, and if this loss cannot be restored, fragmented mitochondria lose their "fusion" capabilities and are degraded [142]. Many of the proteins that control these two process have been characterized and alterations in these processes have been detected in a number of models of familial PD, yielding differences in the size of mitochondria and their ultrastructure [143]. Moreover, a loss of dynamin-1-like protein (DRP1), a key protein in the fission machinery within dopaminergic neurons, causes a Parkinson's like phenotype in affected mice due to degeneration of SN neurons. A staggering 85% of SN neurons had been lost by the age of 1 month in these animals and this loss was due to depletion of the axonal mitochondrial population [144]. Furthermore, mutations in *OPA1* (OMIM 605290) have been linked with parkinsonism, including alterations upon DAT-SPECT scanning [145]. The two heterozygous mutations reported in this paper also caused alterations to the structure and function of mitochondria [145]. In SHSY5Y cells, the overexpression of OPA1 has been shown to protect against the ultrastructural abnormalities induced by treatment with MPP^+, although interestingly this was not related to a reduction of fission [146]. The fusion of mitochondria has been further linked with PD by the finding that mitofusin 1 (MFN1) and MFN2 are ubiquitinated in a Parkin/PINK1 dependent manner [147,148]. The ubiquitination of mitochondrial proteins is a key step in their identification for degradation through mitophagy. Further details of this process have emerged showing that PINK1 phosphorylates MFN2, and this phosphorylation then recruits Parkin, which then ubiquitinates the protein [149]. This study also showed that in cardiomyocytes, a deficiency of MFN2 impedes mitophagy, leading to the accumulation of abnormal mitochondria and respiratory dysfunction [149]. The ubiquitination of the mitofusin proteins is impeded in fibroblasts from individuals with pathogenic *PINK1* or *Parkin* mutations [150]. Interestingly, other proteins important for the fission and fusion of mitochondria are not affected by mutations within these genes [150]. The ubiquitination of the mitofusions will act not only to identify mitochondria for degradation, but will also ensure that such mitochondria are unable to rejoin the mitochondrial network. In addition, as described above, many of the neurotoxins used to generate experimental models of Parkinson's Disease, including rotenone and MPTP, cause the fragmentation of the mitochondrial network, most likely due to their inhibitory effects on mitochondrial complex I [151–153]. In fact, their toxicity might be directly related to their effect on the balance of mitochondrial biogenesis and fission/fusion [154].

4.2. Mitochondrial Distribution

The correct positioning of mitochondria within neurons is required for localized supply of ATP and calcium buffering. By performing these essential tasks mitochondria become integral to the functioning and survival of neurons. The provision of ATP is crucial for the support of neuronal electrical activity, and in line with this, mitochondria are found clustered at sites with high energy demands, for example, at the Nodes of Ranvier in myelinated axons. Their location at such sites supports the function of ion channels such as the Na^+/K^+ ATPase, which is responsible for the restoration of resting membrane potential following an action potential. Furthermore, their distribution changes to mirror alterations in channel distribution, for example, following demyelination [155]. In addition, the positional holding of mitochondria at these locations changes in response to electrical activity. A decline or arrest in electrical activity will increase mitochondrial mobility away from nodes, while conversely, depolarization leads to a movement of mitochondria into these areas to provide ATP to repolarize the membrane (reviewed in Reference [156]).

Localized reliable sources of ATP are also essential for synaptic function. Within the presynaptic terminal, mitochondrial ATP is required for an array of processes, including vesicle recycling, exo and endocytosis of vesicles, and the loading of recycled vesicles with neurotransmitter (reviewed in Reference [157]). As crucial as this energy provision is the ability of mitochondria to buffer calcium (see above). The release of neurotransmitter from presynaptic terminals relies on a number of processes which are modulated by calcium signalling. As such, the concentration of calcium within the presynaptic terminal must be tightly regulated, to control the quantal release of neurotransmitter, the priming of terminals for the next depolarization, and changes in synaptic strength. Calcium buffering might be particularly important for the neurons of the substantia nigra, given their pace-making activity. Blockage of the calcium channel, which governs this activity, forces the neurons to utilize sodium channels to maintain this low frequency activity, which also protects neurons against mitochondrial dysfunction caused by rotenone treatment [158].

Mitochondria can be recruited to synapses, though not all synapses contain mitochondria. Synapses devoid of mitochondria have been found in a number of cell types, including hippocampal neurons, primary cortical neurons, and the DA neurons of the nigrostriatal pathway [159–161]. The number of these "empty" synapses was recently shown to decline in the presence of dopaminergic neuronal degeneration in PD [162]. This suggests two interesting hypotheses, either synapses which lack mitochondria show an increased vulnerability in PD and are the first to be lost, or that in the presence of degenerating neighbors, neurons can populate such synapses with mitochondria and the replenishment with ATP activates them as part of an adaptation to maintain transmission to those post-synaptic sites. In neurons with complex architecture, such as the neurons of the nigrostriatal pathway which have been suggested to have a huge number of pre-synaptic terminals, it may seem obvious that they would not utilize the full synaptic complement but keep some "in reserve" in case of loss of a proportion.

4.3. Mitochondrial Transport

The correct distribution of mitochondria and the maintenance of a healthy functional population within DA neurons relies on efficient transport from sites of genesis or to sites of degradation. The movement of mitochondria along axons relies on motor proteins and microtubules with different proteins mediating retrograde (towards the cell body) and anterograde (towards the terminus) transport. The directionality of mitochondrial movements is controlled by different sets of motors with dynein motors controlling retrograde transport, while anterograde movements are driven by kinesin motors (reviewed in Reference [157]). The transport of mitochondria over long distances within neurons is much more complicated than this and additional protein interactions are required namely between trafficking kinesin binding proteins (TRAKs), kinesin heavy chain isoform 5 (KIF5) and dynein, and the mitochondrial proteins MIRO1 and 2. These outer mitochondrial membrane proteins are responsible for the interaction of mitochondria with these molecular motors. An in-depth discussion of the mechanisms of mitochondrial transport is out of the realm of this review, however, there are a number of excellent reviews which cover this in detail [139,156,157,163].

Previous work has suggested that mitochondria are transported towards the cell body when they have lost their membrane potential, a key signal for their sequestration in autophagosomes, although other studies have been unable to replicate this [164,165]. Many of the interactions involved in these processes have been well characterized, as have the patterns of movement exhibited by mitochondria under normal and disease conditions. In line with the fact that mitochondria are predominantly held at sites where they are required to provide localized ATP or calcium buffering, the majority of mitochondria within neurons are stationary, with only 10–20% of mitochondria being motile in hippocampal neurons [160,166], with over 90% reported as being stationary in cortical and spinal neurons [167–169]. Those mitochondria move through showing a variety of velocities and movements, with some moving in one direction with others seemingly wobbling back and forth. These mitochondrial movements also change with maturation of neurons, with more mitochondria becoming immobile and enriched at sites such as synapses [168].

The docking of mitochondria at discrete sites of the neuron relies on calcium. Localized elevated calcium levels cause mitochondrial stalling. In cultured neurons, mitochondrial mobility is decreased by increasing calcium influx [159,170]. The ability of calcium to cause mitochondrial immobility relies on MIRO and the binding of calcium to the proteins two EF hands. Mutations within these domains leading to impaired calcium binding have been shown to prevent the ability of mitochondria to dock (reviewed in Reference [171]). The importance of calcium for the transport and mobilization of mitochondria is particularly interesting given the importance of calcium for the pace-making activity exhibited by dopaminergic SN neurons (reviewed in Reference [56]). Many studies have investigated mitochondrial trafficking in mouse and cell culture-based models of PD [172,173]. For example, the complex I inhibitor MPP$^+$ alters mitochondrial directionality, increasing the speed of retrograde movement and decreasing the opposing movements. Furthermore, this study also showed that of the mitochondria that were moving, MPP$^+$ caused the stalling of over 50% of these. Interestingly, this study also uncovered that mitochondria within DA neurons were much smaller than those within non-DA axons. This reduction in size in DA neurons may suggest that there are inherent differences in the levels of fission and fusion between DA neurons and other neuronal populations. Differences in transport in these cells may also impede the delivery of mitochondria to synapses and other discrete sites within the neurons [172]. Furthermore, in the DA neurons of the MitoPark mouse (conditional TFAM knockout) the supply of mitochondria to axonal terminals is impaired due to reduced anterograde transport [173].

4.4. Familial PD Genes and Their Association with Mitochondrial Dynamics

The importance of many of the genes associated with PD for mitochondrial dynamics lies in the ability of the proteins they encode to affect the transport of mitochondria. Of all the proteins which have been associated with familial PD, the ones most associated with mitochondrial dynamics, obviously given their roles in mitophagy, are PINK1 and Parkin. Initially thought of as key mediators of mitochondrial degradation through mitophagy, the impact and responsibility of Parkin and PINK1 on the maintenance of mitochondrial integrity is now believed to be more complex. Recent studies have also proposed roles for these two proteins in the mitochondrial unfolded protein response, in the modulation of mitochondrial fission and fusion, and finally in mitochondrial transport and trafficking (reviewed in depth in Reference [174]).

Early studies showed that PINK1, a mitochondrial outer membrane protein, was able to recruit Parkin to mitochondria upon mitochondrial depolarization with the uncoupler carbonyl cyanide m-chlorophenyl hydrazine (CCCP) [78,175]. We now know that PINK1 actively recruits Parkin to mitochondria and phosphorylates it, Parkin is then able to ubiquitinate outer mitochondrial membrane proteins signalling the mitochondrion for destruction. The mitochondrion is then enveloped by an autophagosome and trafficked to the lysosome (reviewed in Reference [176]). *PINK1* and *Parkin* mutations in animal models have been shown to lead to both mitochondrial structural and functional changes, which are often causative of the DA neuron degeneration in these models [177,178]. Parkin overexpression has the ability to rescue many of the phenotypic changes detected in *PINK1* mutants, including the mitochondrial defects and DA loss [177]. Furthermore, the expression of Parkin in cell lines has been shown to drive expression of a number of mitochondria associated proteins, including a number important for mitochondrial dynamics, trafficking, and the ubiquitin proteasome [179].

PINK1 and Parkin have also been linked to mitochondrial dynamics and trafficking through their interaction with a number of proteins essential to these processes. For example, overexpression of PINK1 or Parkin in neurons has been shown to decrease bidirectional mitochondrial movements. PINK1 phosphorylates MIRO, which then causes Parkin mediated degradation and kinesin release [180,181]. The knockdown of PINK1 has been shown to promote anterograde mitochondrial transport in *Drosophila* motor neurons, while conversely, a loss of MIRO in Hela cells was linked to perinuclear mitochondrial clustering and mitochondrial degradation by mitophagy [180]. PINK1 expression in mitochondria has been found to be linked to expression of both MIRO and Milton, with which it forms a complex. Furthermore, the interaction with these proteins can drive the association of PINK1 with mitochondria even in the absence of a PINK1 mitochondrial targeting sequence [182]. Finally, Parkin expression has been found to decrease the amount of mitochondrial movement in hippocampal neurons. This change in mitochondrial movement was also found to be associated with a reduction in axonal mitochondrial density [181].

4.5. Do Mitochondrial Dynamics Drive the Development of Neurodegeneration in PD?

Together these data suggest that many of the proteins that are known to be integral to the development of PD have now been shown to have crucial roles in maintaining the dynamics, distribution, and transport of mitochondria within neurons. We are now beginning to understand more about these dynamic aspects of mitochondria due to improved imaging techniques and models. It is clear, however, that the correct distribution of mitochondria within neurons is as important to their function as the interconnectivity of these organelles. Furthermore, it is not only the movements of functional mitochondria which need to be monitored and controlled, but also the localisation and transport of those which are dysfunctional and require degradation. Disruption of these processes in many models has been linked with impaired neuronal function or even neurodegeneration. With advancing age and in PD the neurons of the SN do accumulate mitochondria which are dysfunctional and may therefore be unable to provide the required level of ATP. Failure to remove these mitochondria from important sites such as the synapse will then lead to further detrimental changes (as described above) and neuronal loss.

5. Mitochondria and Protein Aggregation

Protein aggregation in Parkinson's disease is predominantly driven by alpha-synuclein, a small protein with a propensity to aggregate into oligomeric and fibrillar forms upon damage or mutation. This small protein has been proposed to function to support synaptic transmission, with proposed roles in vesicular packaging, synaptic vesicle trafficking and synaptic plasticity (reviewed in Reference [183]). The interaction of alpha-synuclein with mitochondria has been studied in depth over recent years, particularly since it has been suggested that it may be imported into mitochondria and cause inhibition of complex I [184]. The specific interaction of alpha-synuclein with mitochondrial complex I causes a reduction in its activity. This inhibition can be driven by both wild-type and mutant alpha-synuclein, and by oligomeric and fibrillar forms of the protein [45,185,186]. This functional disruption of mitochondria has most recently been shown to be also driven by an interaction of alpha-synuclein with complex V (ATP synthase) causing alterations in mitochondrial morphology, accompanied by an opening of the permeability transition pore, an increase in oxidative stress, and ultimately, neuronal death [45]. Recent work has highlighted that this capacity to interact with mitochondria may also impact on the ability of mitochondria to import essential proteins from the cytosol [184,187,188]. Alpha-synuclein has been shown to interact with the TOM (translocase of the outer membrane) complex in both tissue and culture-based systems. A blockage of import in this way has previously been shown to be sufficient to drive nigrostriatal degeneration [189].

Alpha-synuclein has been shown to cause fragmentation of the mitochondrial network in a number of models [190–192]. This fragmentation is DRP1 independent, occurs in the presence of both wild-type and mutant forms of the protein, and has been shown to precede the loss of mitochondrial function and neuron death. Interestingly, it has been suggested that the protein has no effect on the structure of the endoplasmic reticulum, the Golgi, or their interactions with the mitochondria. However, a recent study has shown that alpha-synuclein does interact with VAPB, an integral ER protein. This interaction then weakens the association of mitochondria with the ER, causing alteration in calcium buffering and the production of ATP [193]. The effect of alpha-synuclein on the structure of the mitochondria extends beyond merely affecting their fission and fusion with alterations to the ultrastructure of mitochondria also reported. Kamp et al. showed that PINK1, Parkin, and DJ-1 over expression was sufficient to be able to rescue the effect of alpha-synuclein on mitochondrial dynamics [191].

Alpha-synuclein has been suggested to be important for synaptic vesicle trafficking for many years, but recently, mounting evidence has suggested that it also affects the movement of mitochondria around neurons. In neurons exposed to alpha-synuclein, the balance between retrograde and anterograde transport is shifted. Wild type neurons showed a skewed preference for anterograde movement to maintain the axonal mitochondrial populations, and this preference was lost when alpha-synuclein expressed [194]. Kymograph analysis in a zebrafish model confirmed that alpha-synuclein reduced anterograde mitochondrial movements along axons and that the mitochondria within these axons, spent more time in a paused/stationary state [96]. The ability of alpha-synuclein to interrupt mitochondrial trafficking in this manner has been studied in depth, and is driven by its interaction with microtubules and cytoskeletal elements. Alpha-synuclein is capable of binding to a number of these proteins, including kinesin family member 5 (KIF5A), microtubule-associated protein 2 (MAP2), and Tau, with wild type synuclein showing the strongest binding to these proteins, with oligomers and fibrils showing weaker interactions [195]. The effect of alpha-synuclein on microtubule stability affects the distribution of mitochondria to neurites which would have detrimental effects on neuronal health and survival.

Does the Interaction of Alpha-Synuclein with Mitochondria Drive the Development of Neurodegeneration in PD?

Alpha-synuclein, of all the proposed contributors to Parkinson's pathogenesis, perhaps affects the most aspects of mitochondrial function. Alpha-synuclein has been shown to impact mitochondrial function, dynamics, transport, and protein import. Considering that alpha-synuclein aggregation is still one of the pathological hallmarks of PD, this would certainly suggest that in the presence of mitochondrial defects, it may lead to neurodegeneration. However, it is important to consider that studies have reported that Lewy bodies accumulate in neurons which do not have mitochondrial deficiencies, and that not all alpha-synuclein models recapitulate all of the characteristics of PD. Mitochondrial dysfunction, caused by alpha-synuclein or mtDNA mutations, may cause oxidative stress which will further damage alpha-synuclein, causing it to misfold into oligomeric forms. These alpha-synuclein aggregates are then capable of exacerbating mitochondrial dysfunction, as well as interfering with mitochondrial turnover and transport. This would lead to incorrect distribution of mitochondria, impaired calcium buffering, and ATP production increasing the sensitivity of these neurons to loss in Parkinson's.

6. Conclusions

Mitochondrial dysfunction, initially detected as Complex I deficiency, is found within the neurons of the SN, the population of neurons whose loss leads to the development of the motor symptoms associated with this disease. This deficiency may be caused by mtDNA deletions, by alpha-synuclein oligomers, or environmental toxins. A loss of mitochondrial function impedes ATP production and calcium buffering, key processes in the function of these neurons, and exacerbates oxidative stress. Such mitochondria should be targeted for degradation through the mitophagy pathway and replenished with new functional organelles through the PGC1α biogenesis pathway, both of which are affected by advancing age and have been shown to be linked to Parkinson's disease. Furthermore, dysfunctional mitochondria require transport to lysosomes and away from energy demanding sites. Recent evidence has also hinted that the dynamic processes that control the distribution and structure of mitochondria are also linked with PD. All these processes have the ability to cause further accumulation of defective mitochondria if they are themselves impaired.

Therefore, it is clear that alterations in mitochondrial function are important for neuronal survival and are a key driver of neuronal loss in Parkinson's disease (Figure 2). Since the initial description of Complex I deficiency in this disorder, our understanding not only of the complexities of mitochondria but also of the pathways and proteins whose function has an impact on, or is impacted by mitochondrial function, has dramatically increased. However, despite overwhelming evidence to suggest that the function of mitochondria is important for PD pathogenesis, the ability to identify the initial event in the cascade of changes that leads to neurodegeneration remains elusive. While here we have tried to categorize a number of proteins by their primary role (for example PINK1/Parkin as mitophagy proteins), it is becoming clear that many of these proteins have a role to play in a host of other pathways, while many of these also have differential consequences for the mitochondria (for example, the contribution of PINK1/Parkin to mitochondrial dynamics). While current techniques and models are driving this search forward, it is clear that the complex nature of the mitochondria and the role they play in a host of cellular pathways means that they have a large impact on a number of processes (energy provision, calcium buffering, ROS production, etc.). However, since their function is also impacted by changes in many of these pathways, it would seem that for every link between mitochondrial function and a pathway (for example, mitochondrial dynamics), a contrary relationship will then be found between the two processes. Understanding more about these interactions will uncover novel drugs which can modulate them not only to preserve mitochondrial function, but also to protect these organelles against damage and damaging moieties, driving and supporting the hunt for neuroprotective treatments.

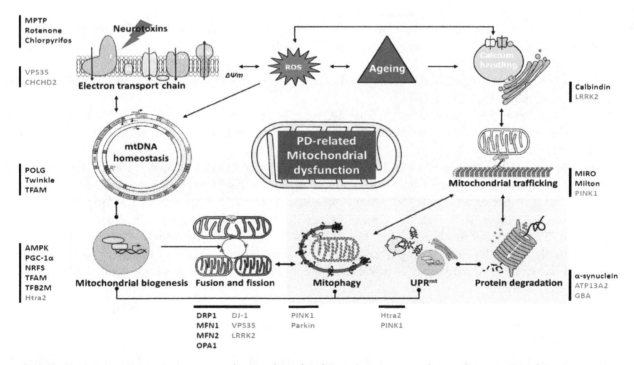

Figure 2. Schematic presentation of mitochondrial involvement in the pathogenesis of Parkinson's disease (PD). This diagram serves to highlight the complex links between the changes in mitochondrial

homeostasis, turnover, quality control and trafficking in cases of PD. These mitochondrial alternations are also intricately associated with the ageing process and impairments of the ubiquitin protease system that are attributed to Lewy body pathology. Lines with dots represent interactive effects, lines with arrows represent regulatory effects. Genes associated with familial PD are shown in blue, while we have also highlighted other proteins and toxins, recently been associated with PD, which impact on mitochondrial function. MPTP: 1-methyl-4-phenyl-1,2,3,6-tetrahydropyridine; VPS35: vacuolar protein sorting 35; CHCHD2: coiled-coil-helix-coiled-coil-helix domain containing 2; TFAM: mitochondrial transcription factor A; AMPK: AMP-activated protein kinase; PGC-1α: peroxisome proliferator-activated receptor γ (PPARγ) coactivator 1α; NRF: nuclear respiratory factors; TFB2M: dimethyladenosine transferase 2; DRP1: dynamin-1-like protein; MFN: mitofusin; LRRK2: Leucine-rich repeat kinase 2; PINK1: phosphatase and tensin homolog (PTEN)-induced putative kinase 1; GBA: lysosomal enzyme glucocerebrosidase; MIRO: mitochondrial Rho GTPase1; $\Delta\Psi$m: mitochondrial membrane potential; ROS: reactive oxygen species; mtDNA: mitochondrial DNA; UPR^{mt}: the mitochondrial unfolded protein response.

Author Contributions: Writing—original draft preparation, C.C. and A.K.R.; writing—review and editing, A.K.R., C.C. and D.M.T.; supervision, A.K.R. and D.M.T.

References

1. Langston, J.W.; Ballard, P.; Tetrud, J.W.; Irwin, I. Chronic Parkinsonism in humans due to a product of meperidine-analog synthesis. *Science* **1983**, *219*, 979–980. [CrossRef] [PubMed]
2. Langston, J.W.; Ballard, P.A., Jr. Parkinson's disease in a chemist working with 1-methyl-4-phenyl-1,2,5,6-tetrahydropyridine. *N. Engl. J. Med.* **1983**, *309*, 310. [PubMed]
3. Levitt, P.; Pintar, J.E.; Breakefield, X.O. Immunocytochemical demonstration of monoamine oxidase B in brain astrocytes and serotonergic neurons. *Proc. Natl. Acad. Sci. USA* **1982**, *79*, 6385–6389. [CrossRef] [PubMed]
4. Schapira, A.H.; Cooper, J.M.; Dexter, D.; Jenner, P.; Clark, J.B.; Marsden, C.D. Mitochondrial complex I deficiency in Parkinson's disease. *Lancet* **1989**, *1*, 1269. [CrossRef]
5. Heikkila, R.E.; Nicklas, W.J.; Vyas, I.; Duvoisin, R.C. Dopaminergic toxicity of rotenone and the 1-methyl-4-phenylpyridinium ion after their stereotaxic administration to rats: Implication for the mechanism of 1-methyl-4-phenyl-1,2,3,6-tetrahydropyridine toxicity. *Neurosci. Lett.* **1985**, *62*, 389–394. [CrossRef]
6. Goldman, S.M. Environmental toxins and Parkinson's disease. *Annu. Rev. Pharmacol. Toxicol.* **2014**, *54*, 141–164. [CrossRef] [PubMed]
7. Nandipati, S.; Litvan, I. Environmental Exposures and Parkinson's Disease. *Int. J. Environ. Res. Public Health* **2016**, *13*, 881. [CrossRef] [PubMed]
8. Betarbet, R.; Sherer, T.B.; MacKenzie, G.; Garcia-Osuna, M.; Panov, A.V.; Greenamyre, J.T. Chronic systemic pesticide exposure reproduces features of Parkinson's disease. *Nat. Neurosci.* **2000**, *3*, 1301–1306. [CrossRef] [PubMed]
9. Nakamura, K.; Bindokas, V.P.; Marks, J.D.; Wright, D.A.; Frim, D.M.; Miller, R.J.; Kang, U.J. The selective toxicity of 1-methyl-4-phenylpyridinium to dopaminergic neurons: The role of mitochondrial complex I and reactive oxygen species revisited. *Mol. Pharmacol.* **2000**, *58*, 271–278. [CrossRef] [PubMed]
10. Richardson, J.R.; Quan, Y.; Sherer, T.B.; Greenamyre, J.T.; Miller, G.W. Paraquat neurotoxicity is distinct from that of MPTP and rotenone. *Toxicol. Sci.* **2005**, *88*, 193–201. [CrossRef] [PubMed]
11. Lotharius, J.; O'Malley, K.L. The parkinsonism-inducing drug 1-methyl-4-phenylpyridinium triggers intracellular dopamine oxidation. A novel mechanism of toxicity. *J. Biol. Chem.* **2000**, *275*, 38581–38588. [CrossRef] [PubMed]
12. Giordano, S.; Lee, J.; Darley-Usmar, V.M.; Zhang, J. Distinct effects of rotenone, 1-methyl-4-phenylpyridinium and 6-hydroxydopamine on cellular bioenergetics and cell death. *PLoS ONE* **2012**, *7*, e44610. [CrossRef] [PubMed]
13. Grunewald, A.; Rygiel, K.A.; Hepplewhite, P.D.; Morris, C.M.; Picard, M.; Turnbull, D.M. Mitochondrial DNA depletion in respiratory chain-deficient Parkinson disease neurons. *Ann. Neurol.* **2016**, *79*, 366–378. [CrossRef] [PubMed]

14. Flones, I.H.; Fernandez-Vizarra, E.; Lykouri, M.; Brakedal, B.; Skeie, G.O.; Miletic, H.; Lilleng, P.K.; Alves, G.; Tysnes, O.B.; Haugarvoll, K.; et al. Neuronal complex I deficiency occurs throughout the Parkinson's disease brain, but is not associated with neurodegeneration or mitochondrial DNA damage. *Acta Neuropathol.* **2018**, *135*, 409–425. [CrossRef] [PubMed]

15. Bury, A.G.; Pyle, A.; Elson, J.L.; Greaves, L.; Morris, C.M.; Hudson, G.; Pienaar, I.S. Mitochondrial DNA changes in pedunculopontine cholinergic neurons in Parkinson disease. *Ann. Neurol.* **2017**, *82*, 1016–1021. [CrossRef] [PubMed]

16. Bender, A.; Krishnan, K.J.; Morris, C.M.; Taylor, G.A.; Reeve, A.K.; Perry, R.H.; Jaros, E.; Hersheson, J.S.; Betts, J.; Klopstock, T.; et al. High levels of mitochondrial DNA deletions in substantia nigra neurons in aging and Parkinson disease. *Nat. Genet.* **2006**, *38*, 515–517. [CrossRef] [PubMed]

17. Kraytsberg, Y.; Kudryavtseva, E.; McKee, A.C.; Geula, C.; Kowall, N.W.; Khrapko, K. Mitochondrial DNA deletions are abundant and cause functional impairment in aged human substantia nigra neurons. *Nat. Genet.* **2006**, *38*, 518–520. [CrossRef] [PubMed]

18. Reeve, A.; Meagher, M.; Lax, N.; Simcox, E.; Hepplewhite, P.; Jaros, E.; Turnbull, D. The impact of pathogenic mitochondrial DNA mutations on substantia nigra neurons. *J. Neurosci.* **2013**, *33*, 10790–10801. [CrossRef] [PubMed]

19. Kann, O.; Huchzermeyer, C.; Kovács, R.; Wirtz, S.; Schuelke, M. Gamma oscillations in the hippocampus require high complex I gene expression and strong functional performance of mitochondria. *Brain* **2010**, *134*, 345–358. [CrossRef] [PubMed]

20. Reeve, A.K.; Krishnan, K.J.; Elson, J.L.; Morris, C.M.; Bender, A.; Lightowlers, R.N.; Turnbull, D.M. Nature of mitochondrial DNA deletions in substantia nigra neurons. *Am. J. Hum. Genet.* **2008**, *82*, 228–235. [CrossRef] [PubMed]

21. Tzoulis, C.; Tran, G.T.; Coxhead, J.; Bertelsen, B.; Lilleng, P.K.; Balafkan, N.; Payne, B.; Miletic, H.; Chinnery, P.F.; Bindoff, L.A. Molecular pathogenesis of polymerase gamma-related neurodegeneration. *Ann. Neurol.* **2014**, *76*, 66–81. [CrossRef] [PubMed]

22. Reeve, A.K.; Park, T.K.; Jaros, E.; Campbell, G.R.; Lax, N.Z.; Hepplewhite, P.D.; Krishnan, K.J.; Elson, J.L.; Morris, C.M.; McKeith, I.G.; Turnbull, D.M. Relationship between mitochondria and α-synuclein: A study of single substantia nigra neurons. *Arch. Neurol.* **2012**, *69*, 385–393. [CrossRef] [PubMed]

23. Dolle, C.; Flones, I.; Nido, G.S.; Miletic, H.; Osuagwu, N.; Kristoffersen, S.; Lilleng, P.K.; Larsen, J.P.; Tysnes, O.B.; Haugarvoll, K.; et al. Defective mitochondrial DNA homeostasis in the substantia nigra in Parkinson disease. *Nat. Commun.* **2016**, *7*, 13548. [CrossRef] [PubMed]

24. Clayton, D.A. Replication of animal mitochondrial DNA. *Cell* **1982**, *28*, 693–705. [CrossRef]

25. Krishnan, K.J.; Reeve, A.K.; Samuels, D.C.; Chinnery, P.F.; Blackwood, J.K.; Taylor, R.W.; Wanrooij, S.; Spelbrink, J.N.; Lightowlers, R.N.; Turnbull, D.M. What causes mitochondrial DNA deletions in human cells? *Nat. Genet.* **2008**, *40*, 275–279. [CrossRef] [PubMed]

26. Fukui, H.; Moraes, C.T. Mechanisms of formation and accumulation of mitochondrial DNA deletions in aging neurons. *Hum. Mol. Genet.* **2009**, *18*, 1028–1036. [CrossRef] [PubMed]

27. Pickrell, A.M.; Pinto, M.; Hida, A.; Moraes, C.T. Striatal dysfunctions associated with mitochondrial DNA damage in dopaminergic neurons in a mouse model of Parkinson's disease. *J. Neurosci.* **2011**, *31*, 17649–17658. [CrossRef] [PubMed]

28. Pinto, M.; Pickrell, A.M.; Wang, X.; Bacman, S.R.; Yu, A.; Hida, A.; Dillon, L.M.; Morton, P.D.; Malek, T.R.; Williams, S.L.; et al. Transient mitochondrial DNA double strand breaks in mice cause accelerated aging phenotypes in a ROS-dependent but p53/p21-independent manner. *Cell Death Differ.* **2017**, *24*, 288–299. [CrossRef] [PubMed]

29. Corral-Debrinski, M.; Horton, T.; Lott, M.T.; Shoffner, J.M.; Beal, M.F.; Wallace, D.C. Mitochondrial DNA deletions in human brain: Regional variability and increase with advanced age. *Nat. Genet.* **1992**, *2*, 324–329. [CrossRef] [PubMed]

30. Cortopassi, G.A.; Shibata, D.; Soong, N.W.; Arnheim, N. A pattern of accumulation of a somatic deletion of mitochondrial DNA in aging human tissues. *Proc. Natl. Acad. Sci. USA* **1992**, *89*, 7370–7374. [CrossRef] [PubMed]

31. Perier, C.; Bender, A.; Garcia-Arumi, E.; Melia, M.J.; Bove, J.; Laub, C.; Klopstock, T.; Elstner, M.; Mounsey, R.B.; Teismann, P.; et al. Accumulation of mitochondrial DNA deletions within dopaminergic neurons triggers neuroprotective mechanisms. *Brain* **2013**, *136*, 2369–2378. [CrossRef] [PubMed]

32. Pyle, A.; Anugrha, H.; Kurzawa-Akanbi, M.; Yarnall, A.; Burn, D.; Hudson, G. Reduced mitochondrial DNA copy number is a biomarker of Parkinson's disease. *Neurobiol. Aging* **2016**, *38*, 216.e7–216.e10. [CrossRef] [PubMed]

33. Pyle, A.; Brennan, R.; Kurzawa-Akanbi, M.; Yarnall, A.; Thouin, A.; Mollenhauer, B.; Burn, D.; Chinnery, P.F.; Hudson, G. Reduced cerebrospinal fluid mitochondrial DNA is a biomarker for early-stage Parkinson's disease. *Ann. Neurol.* **2015**, *78*, 1000–1004. [CrossRef] [PubMed]

34. Lowes, H.; Pyle, A.; Duddy, M.; Hudson, G. Cell-free mitochondrial DNA in progressive multiple sclerosis. *Mitochondrion* **2018**. [CrossRef] [PubMed]

35. Suski, J.M.; Lebiedzinska, M.; Bonora, M.; Pinton, P.; Duszynski, J.; Wieckowski, M.R. Relation between mitochondrial membrane potential and ROS formation. *Methods Mol. Biol.* **2012**, *810*, 183–205. [PubMed]

36. Rigoulet, M.; Yoboue, E.D.; Devin, A. Mitochondrial ROS generation and its regulation: Mechanisms involved in H(2)O(2) signaling. *Antioxid. Redox Signal.* **2011**, *14*, 459–468. [CrossRef] [PubMed]

37. Delcambre, S.; Nonnenmacher, Y.; Hiller, K. Dopamine metabolism and reactive oxygen species production. In *Mitochondrial Mechanisms of Degeneration and Repair in Parkinson's Disease*; Buhlman, L.M., Ed.; Springer: Berlin, Germany, 2016; pp. 25–47.

38. Linnane, A.W.; Marzuki, S.; Ozawa, T.; Tanaka, M. Mitochondrial DNA mutations as an important contributor to ageing and degenerative diseases. *Lancet* **1989**, *1*, 642–645. [CrossRef]

39. Surmeier, D.J.; Guzman, J.N.; Sanchez, J.; Schumacker, P.T. Physiological phenotype and vulnerability in Parkinson's disease. *Cold Spring Harb. Perspect. Med.* **2012**, *2*, a009290. [CrossRef] [PubMed]

40. Vermulst, M.; Bielas, J.H.; Kujoth, G.C.; Ladiges, W.C.; Rabinovitch, P.S.; Prolla, T.A.; Loeb, L.A. Mitochondrial point mutations do not limit the natural lifespan of mice. *Nat. Genet.* **2007**, *39*, 540–543. [CrossRef] [PubMed]

41. Faucheux, B.A.; Martin, M.E.; Beaumont, C.; Hauw, J.J.; Agid, Y.; Hirsch, E.C. Neuromelanin associated redox-active iron is increased in the substantia nigra of patients with Parkinson's disease. *J. Neurochem.* **2003**, *86*, 1142–1148. [CrossRef] [PubMed]

42. Wang, J.-Y.; Zhuang, Q.-Q.; Zhu, L.-B.; Zhu, H.; Li, T.; Li, R.; Chen, S.-F.; Huang, C.-P.; Zhang, X.; Zhu, J.-H. Meta-analysis of brain iron levels of Parkinson's disease patients determined by postmortem and MRI measurements. *Sci. Rep.* **2016**, *6*, 36669. [CrossRef] [PubMed]

43. Smeyne, M.; Smeyne, R.J. Glutathione metabolism and Parkinson's disease. *Free Radic. Biol. Med.* **2013**, *62*, 13–25. [CrossRef] [PubMed]

44. Angelova, P.R.; Horrocks, M.H.; Klenerman, D.; Gandhi, S.; Abramov, A.Y.; Shchepinov, M.S. Lipid peroxidation is essential for alpha-synuclein-induced cell death. *J. Neurochem.* **2015**, *133*, 582–589. [CrossRef] [PubMed]

45. Ludtmann, M.H.R.; Angelova, P.R.; Horrocks, M.H.; Choi, M.L.; Rodrigues, M.; Baev, A.Y.; Berezhnov, A.V.; Yao, Z.; Little, D.; Banushi, B.; et al. α-synuclein oligomers interact with ATP synthase and open the permeability transition pore in Parkinson's disease. *Nat. Commun.* **2018**, *9*, 2293. [CrossRef] [PubMed]

46. Yamada, T.; McGeer, P.L.; Baimbridge, K.G.; McGeer, E.G. Relative sparing in Parkinson's disease of substantia nigra dopamine neurons containing calbindin-D28K. *Brain Res.* **1990**, *526*, 303–307. [CrossRef]

47. German, D.C.; Manaye, K.F.; Sonsalla, P.K.; Brooks, B.A. Midbrain dopaminergic cell loss in Parkinson's disease and MPTP-induced parkinsonism: sparing of calbindin-D28k-containing cells. *Ann. NY Acad. Sci.* **1992**, *648*, 42–62. [CrossRef] [PubMed]

48. David, G.; Barrett, E.F. Stimulation-evoked increases in cytosolic [Ca(2+)] in mouse motor nerve terminals are limited by mitochondrial uptake and are temperature-dependent. *J. Neurosci.* **2000**, *20*, 7290–7296. [PubMed]

49. Billups, B.; Forsythe, I.D. Presynaptic mitochondrial calcium sequestration influences transmission at mammalian central synapses. *J. Neurosci.* **2002**, *22*, 5840–5847. [CrossRef] [PubMed]

50. Wilson, C.J.; Callaway, J.C. Coupled oscillator model of the dopaminergic neuron of the substantia nigra. *J. Neurophysiol.* **2000**, *83*, 3084–3100. [CrossRef] [PubMed]

51. Wiel, C.; Lallet-Daher, H.; Gitenay, D.; Gras, B.; Le Calve, B.; Augert, A.; Ferrand, M.; Prevarskaya, N.; Simonnet, H.; Vindrieux, D.; et al. Endoplasmic reticulum calcium release through ITPR2 channels leads to mitochondrial calcium accumulation and senescence. *Nat. Commun.* **2014**, *5*, 3792. [CrossRef] [PubMed]

52. Mattson, M.P.; Chan, S.L. Calcium orchestrates apoptosis. *Nat. Cell Biol.* **2003**, *5*, 1041. [CrossRef] [PubMed]

53. Ludtmann, M.H.R.; Abramov, A.Y. Mitochondrial calcium imbalance in Parkinson's disease. *Neurosci. Lett.* **2018**, *663*, 86–90. [CrossRef] [PubMed]

54. Liu, Y.; Harding, M.; Pittman, A.; Dore, J.; Striessnig, J.; Rajadhyaksha, A.; Chen, X. Cav1.2 and Cav1.3 L-type calcium channels regulate dopaminergic firing activity in the mouse ventral tegmental area. *J. Neurophysiol.* **2014**, *112*, 1119–1130. [CrossRef] [PubMed]

55. Khaliq, Z.M.; Bean, B.P. Pacemaking in dopaminergic ventral tegmental area neurons: Depolarizing drive from background and voltage-dependent sodium conductances. *J. Neurosci.* **2010**, *30*, 7401–7413. [CrossRef] [PubMed]

56. Surmeier, D.J.; Schumacker, P.T.; Guzman, J.D.; Ilijic, E.; Yang, B.; Zampese, E. Calcium and Parkinson's disease. *Biochem. Biophys. Res. Commun.* **2017**, *483*, 1013–1019. [CrossRef] [PubMed]

57. Lieberman, O.J.; Choi, S.J.; Kanter, E.; Saverchenko, A.; Frier, M.D.; Fiore, G.M.; Wu, M.; Kondapalli, J.; Zampese, E.; Surmeier, D.J.; et al. α-synuclein-dependent calcium entry underlies differential sensitivity of cultured SN and VTA dopaminergic neurons to a parkinsonian neurotoxin. *eNeuro* **2017**, *4*. [CrossRef] [PubMed]

58. Wider, C.; Skipper, L.; Solida, A.; Brown, L.; Farrer, M.; Dickson, D.; Wszolek, Z.K.; Vingerhoets, F.J. Autosomal dominant dopa-responsive parkinsonism in a multigenerational Swiss family. *Parkinsonism Relat. Disord.* **2008**, *14*, 465–470. [CrossRef] [PubMed]

59. Vilarino-Guell, C.; Wider, C.; Ross, O.A.; Dachsel, J.C.; Kachergus, J.M.; Lincoln, S.J.; Soto-Ortolaza, A.I.; Cobb, S.A.; Wilhoite, G.J.; Bacon, J.A.; et al. VPS35 mutations in Parkinson disease. *Am. J. Hum. Genet.* **2011**, *89*, 162–167. [CrossRef] [PubMed]

60. Zhou, L.; Wang, W.; Hoppel, C.; Liu, J.; Zhu, X. Parkinson's disease-associated pathogenic VPS35 mutation causes complex I deficits. *Biochim. Biophys. Acta Mol. Basis Dis.* **2017**, *1863*, 2791–2795. [CrossRef] [PubMed]

61. Tang, F.L.; Liu, W.; Hu, J.X.; Erion, J.R.; Ye, J.; Mei, L.; Xiong, W.C. VPS35 deficiency or mutation causes dopaminergic neuronal loss by impairing mitochondrial fusion and function. *Cell Rep.* **2015**, *12*, 1631–1643. [CrossRef] [PubMed]

62. Cataldi, S.; Follett, J.; Fox, J.D.; Tatarnikov, I.; Kadgien, C.; Gustavsson, E.K. Altered dopamine release and monoamine transporters in Vps35 p.D620N knock-in mice. *NPJ Parkinson's Dis.* **2018**, *4*, 27. [CrossRef] [PubMed]

63. Funayama, M.; Ohe, K.; Amo, T.; Furuya, N.; Yamaguchi, J.; Saiki, S.; Li, Y.; Ogaki, K.; Ando, M.; Yoshino, H.; et al. CHCHD2 mutations in autosomal dominant late-onset Parkinson's disease: A genome-wide linkage and sequencing study. *Lancet Neurol.* **2015**, *14*, 274–282. [CrossRef]

64. Shi, C.H.; Mao, C.Y.; Zhang, S.Y.; Yang, J.; Song, B.; Wu, P.; Zuo, C.T.; Liu, Y.T.; Ji, Y.; Yang, Z.H.; et al. CHCHD2 gene mutations in familial and sporadic Parkinson's disease. *Neurobiol. Aging* **2016**, *38*, 217.e9–217.e13. [CrossRef] [PubMed]

65. Jansen, I.E.; Bras, J.M.; Lesage, S.; Schulte, C.; Gibbs, J.R.; Nalls, M.A.; Brice, A.; Wood, N.W.; Morris, H.; Hardy, J.A.; et al. CHCHD2 and Parkinson's disease. *Lancet Neurol.* **2015**, *14*, 678–679. [CrossRef]

66. Gagliardi, M.; Iannello, G.; Colica, C.; Annesi, G.; Quattrone, A. Analysis of CHCHD2 gene in familial Parkinson's disease from Calabria. *Neurobiol. Aging* **2017**, *50*, 169.e5–169.e6. [CrossRef] [PubMed]

67. Voigt, D.D.; Nascimento, C.M.; de Souza, R.B.; Cabello Acero, P.H.; Campos Junior, M.; da Silva, C.P.; Pereira, J.S.; Rosso, A.L.; Araujo Leite, M.A.; Vasconcellos, L.F.R.; et al. CHCHD2 mutational screening in Brazilian patients with familial Parkinson's disease. *Neurobiol. Aging* **2018**, *74*, 236.e7–236.e8. [CrossRef] [PubMed]

68. Bannwarth, S.; Ait-El-Mkadem, S.; Chaussenot, A.; Genin, E.C.; Lacas-Gervais, S.; Fragaki, K.; Berg-Alonso, L.; Kageyama, Y.; Serre, V.; Moore, D.G.; et al. A mitochondrial origin for frontotemporal dementia and amyotrophic lateral sclerosis through CHCHD10 involvement. *Brain* **2014**, *137*, 2329–2345. [CrossRef] [PubMed]

69. Meng, H.; Yamashita, C.; Shiba-Fukushima, K.; Inoshita, T.; Funayama, M.; Sato, S.; Hatta, T.; Natsume, T.; Umitsu, M.; Takagi, J.; et al. Loss of Parkinson's disease-associated protein CHCHD2 affects mitochondrial crista structure and destabilizes cytochrome c. *Nat. Commun.* **2017**, *8*, 15500. [CrossRef] [PubMed]

70. Longen, S.; Bien, M.; Bihlmaier, K.; Kloeppel, C.; Kauff, F.; Hammermeister, M.; Westermann, B.; Herrmann, J.M.; Riemer, J. Systematic analysis of the twin cx(9)c protein family. *J. Mol. Biol.* **2009**, *393*, 356–368. [CrossRef] [PubMed]

71. Lee, R.G.; Sedghi, M.; Salari, M.; Shearwood, A.J.; Stentenbach, M.; Kariminejad, A.; Goullee, H.; Rackham, O.; Laing, N.G.; Tajsharghi, H.; et al. Early-onset Parkinson disease caused by a mutation in CHCHD2 and mitochondrial dysfunction. *Neurol. Genet.* **2018**, *4*, e276. [CrossRef] [PubMed]

72. Betts-Henderson, J.; Jaros, E.; Krishnan, K.J.; Perry, R.H.; Reeve, A.K.; Schaefer, A.M.; Taylor, R.W.; Turnbull, D.M. Alpha-synuclein pathology and Parkinsonism associated with POLG1 mutations and multiple mitochondrial DNA deletions. *Neuropathol. Appl. Neurobiol.* **2009**, *35*, 120–124. [PubMed]

73. Hudson, G.; Chinnery, P.F. Mitochondrial DNA polymerase-gamma and human disease. *Hum. Mol. Genet.* **2006**, *15*, R244–R252. [CrossRef] [PubMed]

74. Yin, Z.; Pascual, C.; Klionsky, D.J. Autophagy: Machinery and regulation. *Microb. Cell* **2016**, *3*, 588–596. [CrossRef] [PubMed]

75. Andres, A.M.; Stotland, A.; Queliconi, B.B.; Gottlieb, R.A. A time to reap, a time to sow: Mitophagy and biogenesis in cardiac pathophysiology. *J. Mol. Cell Cardiol.* **2015**, *78*, 62–72. [CrossRef] [PubMed]

76. Poole, A.C.; Thomas, R.E.; Andrews, L.A.; McBride, H.M.; Whitworth, A.J.; Pallanck, L.J. The PINK1/Parkin pathway regulates mitochondrial morphology. *Proc. Natl. Acad. Sci. USA* **2008**, *105*, 1638–1643. [CrossRef] [PubMed]

77. Kitada, T.; Asakawa, S.; Hattori, N.; Matsumine, H.; Yamamura, Y.; Minoshima, S.; Yokochi, M.; Mizuno, Y.; Shimiz, N. Mutations in the parkin gene cause autosomal recessive juvenile parkinsonism. *Nature* **1998**, *392*, 605–608. [CrossRef] [PubMed]

78. Vives-Bauza, C.; Zhou, C.; Huang, Y.; Cui, M.; de Vries, R.L.A.; Kim, J.; May, J.; Tocilescu, M.A.; Liu, W.; Ko, H.S.; et al. PINK1-dependent recruitment of Parkin to mitochondria in mitophagy. *Proc. Natl. Acad. Sci. USA* **2010**, *107*, 378–383. [CrossRef] [PubMed]

79. Durcan, T.M.; Fon, E.A. The three 'P's of mitophagy: PARKIN, PINK1, and post-translational modifications. *Genes Dev.* **2015**, *29*, 989–999. [CrossRef] [PubMed]

80. Fu, M.; St-Pierre, P.; Shankar, J.; Wang, P.T.; Joshi, B.; Nabi, I.R. Regulation of mitophagy by the Gp78 E3 ubiquitin ligase. *Mol. Biol. Cell* **2013**, *24*, 1153–1162. [CrossRef] [PubMed]

81. Villa, E.; Proics, E.; Rubio-Patino, C.; Obba, S.; Zunino, B.; Bossowski, J.P.; Rozier, R.M.; Chiche, J.; Mondragon, L.; Riley, J.S.; et al. Parkin-independent mitophagy controls chemotherapeutic response in cancer cells. *Cell Rep.* **2017**, *20*, 2846–2859. [CrossRef] [PubMed]

82. Anderson, S.; Bankier, A.T.; Barrell, B.G.; de Bruijn, M.H.; Coulson, A.R.; Drouin, J.; Eperon, I.C.; Nierlich, D.P.; Roe, B.A.; Sanger, F.; et al. Sequence and organization of the human mitochondrial genome. *Nature* **1981**, *290*, 457–465. [CrossRef] [PubMed]

83. Ventura-Clapier, R.; Garnier, A.; Veksler, V. Transcriptional control of mitochondrial biogenesis: The central role of PGC-1alpha. *Cardiovasc. Res.* **2008**, *79*, 208–217. [CrossRef] [PubMed]

84. Scarpulla, R.C. Metabolic control of mitochondrial biogenesis through the PGC-1 family regulatory network. *Biochim. Biophys. Acta* **2011**, *1813*, 1269–1278. [CrossRef] [PubMed]

85. Gleyzer, N.; Vercauteren, K.; Scarpulla, R.C. Control of mitochondrial transcription specificity factors (TFB1M and TFB2M) by nuclear respiratory factors (NRF-1 and NRF-2) and PGC-1 family coactivators. *Mol. Cell Biol.* **2005**, *25*, 1354–1366. [CrossRef] [PubMed]

86. Scarpulla, R.C. Transcriptional paradigms in mammalian mitochondrial biogenesis and function. *Physiol. Rev.* **2008**, *88*, 611–638. [CrossRef] [PubMed]

87. Zheng, B.; Liao, Z.; Locascio, J.J.; Lesniak, K.A.; Roderick, S.S.; Watt, M.L.; Eklund, A.C.; Zhang-James, Y.; Kim, P.D.; Hauser, M.A.; et al. PGC-1alpha, a potential therapeutic target for early intervention in Parkinson's disease. *Sci. Transl. Med.* **2010**, *2*, 52ra73. [CrossRef] [PubMed]

88. Zahn, J.M.; Sonu, R.; Vogel, H.; Crane, E.; Mazan-Mamczarz, K.; Rabkin, R.; Davis, R.W.; Becker, K.G.; Owen, A.B.; Kim, S.K. Transcriptional profiling of aging in human muscle reveals a common aging signature. *PLoS Genet.* **2006**, *2*, e115. [CrossRef]

89. Kett, L.R.; Dauer, W.T. Endolysosomal dysfunction in Parkinson's disease: Recent developments and future challenges. *Mov. Disord.* **2016**, *31*, 1433–1443. [CrossRef] [PubMed]

90. Reznick, R.M.; Zong, H.; Li, J.; Morino, K.; Moore, I.K.; Yu, H.J.; Liu, Z.X.; Dong, J.; Mustard, K.J.; Hawley, S.A.; et al. Aging-associated reductions in AMP-activated protein kinase activity and mitochondrial biogenesis. *Cell Metab.* **2007**, *5*, 151–156. [CrossRef] [PubMed]

91. Jiang, H.; Kang, S.-U.; Zhang, S.; Karuppagounder, S.; Xu, J.; Lee, Y.-K.; Kang, B.-G.; Lee, Y.; Zhang, J.; Pletnikova, O.; et al. Adult conditional knockout of PGC-1α leads to loss of dopamine neurons. *eNeuro* **2016**, *3*. [CrossRef] [PubMed]

92. Ng, C.H.; Basil, A.H.; Hang, L.; Tan, R.; Goh, K.L.; O'Neill, S.; Zhang, X.; Yu, F.; Lim, K.L. Genetic or pharmacological activation of the Drosophila PGC-1alpha ortholog spargel rescues the disease phenotypes of genetic models of Parkinson's disease. *Neurobiol. Aging* **2017**, *55*, 33–37. [CrossRef] [PubMed]

93. Ye, Q.; Huang, W.; Li, D.; Si, E.; Wang, J.; Wang, Y.; Chen, C.; Chen, X. Overexpression of PGC-1alpha influences mitochondrial signal transduction of dopaminergic neurons. *Mol. Neurobiol.* **2016**, *53*, 3756–3770. [CrossRef] [PubMed]

94. Eschbach, J.; von Einem, B.; Muller, K.; Bayer, H.; Scheffold, A.; Morrison, B.E.; Rudolph, K.L.; Thal, D.R.; Witting, A.; Weydt, P.; et al. Mutual exacerbation of peroxisome proliferator-activated receptor gamma coactivator 1alpha deregulation and alpha-synuclein oligomerization. *Ann. Neurol.* **2015**, *77*, 15–32. [CrossRef] [PubMed]

95. Ciron, C.; Zheng, L.; Bobela, W.; Knott, G.W.; Leone, T.C.; Kelly, D.P.; Schneider, B.L. PGC-1alpha activity in nigral dopamine neurons determines vulnerability to alpha-synuclein. *Acta Neuropathol. Commun.* **2015**, *3*, 16. [CrossRef] [PubMed]

96. O'Donnell, K.C.; Lulla, A.; Stahl, M.C.; Wheat, N.D.; Bronstein, J.M.; Sagasti, A. Axon degeneration and PGC-1alpha-mediated protection in a zebrafish model of alpha-synuclein toxicity. *Dis. Model Mech.* **2014**, *7*, 571–582. [CrossRef] [PubMed]

97. Uldry, M.; Yang, W.; St-Pierre, J.; Lin, J.; Seale, P.; Spiegelman, B.M. Complementary action of the PGC-1 coactivators in mitochondrial biogenesis and brown fat differentiation. *Cell Metab.* **2006**, *3*, 333–341. [CrossRef] [PubMed]

98. St-Pierre, J.; Drori, S.; Uldry, M.; Silvaggi, J.M.; Rhee, J.; Jager, S.; Handschin, C.; Zheng, K.; Lin, J.; Yang, W.; et al. Suppression of reactive oxygen species and neurodegeneration by the PGC-1 transcriptional coactivators. *Cell* **2006**, *127*, 397–408. [CrossRef] [PubMed]

99. Di Giacomo, E.; Benedetti, E.; Cristiano, L.; Antonosante, A.; d'Angelo, M.; Fidoamore, A.; Barone, D.; Moreno, S.; Ippoliti, R.; Ceru, M.P.; et al. Roles of PPAR transcription factors in the energetic metabolic switch occurring during adult neurogenesis. *Cell Cycle* **2017**, *16*, 59–72. [CrossRef] [PubMed]

100. Shin, J.H.; Ko, H.S.; Kang, H.; Lee, Y.; Lee, Y.I.; Pletinkova, O.; Troconso, J.C.; Dawson, V.L.; Dawson, T.M. PARIS (ZNF746) repression of PGC-1alpha contributes to neurodegeneration in Parkinson's disease. *Cell* **2011**, *144*, 689–702. [CrossRef] [PubMed]

101. Peng, K.; Xiao, J.; Yang, L.; Ye, F.; Cao, J.; Sai, Y. Mutual Antagonism of PINK1/Parkin and PGC-1alpha Contributes to Maintenance of Mitochondrial Homeostasis in Rotenone-Induced Neurotoxicity. *Neurotox. Res.* **2018**, *35*, 331–343. [CrossRef] [PubMed]

102. Diot, A.; Morten, K.; Poulton, J. Mitophagy plays a central role in mitochondrial ageing. *Mamm. Genome* **2016**, *27*, 381–395. [CrossRef] [PubMed]

103. Fivenson, E.M.; Lautrup, S.; Sun, N.; Scheibye-Knudsen, M.; Stevnsner, T.; Nilsen, H.; Bohr, V.A.; Fang, E.F. Mitophagy in neurodegeneration and aging. *Neurochem. Int.* **2017**, *109*, 202–209. [CrossRef] [PubMed]

104. Shi, R.; Guberman, M.; Kirshenbaum, L.A. Mitochondrial quality control: The role of mitophagy in aging. *Trends Cardiovasc. Med.* **2018**, *28*, 246–260. [CrossRef] [PubMed]

105. Moreira, O.C.; Estébanez, B.; Martínez-Florez, S.; de Paz, J.A.; Cuevas, M.J.; González-Gallego, H. Mitochondrial Function and mitophagy in the elderly: Effects of exercise. [CrossRef] [PubMed]

106. Reeve, A.; Simcox, E.; Turnbull, D. Ageing and Parkinson's disease: Why is advancing age the biggest risk factor? *Ageing Res. Rev.* **2014**, *14*, 19–30. [CrossRef] [PubMed]

107. Scarffe, L.A.; Stevens, D.A.; Dawson, V.L.; Dawson, T.M. Parkin and PINK1: Much more than mitophagy. *Trends Neurosci.* **2014**, *37*, 315–324. [CrossRef] [PubMed]

108. Zhao, Q.; Wang, J.; Levichkin, I.V.; Stasinopoulos, S.; Ryan, M.T.; Hoogenraad, N.J. A mitochondrial specific stress response in mammalian cells. *EMBO J.* **2002**, *21*, 4411–4419. [CrossRef] [PubMed]

109. Plun-Favreau, H.; Klupsch, K.; Moisoi, N.; Gandhi, S.; Kjaer, S.; Frith, D.; Harvey, K.; Deas, E.; Harvey, R.J.; McDonald, N.; et al. The mitochondrial protease HtrA2 is regulated by Parkinson's disease-associated kinase PINK1. *Nat. Cell Biol.* **2007**, *9*, 1243–1252. [CrossRef] [PubMed]

110. Pridgeon, J.W.; Olzmann, J.A.; Chin, L.-S.; Li, L. PINK1 protects against oxidative stress by phosphorylating mitochondrial chaperone TRAP1. *PLoS Biol.* **2007**, *5*, e172. [CrossRef] [PubMed]

111. Strauss, K.M.; Martins, L.M.; Plun-Favreau, H.; Marx, F.P.; Kautzmann, S.; Berg, D.; Gasser, T.; Wszolek, Z.; Muller, T.; Bornemann, A.; et al. Loss of function mutations in the gene encoding Omi/HtrA2 in Parkinson's disease. *Hum. Mol. Genet.* **2005**, *14*, 2099–2111. [CrossRef] [PubMed]

112. Fitzgerald, J.C.; Zimprich, A.; Carvajal Berrio, D.A.; Schindler, K.M.; Maurer, B.; Schulte, C.; Bus, C.; Hauser, A.K.; Kubler, M.; Lewin, R.; et al. Metformin reverses TRAP1 mutation-associated alterations in mitochondrial function in Parkinson's disease. *Brain* **2017**, *140*, 2444–2459. [CrossRef] [PubMed]

113. Moisoi, N.; Klupsch, K.; Fedele, V.; East, P.; Sharma, S.; Renton, A.; Plun-Favreau, H.; Edwards, R.E.; Teismann, P.; Esposti, M.D.; et al. Mitochondrial dysfunction triggered by loss of HtrA2 results in the activation of a brain-specific transcriptional stress response. *Cell Death Differ.* **2009**, *16*, 449–464. [CrossRef] [PubMed]

114. Costa, A.C.; Loh, S.H.; Martins, L.M. Drosophila Trap1 protects against mitochondrial dysfunction in a PINK1/parkin model of Parkinson's disease. *Cell Death Dis.* **2013**, *4*, e467. [CrossRef] [PubMed]

115. Zhang, L.; Karsten, P.; Hamm, S.; Pogson, J.H.; Müller-Rischart, A.K.; Exner, N.; Haass, C.; Whitworth, A.J.; Winklhofer, K.F.; Schulz, J.B.; et al. TRAP1 rescues PINK1 loss-of-function phenotypes. *Hum. Mol. Genet.* **2013**, *22*, 2829–2841. [CrossRef] [PubMed]

116. Thomas, K.J.; McCoy, M.K.; Blackinton, J.; Beilina, A.; van der Brug, M.; Sandebring, A.; Miller, D.; Maric, D.; Cedazo-Minguez, A.; Cookson, M.R. DJ-1 acts in parallel to the PINK1/parkin pathway to control mitochondrial function and autophagy. *Hum. Mol. Genet.* **2011**, *20*, 40–50. [CrossRef] [PubMed]

117. Wang, X.; Petrie, T.G.; Liu, Y.; Liu, J.; Fujioka, H.; Zhu, X. Parkinson's disease-associated DJ-1 mutations impair mitochondrial dynamics and cause mitochondrial dysfunction. *J. Neurochem.* **2012**, *121*, 830–839. [CrossRef] [PubMed]

118. McCoy, M.K.; Cookson, M.R. DJ-1 regulation of mitochondrial function and autophagy through oxidative stress. *Autophagy* **2011**, *7*, 531–532. [CrossRef] [PubMed]

119. Hsieh, C.H.; Shaltouki, A.; Gonzalez, A.E.; Bettencourt da Cruz, A.; Burbulla, L.F.; St Lawrence, E.; Schule, B.; Krainc, D.; Palmer, T.D.; Wang, X. Functional impairment in Miro degradation and mitophagy is a shared feature in familial and sporadic Parkinson's disease. *Cell Stem Cell* **2016**, *19*, 709–724. [CrossRef] [PubMed]

120. Park, J.-S.; Blair, N.F.; Sue, C.M. The role of ATP13A2 in Parkinson's disease: Clinical phenotypes and molecular mechanisms. *Mov. Disord.* **2015**, *30*, 770–779. [CrossRef] [PubMed]

121. Suleiman, J.; Hamwi, N.; El-Hattab, A.W. ATP13A2 novel mutations causing a rare form of juvenile-onset Parkinson disease. *Brain Dev.* **2018**, *40*, 824–826. [CrossRef] [PubMed]

122. Park, J.S.; Koentjoro, B.; Veivers, D.; Mackay-Sim, A.; Sue, C.M. Parkinson's disease-associated human ATP13A2 (PARK9) deficiency causes zinc dyshomeostasis and mitochondrial dysfunction. *Hum. Mol. Genet.* **2014**, *23*, 2802–2815. [CrossRef] [PubMed]

123. Rayaprolu, S.; Seven, Y.B.; Howard, J.; Duffy, C.; Altshuler, M.; Moloney, C.; Giasson, B.I.; Lewis, J. Partial loss of ATP13A2 causes selective gliosis independent of robust lipofuscinosis. *Mol. Cell Neurosci.* **2018**, *92*, 17–26. [CrossRef] [PubMed]

124. Sato, S.; Koike, M.; Funayama, M.; Ezaki, J.; Fukuda, T.; Ueno, T.; Uchiyama, Y.; Hattori, N. Lysosomal storage of subunit c of mitochondrial ATP Synthase in brain-specific Atp13a2-deficient mice. *Am. J. Pathol.* **2016**, *186*, 3074–3082. [CrossRef] [PubMed]

125. Park, J.S.; Koentjoro, B.; Davis, R.L.; Sue, C.M. Loss of ATP13A2 impairs glycolytic function in Kufor-Rakeb syndrome patient-derived cell models. *Parkinsonism Relat. Disord.* **2016**, *27*, 67–73. [CrossRef] [PubMed]

126. Goker-Alpan, O.; Lopez, G.; Vithayathil, J.; Davis, J.; Hallett, M.; Sidransky, E. The spectrum of parkinsonian manifestations associated with glucocerebrosidase mutations. *Arch. Neurol.* **2008**, *65*, 1353–1357. [CrossRef] [PubMed]

127. Sidransky, E.; Lopez, G. The link between the GBA gene and parkinsonism. *Lancet Neurol.* **2012**, *11*, 986–998. [CrossRef]

128. Gan-Or, Z.; Amshalom, I.; Kilarski, L.L.; Bar-Shira, A.; Gana-Weisz, M.; Mirelman, A.; Marder, K.; Bressman, S.; Giladi, N.; Orr-Utreger, A. Differential effects of severe vs mild GBA mutations on Parkinson disease. *Neurology* **2015**, *84*, 880–887. [CrossRef] [PubMed]

129. Sato, S.; Li, Y.; Hattori, N. Lysosomal defects in ATP13A2 and GBA associated familial Parkinson's disease. *J. Neural Transm.* **2017**, *124*, 1395–1400. [CrossRef] [PubMed]

130. Sun, N.; Youle, R.J.; Finkel, T. The mitochondrial basis of aging. *Mol. Cell* **2016**, *61*, 654–666. [CrossRef] [PubMed]

131. Brunk, U.T.; Terman, A. Lipofuscin: Mechanisms of age-related accumulation and influence on cell function. *Free Radic. Biol. Med.* **2002**, *33*, 611–619. [CrossRef]

132. Dauer, W.; Przedborski, S. Parkinson's disease: Mechanisms and models. *Neuron* **2003**, *39*, 889–909. [CrossRef]

133. Amiri, M.; Hollenbeck, P.J. Mitochondrial biogenesis in the axons of vertebrate peripheral neurons. *Dev. Neurobiol.* **2008**, *68*, 1348–1361. [CrossRef] [PubMed]

134. Lentz, S.I.; Edwards, J.L.; Backus, C.; McLean, L.L.; Haines, K.M.; Feldman, E.L. Mitochondrial DNA (mtDNA) biogenesis: visualization and duel incorporation of BrdU and EdU into newly synthesized mtDNA in vitro. *J. Histochem. Cytochem.* **2010**, *58*, 207–218. [CrossRef] [PubMed]

135. Calkins, M.J.; Reddy, P.H. Assessment of newly synthesized mitochondrial DNA using BrdU labeling in primary neurons from Alzheimer's disease mice: Implications for impaired mitochondrial biogenesis and synaptic damage. *Biochim. Biophys. Acta* **2011**, *1812*, 1182–1189. [CrossRef] [PubMed]

136. Ferguson, S.M. Axonal transport and maturation of lysosomes. *Curr. Opin. Neurobiol.* **2018**, *51*, 45–51. [CrossRef] [PubMed]

137. Hayakawa, K.; Esposito, E.; Wang, X.; Terasaki, Y.; Liu, Y.; Xing, C.; Ji, X.; Lo, E.H. Transfer of mitochondria from astrocytes to neurons after stroke. *Nature* **2016**, *535*, 551. [CrossRef] [PubMed]

138. Davis, C.-h.O.; Kim, K.-Y.; Bushong, E.A.; Mills, E.A.; Boassa, D.; Shih, T.; Kinebuchi, M.; Phan, S.; Zhou, Y.; Bihlmeyer, N.A.; et al. Transcellular degradation of axonal mitochondria. *Proc. Natl. Acad. Sci. USA* **2014**, *111*, 9633–9638. [CrossRef] [PubMed]

139. Lin, M.Y.; Sheng, Z.H. Regulation of mitochondrial transport in neurons. *Exp. Cell Res.* **2015**, *334*, 35–44. [CrossRef] [PubMed]

140. Misgeld, T.; Schwarz, T.L. Mitostasis in neurons: Maintaining mitochondria in an extended cellular architecture. *Neuron* **2017**, *96*, 651–666. [CrossRef] [PubMed]

141. Menzies, F.M.; Fleming, A.; Caricasole, A.; Bento, C.F.; Andrews, S.P.; Ashkenazi, A.; Fullgrabe, J.; Jackson, A.; Jimenez Sanchez, M.; Karabiyik, C.; et al. Autophagy and neurodegeneration: Pathogenic mechanisms and therapeutic opportunities. *Neuron* **2017**, *93*, 1015–1034. [CrossRef] [PubMed]

142. Twig, G.; Elorza, A.; Molina, A.J.; Mohamed, H.; Wikstrom, J.D.; Walzer, G.; Stiles, L.; Haigh, S.E.; Katz, S.; Las, G.; et al. Fission and selective fusion govern mitochondrial segregation and elimination by autophagy. *EMBO J.* **2008**, *27*, 433–446. [CrossRef] [PubMed]

143. Van Laar, V.S.; Berman, S.B. The interplay of neuronal mitochondrial dynamics and bioenergetics: Implications for Parkinson's disease. *Neurobiol. Dis.* **2013**, *51*, 43–55. [CrossRef] [PubMed]

144. Berthet, A.; Margolis, E.B.; Zhang, J.; Hsieh, I.; Zhang, J.; Hnasko, T.S.; Ahmad, J.; Edwards, R.H.; Sesaki, H.; Huang, E.J.; et al. Loss of mitochondrial fission depletes axonal mitochondria in midbrain dopamine neurons. *J Neurosci.* **2014**, *34*, 14304–14317. [CrossRef] [PubMed]

145. Carelli, V.; Musumeci, O.; Caporali, L.; Zanna, C.; La Morgia, C.; Del Dotto, V.; Porcelli, A.M.; Rugolo, M.; Valentino, M.L.; Iommarini, L.; et al. Syndromic parkinsonism and dementia associated with OPA1 missense mutations. *Ann. Neurol.* **2015**, *78*, 21–38. [CrossRef] [PubMed]

146. Ramonet, D.; Perier, C.; Recasens, A.; Dehay, B.; Bove, J.; Costa, V.; Scorrano, L.; Vila, M. Optic atrophy 1 mediates mitochondria remodeling and dopaminergic neurodegeneration linked to complex I deficiency. *Cell Death Differ.* **2013**, *20*, 77–85. [CrossRef] [PubMed]

147. Glauser, L.; Sonnay, S.; Stafa, K.; Moore, D.J. Parkin promotes the ubiquitination and degradation of the mitochondrial fusion factor mitofusin 1. *J. Neurochem.* **2011**, *118*, 636–645. [CrossRef] [PubMed]

148. Gegg, M.E.; Cooper, J.M.; Chau, K.Y.; Rojo, M.; Schapira, A.H.; Taanman, J.W. Mitofusin 1 and mitofusin 2 are ubiquitinated in a PINK1/parkin-dependent manner upon induction of mitophagy. *Hum. Mol. Genet.* **2010**, *19*, 4861–4870. [CrossRef] [PubMed]

149. Chen, Y.; Dorn, G.W., 2nd. PINK1-phosphorylated mitofusin 2 is a Parkin receptor for culling damaged mitochondria. *Science* **2013**, *340*, 471–475. [CrossRef] [PubMed]

150. Rakovic, A.; Grünewald, A.; Kottwitz, J.; Brüggemann, N.; Pramstaller, P.P.; Lohmann, K.; Klein, C. Mutations in PINK1 and parkin impair ubiquitination of mitofusins in human fibroblasts. *PLoS ONE* **2011**, *6*, e16746. [CrossRef] [PubMed]

151. Barsoum, M.J.; Yuan, H.; Gerencser, A.A.; Liot, G.; Kushnareva, Y.; Graber, S.; Kovacs, I.; Lee, W.D.; Waggoner, J.; Cui, J.; et al. Nitric oxide-induced mitochondrial fission is regulated by dynamin-related GTPases in neurons. *EMBO J.* **2006**, *25*, 3900–3911. [CrossRef] [PubMed]

152. Plecita-Hlavata, L.; Lessard, M.; Santorova, J.; Bewersdorf, J.; Jezek, P. Mitochondrial oxidative phosphorylation and energetic status are reflected by morphology of mitochondrial network in INS-1E and HEP-G2 cells viewed by 4Pi microscopy. *Biochim. Biophys. Acta* **2008**, *1777*, 834–846. [CrossRef] [PubMed]

153. Wang, X.; Su, B.; Liu, W.; He, X.; Gao, Y.; Castellani, R.J.; Perry, G.; Smith, M.A.; Zhu, X. DLP1-dependent mitochondrial fragmentation mediates 1-methyl-4-phenylpyridinium toxicity in neurons: Implications for Parkinson's disease. *Aging Cell* **2011**, *10*, 807–823. [CrossRef] [PubMed]

154. Peng, K.; Yang, L.; Wang, J.; Ye, F.; Dan, G.; Zhao, Y.; Cai, Y.; Cui, Z.; Ao, L.; Liu, J.; et al. The interaction of mitochondrial biogenesis and fission/fusion mediated by PGC-1alpha regulates rotenone-induced dopaminergic neurotoxicity. *Mol. Neurobiol.* **2017**, *54*, 3783–3797. [CrossRef] [PubMed]

155. Zambonin, J.L.; Zhao, C.; Ohno, N.; Campbell, G.R.; Engeham, S.; Ziabreva, I.; Schwarz, N.; Lee, S.E.; Frischer, J.M.; Turnbull, D.M.; et al. Increased mitochondrial content in remyelinated axons: Implications for multiple sclerosis. *Brain* **2011**, *134*, 1901–1913. [CrossRef] [PubMed]

156. Schwarz, T.L. Mitochondrial trafficking in neurons. *Cold Spring Harb. Perspect. Biol.* **2013**, *5*. [CrossRef] [PubMed]

157. Devine, M.J.; Kittler, J.T. Mitochondria at the neuronal presynapse in health and disease. *Nat. Rev. Neurosci.* **2018**, *19*, 63–80. [CrossRef] [PubMed]

158. Chan, C.S.; Guzman, J.N.; Ilijic, E.; Mercer, J.N.; Rick, C.; Tkatch, T.; Meredith, G.E.; Surmeier, D.J. 'Rejuvenation' protects neurons in mouse models of Parkinson's disease. *Nature* **2007**, *447*, 1081–1086. [CrossRef] [PubMed]

159. Chang, D.T.; Honick, A.S.; Reynolds, I.J. Mitochondrial trafficking to synapses in cultured primary cortical neurons. *J. Neurosci.* **2006**, *26*, 7035–7045. [CrossRef] [PubMed]

160. Kang, J.S.; Tian, J.H.; Pan, P.Y.; Zald, P.; Li, C.; Deng, C.; Sheng, Z.H. Docking of axonal mitochondria by syntaphilin controls their mobility and affects short-term facilitation. *Cell* **2008**, *132*, 137–148. [CrossRef] [PubMed]

161. Obashi, K.; Okabe, S. Regulation of mitochondrial dynamics and distribution by synapse position and neuronal activity in the axon. *Eur. J. Neurosci.* **2013**, *38*, 2350–2363. [CrossRef] [PubMed]

162. Reeve, A.K.; Grady, J.P.; Cosgrave, E.M.; Bennison, E.; Chen, C.; Hepplewhite, P.D.; Morris, C.M. Mitochondrial dysfunction within the synapses of substantia nigra neurons in Parkinson's disease. *NPJ Parkinson's Dis.* **2018**, *4*, 9. [CrossRef] [PubMed]

163. Barnhart, E.L. Mechanics of mitochondrial motility in neurons. *Curr. Opin. Cell Biol.* **2016**, *38*, 90–99. [CrossRef] [PubMed]

164. Miller, K.E.; Sheetz, M.P. Axonal mitochondrial transport and potential are correlated. *J. Cell Sci.* **2004**, *117*, 2791–2804. [CrossRef] [PubMed]

165. Verburg, J.; Hollenbeck, P.J. Mitochondrial membrane potential in axons increases with local nerve growth factor or semaphorin signaling. *J. Neurosci.* **2008**, *28*, 8306–8315. [CrossRef] [PubMed]

166. Chen, Y.; Sheng, Z.H. Kinesin-1-syntaphilin coupling mediates activity-dependent regulation of axonal mitochondrial transport. *J. Cell Biol.* **2013**, *202*, 351–364. [CrossRef] [PubMed]

167. Sorbara, C.D.; Wagner, N.E.; Ladwig, A.; Nikic, I.; Merkler, D.; Kleele, T.; Marinkovic, P.; Naumann, R.; Godinho, L.; Bareyre, F.M.; et al. Pervasive axonal transport deficits in multiple sclerosis models. *Neuron* **2014**, *84*, 1183–1190. [CrossRef] [PubMed]

168. Lewis, T.L., Jr.; Turi, G.F.; Kwon, S.K.; Losonczy, A.; Polleux, F. Progressive decrease of mitochondrial motility during maturation of cortical axons in vitro and in vivo. *Curr. Biol.* **2016**, *26*, 2602–2608. [CrossRef] [PubMed]

169. Smit-Rigter, L.; Rajendran, R.; Silva, C.A.; Spierenburg, L.; Groeneweg, F.; Ruimschotel, E.M.; van Versendaal, D.; van der Togt, C.; Eysel, U.T.; Heimel, J.A.; et al. Mitochondrial dynamics in visual cortex are limited in vivo and not affected by axonal structural plasticity. *Curr. Biol.* **2016**, *26*, 2609–2616. [CrossRef] [PubMed]

170. Rintoul, G.L.; Filiano, A.J.; Brocard, J.B.; Kress, G.J.; Reynolds, I.J. Glutamate decreases mitochondrial size and movement in primary forebrain neurons. *J. Neurosci.* **2003**, *23*, 7881–7888. [CrossRef] [PubMed]

171. Sheng, Z.H.; Cai, Q. Mitochondrial transport in neurons: Impact on synaptic homeostasis and neurodegeneration. *Nat. Rev. Neurosci.* **2012**, *13*, 77–93. [CrossRef] [PubMed]

172. Kim-Han, J.S.; Antenor-Dorsey, J.A.; O'Malley, K.L. The parkinsonian mimetic, MPP+, specifically impairs mitochondrial transport in dopamine axons. *J. Neurosci.* **2011**, *31*, 7212–7221. [CrossRef] [PubMed]

173. Sterky, F.H.; Lee, S.; Wibom, R.; Olson, L.; Larsson, N.G. Impaired mitochondrial transport and Parkin-independent degeneration of respiratory chain-deficient dopamine neurons in vivo. *Proc. Natl. Acad. Sci. USA* **2011**, *108*, 12937–12942. [CrossRef] [PubMed]

174. Pickrell, A.M.; Youle, R.J. The roles of PINK1, parkin, and mitochondrial fidelity in Parkinson's disease. *Neuron* **2015**, *85*, 257–273. [CrossRef] [PubMed]

175. Narendra, D.; Tanaka, A.; Suen, D.F.; Youle, R.J. Parkin is recruited selectively to impaired mitochondria and promotes their autophagy. *J. Cell Biol.* **2008**, *183*, 795–803. [CrossRef] [PubMed]

176. McWilliams, T.G.; Muqit, M.M. PINK1 and Parkin: Emerging themes in mitochondrial homeostasis. *Curr. Opin. Cell Biol.* **2017**, *45*, 83–91. [CrossRef] [PubMed]

177. Park, J.; Lee, S.B.; Lee, S.; Kim, Y.; Song, S.; Kim, S.; Bae, E.; Kim, J.; Shong, M.; Kim, J.M.; et al. Mitochondrial dysfunction in Drosophila PINK1 mutants is complemented by parkin. *Nature* **2006**, *441*, 1157–1161. [CrossRef] [PubMed]

178. Gispert, S.; Ricciardi, F.; Kurz, A.; Azizov, M.; Hoepken, H.H.; Becker, D.; Voos, W.; Leuner, K.; Muller, W.E.; Kudin, A.P.; et al. Parkinson phenotype in aged PINK1-deficient mice is accompanied by progressive mitochondrial dysfunction in absence of neurodegeneration. *PLoS ONE* **2009**, *4*, e5777. [CrossRef] [PubMed]

179. Chan, N.C.; Salazar, A.M.; Pham, A.H.; Sweredoski, M.J.; Kolawa, N.J.; Graham, R.L.; Hess, S.; Chan, D.C. Broad activation of the ubiquitin-proteasome system by Parkin is critical for mitophagy. *Hum. Mol. Genet.* **2011**, *20*, 1726–1737. [CrossRef] [PubMed]

180. Liu, S.; Sawada, T.; Lee, S.; Yu, W.; Silverio, G.; Alapatt, P.; Millan, I.; Shen, A.; Saxton, W.; Kanao, T.; et al. Parkinson's disease–associated kinase PINK1 regulates miro protein level and axonal transport of mitochondria. *PLoS Genet.* **2012**, *8*, e1002537. [CrossRef] [PubMed]

181. Wang, X.; Winter, D.; Ashrafi, G.; Schlehe, J.; Wong, Y.L.; Selkoe, D.; Rice, S.; Steen, J.; LaVoie, M.J.; Schwarz, T.L. PINK1 and Parkin target Miro for phosphorylation and degradation to arrest mitochondrial motility. *Cell* **2011**, *147*, 893–906. [CrossRef] [PubMed]

182. Weihofen, A.; Thomas, K.J.; Ostaszewski, B.L.; Cookson, M.R.; Selkoe, D.J. Pink1 forms a multiprotein complex with Miro and Milton, linking Pink1 function to mitochondrial trafficking. *Biochemistry* **2009**, *48*, 2045–2052. [CrossRef] [PubMed]

183. Villar-Pique, A.; Lopes da Fonseca, T.; Outeiro, T.F. Structure, function and toxicity of alpha-synuclein: The Bermuda triangle in synucleinopathies. *J. Neurochem.* **2016**, *139*, 240–255. [CrossRef] [PubMed]

184. Devi, L.; Raghavendran, V.; Prabhu, B.M.; Avadhani, N.G.; Anandatheerthavarada, H.K. Mitochondrial import and accumulation of alpha-synuclein impair complex I in human dopaminergic neuronal cultures and Parkinson disease brain. *J. Biol. Chem.* **2008**, *283*, 9089–9100. [CrossRef] [PubMed]

185. Reeve, A.K.; Ludtmann, M.H.; Angelova, P.R.; Simcox, E.M.; Horrocks, M.H.; Klenerman, D.; Gandhi, S.; Turnbull, D.M.; Abramov, A.Y. Aggregated alpha-synuclein and complex I deficiency: Exploration of their relationship in differentiated neurons. *Cell Death Dis.* **2015**, *6*, e1820. [CrossRef] [PubMed]

186. Chinta, S.J.; Mallajosyula, J.K.; Rane, A.; Andersen, J.K. Mitochondrial alpha-synuclein accumulation impairs complex I function in dopaminergic neurons and results in increased mitophagy in vivo. *Neurosci. Lett.* **2010**, *486*, 235–239. [CrossRef] [PubMed]

187. Bender, A.; Desplats, P.; Spencer, B.; Rockenstein, E.; Adame, A.; Elstner, M.; Laub, C.; Mueller, S.; Koob, A.O.; Mante, M.; et al. TOM40 mediates mitochondrial dysfunction induced by alpha-synuclein accumulation in Parkinson's disease. *PLoS ONE* **2013**, *8*, e62277. [CrossRef] [PubMed]

188. Di Maio, R.; Barrett, P.J.; Hoffman, E.K.; Barrett, C.W.; Zharikov, A.; Borah, A.; Hu, X.; McCoy, J.; Chu, C.T.; Burton, E.A.; et al. α-Synuclein binds to TOM20 and inhibits mitochondrial protein import in Parkinson's disease. *Sci. Transl. Med.* **2016**, *8*, 342ra78. [CrossRef] [PubMed]

189. Yano, H.; Baranov, S.V.; Baranova, O.V.; Kim, J.; Pan, Y.; Yablonska, S.; Carlisle, D.L.; Ferrante, R.J.; Kim, A.H.; Friedlander, R.M. Inhibition of mitochondrial protein import by mutant huntingtin. *Nat. Neurosci.* **2014**, *17*, 822–831. [CrossRef] [PubMed]

190. Nakamura, K.; Nemani, V.M.; Azarbal, F.; Skibinski, G.; Levy, J.M.; Egami, K.; Munishkina, L.; Zhang, J.; Gardner, B.; Wakabayashi, J.; et al. Direct membrane association drives mitochondrial fission by the Parkinson disease-associated protein alpha-synuclein. *J. Biol. Chem.* **2011**, *286*, 20710–20726. [CrossRef] [PubMed]

191. Kamp, F.; Exner, N.; Lutz, A.K.; Wender, N.; Hegermann, J.; Brunner, B.; Nuscher, B.; Bartels, T.; Giese, A.; Beyer, K.; et al. Inhibition of mitochondrial fusion by alpha-synuclein is rescued by PINK1, Parkin and DJ-1. *EMBO J.* **2010**, *29*, 3571–3589. [CrossRef] [PubMed]

192. Guardia-Laguarta, C.; Area-Gomez, E.; Rub, C.; Liu, Y.; Magrane, J.; Becker, D.; Voos, W.; Schon, E.A.; Przedborski, S. Alpha-Synuclein is localized to mitochondria-associated ER membranes. *J. Neurosci.* **2014**, *34*, 249–259. [CrossRef] [PubMed]

193. Paillusson, S.; Gomez-Suaga, P.; Stoica, R.; Little, D.; Gissen, P.; Devine, M.J.; Noble, W.; Hanger, D.P.; Miller, C.C.J. Alpha-Synuclein binds to the ER-mitochondria tethering protein VAPB to disrupt Ca(2+) homeostasis and mitochondrial ATP production. *Acta Neuropathol.* **2017**, *134*, 129–149. [CrossRef] [PubMed]

194. Pozo Devoto, V.M.; Dimopoulos, N.; Alloatti, M.; Pardi, M.B.; Saez, T.M.; Otero, M.G.; Cromberg, L.E.; Marín-Burgin, A.; Scassa, M.E.; Stokin, G.B.; et al. αSynuclein control of mitochondrial homeostasis in human-derived neurons is disrupted by mutations associated with Parkinson's disease. *Sci. Rep.* **2017**, *7*, 5042. [CrossRef] [PubMed]

195. Prots, I.; Veber, V.; Brey, S.; Campioni, S.; Buder, K.; Riek, R.; Bohm, K.J.; Winner, B. Alpha-Synuclein oligomers impair neuronal microtubule-kinesin interplay. *J. Biol. Chem.* **2013**, *288*, 21742–21754. [CrossRef] [PubMed]

13

CoQ10 and Aging

Isabella Peixoto de Barcelos [1] and Richard H. Haas [1,2,*]

[1]   Department of Neurosciences, University of California San Diego, San Diego, CA 92093-0935, USA;
      ibarcelos@ucsd.edu
[2]   Department of Pediatrics, University of California San Diego, San Diego, CA 92093-0935, USA
*   Correspondence: rhaas@ucsd.edu

Abstract: The aging process includes impairment in mitochondrial function, a reduction in anti-oxidant activity, and an increase in oxidative stress, marked by an increase in reactive oxygen species (ROS) production. Oxidative damage to macromolecules including DNA and electron transport proteins likely increases ROS production resulting in further damage. This oxidative theory of cell aging is supported by the fact that diseases associated with the aging process are marked by increased oxidative stress. Coenzyme Q10 (CoQ_{10}) levels fall with aging in the human but this is not seen in all species or all tissues. It is unknown whether lower CoQ_{10} levels have a part to play in aging and disease or whether it is an inconsequential cellular response to aging. Despite the current lay public interest in supplementing with CoQ_{10}, there is currently not enough evidence to recommend CoQ_{10} supplementation as an anti-aging anti-oxidant therapy.

Keywords: coenzyme Q10; aging; age-related diseases; mitochondrial dysfunction

1. Introduction

CoQ_{10} was first described in 1955, named ubiquitous quinone, a small lipophilic molecule located widely in cell membranes [1], and in 1957 its function as an electron carrier in the mitochondrial electron transport chain was reported [2]. The role in human disease was unknown for 20 years until in 1986 a benefit of CoQ_{10} treatment was reported in Kearns–Sayre syndrome [3]. Initially, therapeutic use of CoQ_{10} was focused on the oxidative phosphorylation (OXPHOS) defects in which there is documented CoQ_{10} deficiency [4] and in the group of CoQ_{10} synthesis disorders [5]. These conditions provided evidence for efficacy and safety of treatment with CoQ_{10} [6]. Subsequent larger-scale trials in Parkinson disease [7] and other neurodegenerative diseases have shown safety but no convincing benefit.

In the last decade, CoQ_{10} functions in membranes throughout the cell where antioxidant and signaling roles predominate have been of increasing interest [8]. There is growing evidence that oxidative stress is a major component of cellular senescence [9]. This multifactorial process involves DNA injury [10], protein and lipid damage, and activation of signaling pathways associated with aging [11]. Recently, the CoQ_{10} antioxidant effect has been shown to reduce markers for cardiovascular disease (CVD) and inflammation, the main components of atherosclerotic vascular disease [12].

It is suggested that CoQ_{10} supplementation can improve the symptoms of mitochondrial diseases and of aging because of an improvement in bioenergetics [12,13].

Our objective is to review, from a translational perspective, data regarding the association of CoQ_{10} and aging. Are the aging process and mitochondrial progressive failure related and can CoQ_{10} supplementation decelerate aging?

2. CoQ₁₀

2.1. What Is It?

Coenzyme Q10, CoQ$_{10}$ or ubiquinone (2,3 dimethoxy-5-methyl-6-decaprenyl-1,4-benzoquinone) is a small lipophilic structure, composed of a benzoquinone ring and an isoprenoid side-chain and it is found universally in cell membranes. In humans, synthesis occurs utilizing a collection of enzymes (complex Q) located in the mitochondrial matrix membrane [14]. The benzoquinone ring is derived from 4-hydroxybenzoic acid, while 10 isoprenes are derived from mevalonic acid (from the cholesterol synthesis pathway). The quinone ring is the functional group in the molecule, responsible for carrying electrons to complex III. CoQ$_{10}$ (ubiquinone) is reversely reduced to ubiquinol. The polyisoprenoid tail is very lipophilic and localizes to hydrophobic membranes. The length of the isoprenyl chain is variable between species with 10 isoprenes forming human CoQ$_{10}$ whilst rodents predominantly have CoQ$_9$ [15].

2.2. Function

CoQ$_{10}$ is widely distributed in all cell membranes and forms a critical component of the electron transport chain (ETC) transporting electrons between complexes I/II and III [13]. In rat liver the largest ubiquinone (CoQ$_9$) concentration is found in the Golgi vesicles (2.62 µg/mg) followed by mitochondrial matrix membrane and lysosomes (with levels of 1.86 in each structure) [16].

The major function of ubiquinone is in the mitochondrial ETC. CoQ$_{10}$ accepts electrons from different donors, including complex I (reduced nicotinamide adenine dinucleotide [NADH]-coenzyme Q oxidoreductase), complex II (succinate dehydrogenase), the oxidation of fatty acids and branched-chain amino acids via flavin-linked dehydrogenases and electron transfer factor Q oxidoreductase (ETF-QO) to complex III (ubiquinone-cytochrome c oxidoreductase) [17,18]. CoQ$_{10}$ cycles between its three chemical forms: completely oxidized (ubiquinone), a semi-oxidized intermediate free radical (semiquinone) and a completely reduced form (ubiquinol) as shown in Figure 1 [19,20]. By moving within the mitochondrial membrane, the proton-motive Q cycle allows proton pumping at complex III helping to generate the proton motive force for adenosine triphosphate (ATP) production.

Figure 1. Redox forms of CoQ$_{10}$, ubiquinone (oxidized form), ubiquinol (reduced form), and semiquinone (semi-oxidized). The Q cycle within the matrix membrane allows proton transfer from the mitochondrial matrix to the intermembrane space helping to generate the electrochemical gradient for ATP production.

The interaction of the CoQ pool with the ETC has in recent years been shown to be more complex with the recognition that mitochondrial supercomplexes composed mostly of complexes I/III, I/III/IV, and III/IV interact physically forming respirasomes. It seems likely that both single complexes within the matrix membrane and supercomplexes coexist in a dynamic state. The factors controlling assembly and disassembly of supercomplexes are not known although cardiolipin appears to play a role. There is evidence that in the I/III supercomplex intercomplex binding of CoQ shuttles electrons from complex I to III. This bound CoQ may be in equilibrium with the free CoQ pool. [21].

CoQ10 supplementation has been shown to have epigenetic effects in genes involved with signaling, intermediary metabolism, transport, transcription control, disease mutation, phosphorylation, and embryonal development indicating a role in modulation of gene expression [22,23].

In addition to its major function in the ETC, CoQ_{10} has an important anti-oxidant role stabilizing the plasma membrane and other intracellular membranes protecting membrane phospholipids from peroxidation [13]. Ubiquinone and semiquinone are also involved with recycling of other anti-oxidant molecules, reducing α-tocopherol and ascorbate contributing to redox balance in the cell. Diminished CoQ_{10} levels in aging likely contribute to membrane peroxidation injury. There is evidence that part of its anti-oxidant effect occurs by enhancing the enzymatic activity of the antioxidant proteins superoxide dismutase and glutathione peroxidase [24]. Recent publications associate ubiquinol with protection of plasma low density lipoproteins (LDL) from oxidation, an important anti-atherogenic effect [25]. The pro-oxidant role of CoQ_{10} is a signaling function involved in gene expression but the mechanism of this function is not fully understood [26,27]. Other functions include modulation of the permeability transition pore, thus playing a role in apoptosis [28]. CoQ_{10}'s main functions are summarized in Figure 2.

Figure 2. The Multiple Roles of Ubiquinone in the Cell.

Chronic inflammation is a frequent aging-related problem. CoQ_{10}, by reduction of free radicals, reduces the activation of NF-κB (nuclear factor kappa-light-chain-enhancer of activated B cells) cells and consequently reduces the release of pro-inflammatory cytokines mainly tumor necrosis factor alpha (TNF-α) and interleukin 6 (IL-6) [29]. Aging-related reduced CoQ_{10} levels may contribute to inflammation and there is accumulating evidence of secondary anti-inflammatory effects of CoQ_{10} supplementation. A recent meta-analysis provided evidence that CoQ_{10} supplementation significantly reduced the inflammatory markers CRP (C-reactive protein), IL-6 and TNF-α [30]. Another recent publication reported that patients with metabolic diseases (obesity, type 2 diabetes, metabolic syndrome, cardiovascular disease, and nonalcoholic fatty liver disease) had a significant decrease in TNF-α plasma levels with CoQ_{10} supplementation but not CRP or IL-6 [31]. CoQ_{10} was found to have an anti-inflammatory function via epigenetic effects on expression of genes related to NFkappaB1 (NFk-B1) [32]. CoQ_{10} has a hepatoprotective and neuroprotective effect in a rat model of non-alcoholic steatohepatitis [33] apparently through an adenosine 5′ monophosphate-activated protein kinase (AMPK) activation mechanism and in humans a randomized trial showed that supplementation of CoQ_{10} improved biomarkers for inflammation in nonalcoholic fatty liver disease (NAFLD) [34]. CoQ_{10} supplementation in patients with antiphospholipid syndrome has been found to attenuate levels of pro-inflammatory and thrombotic markers, with evidence of endothelial and mitochondrial function improvement [35]. In Down syndrome patients, chronic neuro-inflammatory changes have been proposed as a possible accelerator of Alzheimer disease [36]. These include high levels of interleukin 6 and tumor necrosis factor α along with decreased levels of CoQ_{10}. A positive correlation between CoQ_{10} and intelligence quotient levels was also reported [37]. CoQ_{10} treatment in Down syndrome cells is associated with improved DNA repair mechanisms and DNA protection [38].

Cardiovascular disease is a common aging-related problem. There is a considerable body of evidence supporting a role for CoQ_{10} in cardiovascular function including a correlation of low endomyocardial levels with severity of heart failure and an improvement in cardiac contractility with CoQ_{10} treatment [39]. Improvement in lipid profiles (a major contributor to cardiovascular disease) has been reported with CoQ_{10} treatment [40].

CoQ_{10} has other important functions, participating in metabolic pathways as an electron receptor: (1) CoQ_{10} is a co-factor for dihydro-orotate dehydrogenase, an enzyme involved in the de novo pyrimidine biosynthesis [41]. (2) During the process of sulfide oxidation CoQ_{10} accepts electrons from the enzyme sulfide-quinone reductase to convert sulfide into thiosulfate [42]. (3) The oxidation from choline to glycine is catalyzed by choline dehydrogenase in the inner mitochondrial membrane, and CoQ_{10} is proposed to be the electron acceptor for this reaction [43]. (4) Proline dehydrogenase donates electrons from FAD and NAD+ to CoQ_{10} during process of synthesis of proline and arginine [21,44].

2.3. Sources of CoQ_{10}

2.3.1. Internal Biosynthesis

CoQ_{10} is the only lipid-soluble antioxidant synthetized by the human body [13]. The majority of CoQ_{10} comes from the internal synthesis, from tyrosine or phenylalanine (benzoquinone ring) and mevalonic acid (isoprenoid side-chain). Synthesis occurs in all tissues studied. In humans synthesis occurs utilizing a collection of enzymes (complex Q) located in the mitochondrial matrix membrane and in the endoplasmic reticulum The mevalonic acid pathway is responsible for cholesterol synthesis with 3-hydroxy-3-methyl-glutaryl-coenzyme A (HMG-CoA) reductase (the site of statin inhibition) as the regulatory step. CoQ_{10} derived from dietary intake becomes more important with aging as endogenous production decreases [13].

At least 14 genes are involved in CoQ_{10}'s biosynthesis in yeast with 18 genes so far reported in humans. Many are homologues of genes identified in c. cerevisiae. These synthetic proteins are nuclear encoded and require mitochondrial targeting sequences for entry into the matrix or the inner mitochondrial membrane [14]. There is assembly of many of the components into a 'supercomplex' termed Complex Q in the mammal. Mitochondrial synthesis is thought to occur in all cells containing mitochondria but also in other organelles including the endoplasmic reticulum and peroxisomes [45]. Figure 3 summarizes the mammalian CoQ_{10} biosynthesis pathway.

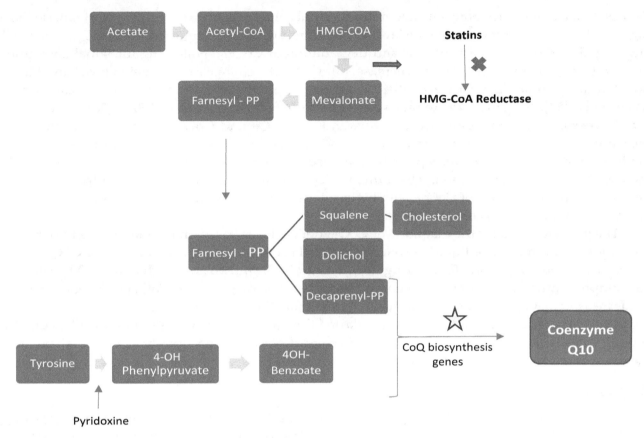

Figure 3. Schematic representation of CoQ biosynthesis. The isoprenoid side-chain derives from the cholesterol and dolichol synthetic pathway from mevalonate, the benzoquinone ring is derived from tyrosine metabolism. The star symbolizes the genes involved in the final synthesis of CoQ_{10}.

2.3.2. External Sources

CoQ_{10} is widely found in many animal protein sources (pork, lamb, beef, chicken, fish), vegetables (spinach, pea, broccoli, cauliflower), fruits (orange, strawberry, apple) and cereals (rye, wheat) [13]. Heart, chicken leg, herring, and trout contain particularly high amounts of CoQ_{10}. Daily intake between 3 and 5 mg is considered adequate and whilst external supplementation increases plasma levels, supplementation was not thought to increase tissue levels of CoQ_{10} in tissues with normal synthetic capacity [46], although evidence of treatment efficacy in a variety of human diseases does suggest that tissue uptake can occur [13,47].

2.3.3. Absorption and Transport

CoQ_{10} absorption is slow and occurs in the small intestine; in its reduced form, ubiquinol is 3 to 4 times better absorbed than the oxidized form, ubiquinone [48]. The absorption of CoQ_{10} can be increased if administered with food intake, mainly with lipids because of its lipophilic structure [13,49]. After absorption by the enterocytes, CoQ_{10} passes through lymphatic vessels and reaches the plasma, where it circulates bound to lipoproteins (LDL). Because of this, plasma measurements of CoQ_{10} should be corrected for lipoproteins levels. Between 80 and 95% of plasma circulating CoQ_{10} is in the reduced ubiquinol form. [48,50].

2.4. Tissue Levels and Distribution of CoQ_{10}

Although the major CoQ_{10} plasma form is ubiquinol, laboratory measurements, in general, report the CoQ_{10} total level [50]. Lymphocyte and platelet levels may give some insight into levels in less accessible tissues such as heart, muscle, and brain [51]. The CoQ_{10} level varies in different tissues.

Tissues with a higher metabolic rate and mitochondrial content (heart, kidney, liver, and muscle) have high levels of CoQ_{10}, for example the level is 8 µg/g in lung and 114 µg/g in heart [13]. Tissue levels largely reflect the results of synthesis and degradation of CoQ_{10}. Following intestinal absorption, liver and lipoprotein concentrations increase, but without a change in the level in heart and kidney noted in early studies [52]. However, there is some evidence that chronic administration can increase tissue levels [53]. In a study where rats were chronically fed a large dose of 150 mg/kg/day of CoQ_{10} for 13 weeks, small but significant increases in both CoQ_9 and CoQ_{10} were found in all tissues measured [54]. No such data exist for young or aged human tissues; however, the accumulated evidence of benefit of CoQ_{10} therapy in human disease states does suggest that tissue levels can be increased by oral administration. The number, size, and structure of the mitochondria in each cell determines the tissue level of CoQ_{10} with highest levels found in tissues with high energy demands and a high mitochondrial content [13,48].

The gold standard for the diagnosis of CoQ_{10} deficiency is based on the measurement of muscle level by high-performance liquid chromatography (HLPC) [55,56]. Plasma levels of CoQ_{10} range between 0.40 and 1.91 µmol/L (0.34–1.65 µg/mL) in controls [57] but do not match tissue levels, reflecting consumption much more than endogenous synthesis. The diagnosis of CoQ_{10} deficiency requires tissue measurement [58]. There is evidence suggesting that the CoQ_{10} level in mononuclear cells can be correlated to muscle measurements [45,56]. Plasma CoQ_{10} levels are increased in some physiological conditions (cold adaptation and exercise) and in some diseases (paraneoplastic nodules, Alzheimer's disease, and prion disease). Levels are decreased in aging. [45].

2.5. Causes of Reduction

Conditions associated with CoQ_{10} deficiency can be divided into three main groups: (1) CoQ_{10} nutritional deficiency, including intake of CoQ_{10} itself and nutrients and vitamins necessary for its synthesis (vitamin B6 is a cofactor in the pathway of CoQ_{10} biosynthesis); (2) CoQ_{10} synthesis genes (*COQ* family genes: *COQ1* and the Complex Q genes including the mammalian homolog of the yeast Coq11 gene; the Complex I subunit *NDUFA9*), and acquired disorders impairing CoQ_{10} synthesis (statin use) [59–61]; and (3) medical conditions associated with decreased levels of CoQ_{10} [45,46]. In this last category, a variety of conditions have been reported with low CoQ_{10} including neurodegenerative disorders Friedreich's ataxia, Nieman–Pick type C disease, and Parkinson Disease. In other disorders such as Alzheimer disease, diabetes, cancer, fibromyalgia, and cardiovascular diseases, elevations in plasma CoQ_{10} levels may be a stress response. [45,46]. Defects in genes which may be associated with reduced CoQ_{10} levels can be included in this group (*APTX, ETFDH, BRAF*).

Special attention should be given to the important observation that CoQ_{10} deficiency is potentially reversible if the supplementation starts before the appearance of the symptoms, when brain and kidney have not sustained permanent damage [46,62].

2.6. Supplementation

2.6.1. Dosing

A recent trend over the last few years has been to supplement adult patients with mitochondrial diseases with high doses of oral CoQ_{10} or ubiquinol, up to 1200 mg/day or higher. For the pediatric population, doses between 5 and 10 mg/kg/day of ubiquinol are recommended [63]. For a dose of 10 mg/kg/day, plasma levels range between 5 and 10 µg/mL 3–4 weeks after the beginning of the supplementation [53,63,64]. As explained above, there are important differences in bioavailability of the different formulations of CoQ_{10} used; ubiquinol (the reduced form) is 3 to 4 times better absorbed than ubiquinone (oxidized form) [48]. Primary CoQ_{10} diseases tend to respond to supplementation but may require very high doses. Also, some patients with secondary CoQ_{10} dysfunction were reported to improve some symptoms with CoQ_{10} supplementation. Examples are cardiomyopathy in organic acidurias (25 mg/kg/day with improvement in the cardiomyopathy) [65], glutaric acidemia type II

(500 mg per day of CoQ_{10} along with riboflavin with improvement in strength, lactate, and creatine kinase levels) [59], ataxia oculomotor apraxia type 1 (200–600 mg with reported improvement in strength, ataxia, and cessation of seizures in one patient) [60], GLUT-1 deficiency (30 mg/kg/day with improvement in the ataxia and nystagmus) [66].

Exogenous administration of CoQ_{10} reportedly does not raise tissue levels above normal in healthy young individuals, except for two tissues (liver and spleen) [13]; however, this traditional view may be wrong given the improvement in multi-organ symptoms in a variety of disorders with mitochondrial dysfunction when treated with CoQ [67].

2.6.2. Safety and Adverse Events

Although the majority of studies have not shown convincing enough scientific evidence to support treatment with CoQ_{10} in specific diseases, they do provide evidence that oral supplementation is safe and well tolerated. One of the largest trials was a phase III randomized, placebo-controlled, double-blind clinical trial at 67 North American sites by the Parkinson Study Group using doses of CoQ_{10} up to 2400 mg/day demonstrated the safety of this dose [7]. Evidence suggests that supplementation does not inhibit endogenous production [13]. Previous studies had reported only mild side effects such as gastrointestinal symptoms, mainly nausea, with CoQ_{10} supplementation [13,68].

3. Aging

3.1. Physiology of Mitochondrial Involvement in the Process of Aging

Human aging is a normal multifactorial process resulting from the interaction of genetic and environmental factors. It is characterized by multi-organ system functional decline in association with the risk of age-related diseases (dementia, neurodegenerative disorders, osteoporosis, arthritis, diabetes, cardiovascular disease, age-related hearing loss, and cancer) [13,68–71].

A common hypothesis to explain some of the pathophysiology of age and degenerative diseases is an oxidative imbalance between the production of reactive oxygen species (hydrogen peroxide: $H2O2$, the oxygen-derived free radicals superoxide: $O2\bullet-$, and hydroxyl radical: $HO\bullet$), and antioxidant mechanisms such as superoxide dismutase, catalase, glutathione peroxidase, ascorbic acid, tocopherol, glutathione, and CoQ_{10}, leading to a state of oxidative stress [72–80]. A number of animal models support this theory with shortened survival in mice lacking superoxide dismutase 1 (SOD1) and a lethal phenotype in mice lacking superoxide dismutase 2 (SOD2) [81,82].

As mitochondria are the main source of reactive oxygen species (ROS) production though OXPHOS supercomplex activity in the cristae of the inner mitochondrial membrane (mainly at complex I and III), this organelle is the major target of ROS damage. Mitochondrial DNA (mtDNA) is particularly vulnerable with a high mutation rate and limited mtDNA repair mechanisms [69,74]. The continuous production and accumulation of mitochondrial ROS is the basis for "the free radical theory of aging" [70,71]. Although the accumulation of ROS has a major effect on DNA (strand breaks, oxidation of bases, damage in sites coding for ETC proteins), other structures of the cell are also damaged: lipids, membranes, proteins (leading to dysfunction of the ETC, inadequate ATP production, and further ROS production) [72–75]. There is evidence that impaired mitochondrial machinery produces more oxidative stress and more ROS production, resulting in a vicious cycle [76,83]. Electrons leaking from impaired OXPHOS react with oxygen molecules to form the free radical superoxide [80]. There is also an effect on mitochondrial dynamics with impairment of fission, contributing to mitochondrial enlargement, which reduces recycling through mitophagy leading to a reduction in ATP generation [73]. Impairment of the mitochondrial–lysosomal axis occurs with aging, with accumulation of lipofuscin inside lysosomes with senescence. Lipofuscin accumulation is postulated to limit the ability of lysosomes to participate in mitophagy [73].

Considerable evidence supports the relationship between ROS accumulation and mitochondrial dysfunction leading to aging (the mitochondrial free radical theory of aging): ROS production increases in aged humans and animals [70,84], imbalance in the levels of pro and anti-oxidant substances occurs [85] with high levels of oxidized and damaged macromolecules (proteins, lipids, and DNA) [86]. There seems to be a convincing relationship between high ROS levels and longevity in humans and animals [87]; however, the exact role of ROS remains unclear as some animal models report a failure to increase longevity with ROS reduction and others link high levels of ROS and longevity. It remains unclear what the contribution of ROS generation is versus epigenetic factors modulating genes related to the protection from effects of aging [77,88,89]. Evidence against the oxidative theory of aging comes from some animal models where longevity is unaffected by increased ROS production. Some of these studies are detailed below.

Growing evidence supports the idea that increased levels of ROS are associated with the specific biochemical pathway that improves longevity, at least in some species [90]. C. elegans, a nematode mutant model clk-1 (COQ7 equivalent gene in humans), has higher longevity associated with higher ROS production. C. elegans with a point mutation in the gene isp-1, responsible for an iron-sulfur mitochondrial complex, also demonstrate an increase in life span [91]. These observations point out the multiple roles of ROS particularly as signaling molecules triggering protective pathways. Some mouse models of defective CoQ synthesis are difficult to square with the oxidative theory of aging. Mice with only one copy of the gene Mclk1 (equivalent of mammals COQ7 and C. elegans clk-1 model) have higher production of ROS in the mitochondria (although a normal level of total ROS in the body), a higher level of protection of the immune system (from some infections and also tumorigenesis) and increased longevity [92]. Homozygous knockout of the Mclk1 gene is embryonic lethal but utilizing a Tamoxifen dependent transgene mouse KO activated at 2 months of age a multisystemic disorder (heart, kidneys, and skeletal muscles) with a decline in ubiquinol levels is produced. At 8 months this "ubiquinol deficit" animal presented normal levels of some factors associated with oxidative stress (catalase, F_2-isoprostanes, DNA oxidative damage, SOD1, and SOD2). Diet supplementation at 9 months with an analogue of the ubiquinol precursor 4-hydroxybenzoic acid rescued the clinical phenotype [93]. Another mouse model heterozygous for the Sod2 gene (with decreased Mn-superoxide dismutase activity) does show oxidative injury (increased tumor incidence and DNA damage) but does not decrease longevity [94]. The concept that mitochondrial dysfunction may be a consequence of aging factors rather than a cause is also supported by observations of sarcopenia in rat and human muscles with other factors such as denervation playing a role [95].

Further studies are needed to understand the balance of ROS as an agent of oxidative injury and its signaling epigenetic role modulating genes related to the protection of effects of aging. It may be that after the saturation of the mechanisms of protection, the ROS-stress protective cascade can no longer prevent oxidative damage [88].

It is not surprising that given the contradictory evidence for a central role for ROS in aging, evidence supporting the utility of anti-oxidant therapies in aging (such as CoQ_{10}) remains unclear.

3.2. CoQ_{10} and Aging, CoQ_{10} Deficiency in Advanced Age, Evidence for Beneficial Supplementation

Published results from various research groups about CoQ levels and lifespan are often at variance, model dependent and do not support a similar pattern in all species [96–98].

3.2.1. C. elegans

Studies in the nematode C. elegans have produced unexpected results compared to mammals. As discussed above, a nematode mutant model clk-1 (mammals COQ7 equivalent gene), with low production of CoQ_8, has an extension in longevity compared with the wild strain but requires dietary Q supplementation [99]. This diet does trigger a Dauer long-lived larval anerobic state. Other studies with CoQ gene knockouts confirm that deficiency in CoQ (less than 50%) also leads to an increase in lifespan, and a possible explanation is that less ROS production occurs in the case of moderate CoQ deficiency [100,101], but with more severe depletion of CoQ, longevity would be affected [100,102]. This finding was also confirmed in human cells, with two different studies from the same group reporting that fibroblasts with mutations on *PDSS2* (homologue of yeast coq1) with less than 12 and 20% of CoQ$_{10}$ of control cells had decreased synthesis of ATP without increase in the levels of ROS. However, when the defect was of 30%, with partial defect in the synthesis of ATP the levels of ROS were higher. The explanation proposed centered on the severity of the deficiency of coenzyme Q as an oxphos modulator [103,104].

3.2.2. Rodent Models

A diet supplemented with Ubiquinol-10 in the senescence-accelerated mouse prone 1 (SAMP1) reduced markers of oxidative stress (ratio of reduced and oxidized glutathione—GSH/GSSG), decelerated the normal decline in expression of genes (*Sirt1*, *Sirt3*, and *Pgc-1a*, and *Ppara*), and their respective proteins related to mitochondrial function during aging [105]. This treatment also increased auditory brainstem response hearing loss. The proposed mechanism of CoQ$_{10}$ benefit as an anti-oxidant agent in this aging mouse is through cyclic adenosine monophosphate (cAMP). There is an enhancement in sirtuin genes, and PGC-1α (peroxisome proliferator-activated receptor gamma coactivator 1-alpha) with increased complex I and IV activity and reduce oxidative stress. Despite all these beneficial effects, there was no significant change in the overall lifespans compared to the control animals [105]. These findings of increased cAMP, SIRT1 (sirtuin 1) expression, and PGC-1α in reducing parameters of oxidative stress and increasing mitochondrial function were also confirmed in other experiments with ubiquinol supplementation in senescence-accelerated mice, with added benefits in obesity, insulin resistance, and metabolic syndrome, (hypothesized mechanism in Figure 4 [106]). PPARα (peroxisome proliferator-activated receptors) signaling and lipid metabolism gene expression changes in liver of C57BL6J mice was reported after one-week supplementation with ubiquinol (250 mg/kg BW/day) [23].

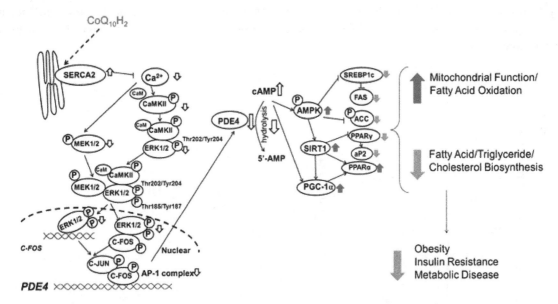

Figure 4. Proposed mechanism by which ubiquinol improves metabolic function and inhibits insulin resistance in KKAy mice (a mouse model of obesity and diabetes). Ubiquinol inhibited phosphorylation of CaMKII (Ca2+/calmodulin-dependent protein kinase II) in the liver resulting in inhibition of C-FOS transcriptional activity and inhibition of PDE4 gene expression. Increased cAMP increases AMPK (AMP-activated protein kinase) activity resulting in SIRT1 and PGC-1α increased mitochondrial function and inhibition of lipid synthesis. (Adapted from Xu H. et al. 2017 [106] with permission).

Interestingly mice with a single copy of the Coq7 synthesis gene demonstrated increased longevity [107]. However the mechanism is unclear and several studies report that dietary supplementation with CoQ$_{10}$ or ubiquinol in various rat models improves mechanisms involved with mitochondrial biogenesis, including parameters of oxidative stress [105,108–111].

3.2.3. Mammals and Tissue CoQ levels

In mammals there is a tendency to ubiquinone to be reduced with age, but this finding depends on the tissue investigated and also the species [97]. Early studies suggested that tissue levels of ubiquinol were endogenously produced with little change with dietary supplementation except in liver and spleen; however, subsequent studies in rodents confirm that oral supplementation with CoQ_{10} does increase tissue levels of both CoQ_{10} and CoQ_9 in skeletal muscle, heart, and kidney [26], and when high doses (200 mg/kg) are used for 2 months in rats, brain levels are increased and are neuroprotective [112].

In humans, there is also a lack of consistent data. One study did not find a relationship between aging and CoQ_{10} plasma levels in elderly women [113]. Others report that plasma and tissue levels change over time, with a peak in pancreas and adrenal by 1 year of age and in the brain, heart, and lung by 20 years. After this peak, levels decrease over time [114]. A decrease in brain CoQ_{10} was confirmed in other studies [115,116]. Only 50% of the myocardial CoQ_{10} endogenous production remains by the age of 80 [114]. Serum total CoQ_{10} and ascorbic acid levels were decreased in centenarians compared with 76-year-old controls. An elevation of the CoQ_{10} binding protein prosaposin was also noted presumably in an attempt to compensate for low CoQ_{10} levels [117]. The authors conclude that CoQ_{10} supplementation could be beneficial for centenarians. However, it is not known if low tissue and plasma CoQ_{10} levels contribute to or are a side effect of aging.

Reduction of CoQ_{10} with age is postulated to result from reduction in biosynthesis coupled with an increase in degradation attributed to age-related modification in lipid membranes, which alters quinone behavior [118]. This reduction of CoQ_{10} levels has a tissue/organ specificity with reported high levels of CoQ_{10} in the brain mitochondria from old rats [26], and reduced level in the muscle [98]. A recent paper showed age-related reduction in mitochondrial respiration parameters and ATP production in epithelial cells, rescued with CoQ_{10} administration. Both cited that parameters decrease as age increases, as seen in Figure 5, with the estimate of 10% reduction in mitochondrial respiration every ten years [70].

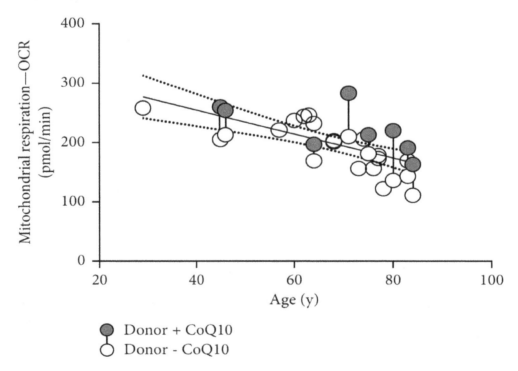

Figure 5. Age-related decline in the oxygen consumption rate in epithelial tissue measured 16 h after collection in a Seahorse XF analyzer. The gray circles show treated samples, the white circles untreated samples, and the connected circles represent samples from the same donor. Significant improvement with 100 μM CoQ_{10} incubation. (Adapted from Schniertshauer et al. 2018 [70] with permission).

High CoQ_{10} concentration was reported to be associated with higher physical activity, lipid peroxidation, and lower oxidized LDL levels in elderly people. The same publication describes higher levels of plasma CoQ_{10} in elderly (more than 50 years old) people compared with young (less than 30 years) [119]. The same group confirmed lower lipid peroxidation and lower oxidized LDL in young adults and also showed that CoQ_{10} is lower in obese elderly patients [120].

In another study, prolonged CoQ_{10} supplementation for 4 years in community-dwelling elderly was associated not only with an improvement in health-related quality of life but more importantly with a lower "more days out of hospital" rate. In this study, subjects were co-supplemented with selenium [121].

Although the association between CoQ_{10} and muscle power is not well established, one study showed a positive relation between CoQ_{10}/cholesterol levels and hand grip, and lower ubiquinol levels in patients with less muscle strength. This study was undertaken to evaluate a possible relationship between low levels of CoQ_{10} and ubiquinol in sarcopenia [122].

Despite the multiple reports on the effects of CoQ_{10} supplementation on aging-related oxidative markers, reduction in biomarkers related to inflammation and in DNA repair mechanisms reports there is a great need for more controlled studies in an older population to determine effectiveness of CoQ_{10} as an anti-aging therapy [97] and also to determine the tissue CoQ_{10} levels in the human species during senescence.

3.3. CoQ_{10} and Specific Conditions Associated with Age

The case for beneficial effects of CoQ_{10} or ubiquinol supplementation is stronger for a number of aging-related diseases many of which have documented mitochondrial dysfunction or CoQ_{10} deficiency. Despite this, the majority of studies proving therapeutic effects of CoQ_{10} supplementation were carried out in animal models [25].

Early studies were carried out with CoQ_{10} although often information on the formulation used is lacking (it is known that ubiquinol can be 3 to 4 times better absorbed than ubiquinone). Also, the doses used in most of the studies were lower than the doses studied for primary CoQ_{10} deficiency (up to 1200 mg/day) and in secondary CoQ_{10} deficiency studies. The formulation and absorption will affect studies of treatment efficacy. A colloidal-Q10 formulation has been shown to have a better enteral absorption and bioavailability in human tissues, and also the vehicle of the active ingredient can impact the results of trials [123].

3.3.1. Neurodegenerative Disorders

Neurodegenerative diseases involve neuro-inflammation and oxidative stress, with ROS accumulation and mitochondrial dysfunction [83,124,125].

The data supporting mitochondrial cofactor supplementation in aging and the aging-related diseases, including Alzheimer disease, Parkinson disease, amyotrophic lateral sclerosis, and multiple sclerosis, are addressed in focused review articles in this supplement. A systematic review published in 2014 reviewed 16 articles and concluded that there is no available data from randomized controlled trials (RCTs) to support the use of mitochondrial supplements for Parkinson disease, atypical Parkinsonism, Huntington disease, and Friedreich ataxia [126].

Previous studies have shown that patients with Lewy's body disease and amyotrophic lateral sclerosis have lower CoQ_{10} plasma levels and Alzheimer disease patients have reduced levels of CoQ_{10} in the cerebral spinal fluid [127,128].

In Huntington disease, increased levels of cortical lactate were observed, which were normalized after 2 months of Coenzyme Q_{10} oral supplementation at a dose of 360 mg/day. In another publication, after discontinuation of the supplement, the lactate levels rose again [67,124]. This study does provide evidence for CNS penetration of administered CoQ_{10} in humans. These and other data lead to a multicenter RCT with 609 patients, which could not identify a benefit in Functional Capacity Score and time to death after 60 months of 2400 mg per day of CoQ_{10} supplementation compared to placebo [129]. Thus, currently, there is insufficient evidence to support CoQ_{10} supplementation as a treatment to delay neurodegeneration in Huntington disease even in the early stages of the disease.

A similar situation occurred in Parkinson disease. An early study found that patients had decreased levels of α-tocopherol and CoQ_{10} in plasma and cerebrospinal fluid with increased levels of lipoprotein oxidation compared to controls in a 2004 study of 161 subjects. [130]. Mitochondrial complexes I and II/III were reduced in platelet mitochondria from early Parkinson disease patients [131]. A more recent study confirmed the association of Parkinson's disease and CoQ_{10} deficiency using Functional Intracellular Assay, when compared to matched controls for age and gender [132]. A phase 2 study in 80 subjects at early or mid-stage Parkinson disease showed a beneficial effect from supplementation with CoQ_{10} in progressive doses of 300, 600, 1200 mg/day for 16 months. There was an improvement in the ADL UPDRS (Activity Of Daily Living Unified Parkinson Disease Rating Scale) and Schwab and England scales compared to placebo (+11.99), with highest dose (+6.69) having the best effect [133]. This lead to a phase III randomized, placebo-controlled, double-blind clinical trial at 67 North American sites by the Parkinson Study Group which used doses up to 2400 mg/day of CoQ_{10} vitamin E in the dose of 1200 IU/d (to enhance the absorption of the lipophilic coenzyme) however this large study did not find convincing evidence to support CoQ_{10} treatment for this disease [7]. A systematic review and meta-analysis from 2016 could not find sufficient evidence in five selected RCTs to support the use of ubiquinone (300 mg/day to 2400 mg/day) to decelerate the progression of Parkinson's disease or improve symptoms [134].

In aged, cognitively impaired mice, CoQ_{10} supplementation does improve special learning and attenuates oxidative damage [135]. In Alzheimer Disease, the Alzheimer's Disease Cooperative Study could not identify benefits in the levels of oxidative stress and neurodegeneration biomarkers in CSF (cerebrospinal fluid) with a dose of 400 mg of CoQ_{10} 3 times/day for 16 weeks for patients [136]. To date, chronic large-scale trials of CoQ_{10} have not been carried out in Alzheimer disease.

3.3.2. Cardiovascular Disease

A meta-analysis reviewed randomized controlled trials in healthy adults; two trials reported reduction in systolic blood pressure, and no evidence for reduction in diastolic blood pressure was reported. Another trial included in this meta-analysis failed to show an effect of CoQ_{10} supplementation on the lipid profile (LDL: low-density lipoprotein cholesterol, HDL: high-density lipoprotein cholesterol, and triglycerides) [137]. Another meta-analysis from 2016 concluded that there is not enough evidence to support CoQ_{10} use to treat hypertension [138]. For dyslipidemia, no relationship was found between CoQ levels in hyperlipidemic and normolipidemic, older women and no association with body mass index was found [139]. Statins are well known to reduce CoQ_{10} levels because of inhibition of 3-hydroxy-3-methylglutaryl-coenzyme A (HMG-CoA) reductase. This enzyme is the first step in the mevalonic acid synthesis pathway, which is necessary for the synthesis of cholesterol but also the isoprenoid side-chain of CoQ_{10} [140].

Patients with mitochondrial myopathy do not tolerate statin treatment, often developing exercise intolerance and myalgia when treated with statins. These symptoms may improve with CoQ_{10} oral supplementation [141–143]. Statins were also found related to a reduction in complex III activity. However, the exact mechanism for the mitochondrial myotoxicity of statins is not well understood and other factors than CoQ_{10} can be involved, such as genetic polymorphisms [144].

There is evidence that cardiac function in the elderly may be improved by CoQ_{10} treatment. This effect may be related to the documented fall in cardiac CoQ_{10} levels in the aged heart [114]. A meta-analysis reviewed eight clinical trials and concluded that patients submitted to cardiopulmonary bypass have a decreased requirement for ionotropic drugs and a reduced chance of ventricular arrhythmia if receiving CoQ_{10} supplementation [145].

The best case for CoQ_{10} supplementation is in cardiovascular disease. It was recently reported that 12 years after a 4-year double-blind treatment protocol in the elderly co-supplemented with selenium (200 μg) and CoQ_{10} (200 mg/day) (ubiquinone in a softgel vehicle of vegetable oils) the treated subjects still had a reduced cardiovascular mortality (38.7% in placebo-treated group versus 28.1% in CoQ-treated group) [146]. The Q-SYMBIO trial enrolled 420 patients and showed that CoQ_{10} 100 mg 3 times daily for 2 years plus standard therapy reduced the risk of cardiovascular events, in this study measured as cardiovascular mortality (16% in placebo and 9% in the treated group) and hospitalization for heart failure compared to placebo, and also a positive change in the New York Heart Association (NYHA) functional classification (26% in placebo and 15% in the treated group) [147]. A recent review of the use of CoQ_{10} in heart failure is recommended [39].

3.3.3. Endothelial Dysfunction

Endothelial function may be a risk factor for coronary artery disease and atherosclerosis. CoQ_{10} together with a Mediterranean diet was shown to improve markers of endothelial function in elderly patients [148,149].

3.3.4. Renal Disease

Although ubiquinol can improve the endothelial dysfunction associated with the diabetic kidney disease (systolic blood pressure and urinary albumin) [150], and a trial with CoQ_{10} supplementation (1200 mg/day in dialysis patients) identified a reduction in a plasma indicator of oxidative stress (F2-isoprostane) [151], a meta-analysis failed to prove CoQ_{10} efficacy in avoiding the progression of diabetic kidney disease [152].

3.3.5. Inflammation

Many aging-related diseases share a common physiologic pathway of chronic inflammation leading to oxidative stress, such as cardiovascular diseases, diabetes, cancer, and chronic kidney disease.

A recent meta-analysis reports a reduction in the plasma inflammatory biomarkers, C-reactive protein, IL-6, and TNF-α, after CoQ_{10} supplementation (60 to 500 mg/day, formulations described as CoQ10 or ubiquinol), for 1 week to 4 months in different inflammatory disorders (cardio and cerebral vascular disease, multiple sclerosis, obesity, renal failure, rheumatoid arthritis, diabetes, and fatty liver disease). The same review reports that CoQ_{10} decreases other biomarkers for inflammation and inflammatory cytokines [30]. Although CoQ_{10} treatment has been shown to improve markers of inflammation, a benefit of chronic treatment for the diseases associated with inflammation has not been demonstrated.

CoQ_{10} (100 mg/day) supplementation for 2 months decreased the levels of TFN-α in rheumatoid arthritis patients compared to placebo, [153]. A more recent systematic review and meta-analysis reported CoQ_{10} supplementation between 60 to 300 mg/day (no extra information about formulations) was associated with a slightly drop in C-reactive protein levels and a significant decrease in in IL-6 levels [154].

Down syndrome patients have an abnormal pro-inflammatory profile (increased IL-6 and TNF-α) [36,37] and reduced CoQ_{10} levels, and supplementation reduced markers of oxidative stress and mitochondrial dysfunction [38,155].

3.3.6. Osteoporosis

Animal and human studies have demonstrated that benefits of CoQ_{10} supplementation have a beneficial profile for osteoporosis [156–158].

3.3.7. Cancer

There is evidence of the relationship between some cancers and reduced CoQ_{10} levels in blood, particularly breast cancer [159], myeloma [160], melanoma [161], and follicular and papillary thyroid carcinomas [162]. There is also evidence that CoQ_{10} supplementation modulates phospholipid hydroperoxide glutathione peroxidase gene expression, free radical production, and can decelerate the growth of tumor cells in a prostate cancer line (PC3 line) [163].

4. Conclusions

There is still much to be learned about the pathophysiology of the process of aging. There are well documented reductions of tissue CoQ_{10} in senescence. It is not known if low CoQ_{10} is an effect of aging, perhaps matching the fall in mitochondrial electron transport function or a contributing cause to the aging process. There is accumulating evidence that some diseases of aging may benefit from supplemental ubiquinol or CoQ_{10} treatment. Studies to date have supported the safety and the potential of CoQ_{10} in reducing oxidative stress biomarkers. There remains a lack of adequate large-scale clinical trials preferably utilizing ubiquinol as the better absorbed form of CoQ_{10}. Despite the lack of evidence, large numbers of people in the population are taking CoQ_{10} and other vitamins and cofactors in the hope that these agents will slow senescence and expand longevity.

Acknowledgments: Thank you to the many patients and families who have taught the authors so much including their experiences with CoQ_{10} treatment.

References

1. Festenstein, G.N.; Heaton, F.W.; Lowe, J.S.; Morton, R.A. A constituent of the unsaponifiable portion of animal tissue lipids (λmax. Mμ.). *Biochem. J.* **1955**, *59*, 558–566. [CrossRef] [PubMed]

2. Crane, F.L. Electron transport and cytochromes of sub-cellular particles from cauliflower buds. *Plant Physiol.* **1957**, *32*, 619–625. [CrossRef]

3. Ogasahara, S.; Nishikawa, Y.; Yorifuji, S.; Soga, F.; Nakamura, Y.; Takahashi, M.; Hashimoto, S.; Kono, N.; Tarui, S. Treatment of Kearns-Sayre syndrome with coenzyme Q10. *Neurology* **1986**, *36*, 45–53. [CrossRef]

4. Miles, M.V.; Miles, L.; Tang, P.H.; Horn, P.S.; Steele, P.E.; DeGrauw, A.J.; Wong, B.L.; Bove, K.E. Systematic evaluation of muscle coenzyme Q10 content in children with mitochondrial respiratory chain enzyme deficiencies. *Mitochondrion* **2008**, *8*, 170–180. [CrossRef] [PubMed]

5. Hirano, M.; Garone, C.; Quinzii, C.M. CoQ(10) deficiencies and MNGIE: Two treatable mitochondrial disorders. *Biochim. Biophys. Acta* **2012**, *1820*, 625–631. [CrossRef] [PubMed]

6. Marin, S.E.; Haas, R.H. Coenzyme Q10 and the Treatment of Mitochondrial Disease. In *Coenzyme Q10: From Fact to Fiction*; Hargreaves, I.P., Hargreaves, A.K., Eds.; Nova Science Publishers: Hauppauge, NY, USA, 2015; pp. 85–108.

7. Parkinson Study Group QE3 Investigators; Beal, M.F.; Oakes, D.; Shoulson, I.; Henchcliffe, C.; Galpern, W.R.; Haas, R.; Juncos, J.L.; Nutt, J.G.; Voss, T.S.; et al. A randomized clinical trial of high-dosage coenzyme Q10 in early Parkinson disease: No evidence of benefit. *JAMA Neurol* **2014**, *71*, 543–552. [PubMed]

8. Navas, P.; Villalba, J.M.; de Cabo, R. The importance of plasma membrane coenzyme Q in aging and stress responses. *Mitochondrion* **2007**, *7*, S34–S40. [CrossRef] [PubMed]

9. Huo, J.; Xu, Z.; Hosoe, K.; Kubo, H.; Miyahara, H.; Dai, J.; Mori, M.; Sawashita, J.; Higuchi, K. Coenzyme Q10 prevents senescence and dysfunction caused by oxidative stress in vascular endothelial cells. *Oxid. Med. Cell. Longev.* **2018**, *2018*, 1–15. [CrossRef] [PubMed]

10. Zhang, W.; Hui, R.; Yang, S. Telomeres, cardiovascular aging, and potential intervention for cellular senescence. *Sci. China Life Sci.* **2014**, *57*, 858–862. [CrossRef] [PubMed]

11. Davalli, P.; Mitic, T.; Caporali, A.; Lauriola, A.; D'Arca, D. Ros, cell senescence, and novel molecular mechanisms in aging and age-related diseases. *Oxid. Med. Cell. Longev.* **2016**, *2016*. [CrossRef] [PubMed]

12. Hernández-Camacho, J.D.; Bernier, M.; López-Lluch, G.; Navas, P. Coenzyme Q10 supplementation in aging and disease. *Front. Physiol.* **2018**. [CrossRef] [PubMed]

13. Gutierrez-Mariscal, F.M.; Yubero-Serrano, E.M.; Villalba, J.M.; Lopez-Miranda, J. Coenzyme Q10: From bench to clinic in aging diseases, a translational review. *Crit. Rev. Food Sci. Nutr.* **2018**. [CrossRef]

14. Awad, A.M.; Bradley, M.C.; Fernandez-Del-Rio, L.; Nag, A.; Tsui, H.S.; Clarke, C.F. Coenzyme Q10 deficiencies: Pathways in yeast and humans. *Essays Biochem.* **2018**, *62*, 361–376. [CrossRef]

15. Gale, P.H.; Erickson, R.E.; Page, A.C., Jr.; Folkers, K. Coenzyme Q. Li. New data on the distribution of coenzyme Q in nature. *Arch. Biochem. Biophys.* **1964**, *104*, 169–172. [CrossRef]

16. Kalen, A.; Norling, B.; Appelkvist, E.L.; Dallner, G. Ubiquinone biosynthesis by the microsomal fraction from rat liver. *Biochim. Biophys. Acta* **1987**, *926*, 70–78. [CrossRef]

17. Lenaz, G.; Fato, R.; Di Bernardo, S.; Jarreta, D.; Costa, A.; Genova, M.L.; Parenti Castelli, G. Localization and mobility of coenzyme Q in lipid bilayers and membranes. *BioFactors* **1999**, *9*, 87–93. [CrossRef]

18. Olson, R.E.; Rudney, H. Biosynthesis of ubiquinone. *Vitam Horm* **1983**, *40*, 1–43. [PubMed]

19. Alcazar-Fabra, M.; Navas, P.; Brea-Calvo, G. Coenzyme Q biosynthesis and its role in the respiratory chain structure. *Biochim. Biophys. Acta* **2016**, *1857*, 1073–1078. [CrossRef]

20. Lenaz, G.; Fato, R.; Castelluccio, C.; Genova, M.L.; Bovina, C.; Estornell, E.; Valls, V.; Pallotti, F.; Parenti Castelli, G. The function of coenzyme Q in mitochondria. *Clin. Investig.* **1993**, *71*, S66–S70. [CrossRef]

21. Enriquez, J.A.; Lenaz, G. Coenzyme Q and the respiratory chain: Coenzyme Q pool and mitochondrial supercomplexes. *Mol. Syndromol.* **2014**, *5*, 119–140. [CrossRef] [PubMed]

22. Groneberg, D.A.; Kindermann, B.; Althammer, M.; Klapper, M.; Vormann, J.; Littarru, G.P.; Doring, F. Coenzyme Q10 affects expression of genes involved in cell signalling, metabolism and transport in human caco-2 cells. *Int. J. Biochem. Cell Biol.* **2005**, *37*, 1208–1218. [CrossRef] [PubMed]

23. Schmelzer, C.; Kitano, M.; Hosoe, K.; Döring, F. Ubiquinol affects the expression of genes involved in pparα signalling and lipid metabolism without changes in methylation of CpG promoter islands in the liver of mice. *J. Clin. Biochem. Nutr.* **2012**, *50*, 119–126. [CrossRef]

24. Blatt, T.; Littarru, G.P. Biochemical rationale and experimental data on the antiaging properties of CoQ(10) at skin level. *BioFactors* **2011**, *37*, 381–385. [CrossRef]

25. Lopez-Lluch, G.; Rodriguez-Aguilera, J.C.; Santos-Ocana, C.; Navas, P. Is coenzyme Q a key factor in aging? *Mech. Ageing Dev.* **2010**, *131*, 225–235. [CrossRef] [PubMed]

26. Sohal, R.S.; Kamzalov, S.; Sumien, N.; Ferguson, M.; Rebrin, I.; Heinrich, K.R.; Forster, M.J. Effect of coenzyme Q10 intake on endogenous coenzyme Q content, mitochondrial electron transport chain, antioxidative defenses, and life span of mice. *Free Radic. Biol. Med.* **2006**, *40*, 480–487. [CrossRef]

27. Crane, F.L. Discovery of ubiquinone (coenzyme Q) and an overview of function. *Mitochondrion* **2007**, *7*, S2–S7. [CrossRef]

28. Belliere, J.; Devun, F.; Cottet-Rousselle, C.; Batandier, C.; Leverve, X.; Fontaine, E. Prerequisites for ubiquinone analogs to prevent mitochondrial permeability transition-induced cell death. *J. Bioenerg. Biomembr.* **2012**, *44*, 207–212. [CrossRef] [PubMed]

29. Olivieri, F.; Lazzarini, R.; Babini, L.; Prattichizzo, F.; Rippo, M.R.; Tiano, L.; Di Nuzzo, S.; Graciotti, L.; Festa, R.; Bruge, F.; et al. Anti-inflammatory effect of ubiquinol-10 on young and senescent endothelial cells via mir-146a modulation. *Free Radic. Biol. Med.* **2013**, *63*, 410–420. [CrossRef] [PubMed]

30. Fan, L.; Feng, Y.; Chen, G.C.; Qin, L.Q.; Fu, C.L.; Chen, L.H. Effects of coenzyme Q10 supplementation on inflammatory markers: A systematic review and meta-analysis of randomized controlled trials. *Pharmacol. Res.* **2017**, *119*, 128–136. [CrossRef]

31. Zhai, J.; Bo, Y.; Lu, Y.; Liu, C.; Zhang, L. Effects of coenzyme Q10 on markers of inflammation: A systematic review and meta-analysis. *PLoS ONE* **2017**, *12*, e0170172. [CrossRef]

32. Schmelzer, C.; Lindner, I.; Rimbach, G.; Niklowitz, P.; Menke, T.; Doring, F. Functions of coenzyme Q10 in inflammation and gene expression. *BioFactors* **2008**, *32*, 179–183. [CrossRef]

33. Saleh, D.O.; Ahmed, R.F.; Amin, M.M. Modulatory role of co-enzyme Q10 on methionine and choline deficient diet-induced non-alcoholic steatohepatitis (nash) in albino rats. *Appl. Physiol. Nutr. Metabol.* **2017**, *42*, 243–249. [CrossRef]

34. Farhangi, M.A.; Alipour, B.; Jafarvand, E.; Khoshbaten, M. Oral coenzyme Q10 supplementation in patients with nonalcoholic fatty liver disease: Effects on serum vaspin, chemerin, pentraxin 3, insulin resistance and oxidative stress. *Arch. Med. Res.* **2014**, *45*, 589–595. [CrossRef]

35. Perez-Sanchez, C.; Aguirre, M.A.; Ruiz-Limon, P.; Abalos-Aguilera, M.C.; Jimenez-Gomez, Y.; Arias-de la Rosa, I.; Rodriguez-Ariza, A.; Fernandez-Del Rio, L.; Gonzalez-Reyes, J.A.; Segui, P.; et al. Ubiquinol effects on antiphospholipid syndrome prothrombotic profile: A randomized, placebo-controlled trial. *Arterioscler. Thromb. Vasc. Biol.* **2017**, *37*, 1923–1932. [CrossRef]

36. Wilcock, D.M.; Griffin, W.S. Down's syndrome, neuroinflammation, and Alzheimer neuropathogenesis. *J. Neuroinflamm.* **2013**, *10*, 84. [CrossRef] [PubMed]

37. Zaki, M.E.; El-Bassyouni, H.T.; Tosson, A.M.; Youness, E.; Hussein, J. Coenzyme Q10 and pro-inflammatory markers in children with Down syndrome: Clinical and biochemical aspects. *J. Pediatr.* **2017**, *93*, 100–104. [CrossRef]

38. Tiano, L.; Carnevali, P.; Padella, L.; Santoro, L.; Principi, F.; Bruge, F.; Carle, F.; Gesuita, R.; Gabrielli, O.; Littarru, G.P. Effect of coenzyme Q10 in mitigating oxidative DNA damage in Down syndrome patients, a double blind randomized controlled trial. *Neurobiol. Aging* **2011**, *32*, 2103–2105. [CrossRef]

39. Sharma, A.; Fonarow, G.C.; Butler, J.; Ezekowitz, J.A.; Felker, G.M. Coenzyme Q10 and heart failure: A state-of-the-art review. *Circ. Heart Fail.* **2016**, *9*, e002639. [CrossRef]

40. Jorat, M.V.; Tabrizi, R.; Mirhosseini, N.; Lankarani, K.B.; Akbari, M.; Heydari, S.T.; Mottaghi, R.; Asemi, Z. The effects of coenzyme Q10 supplementation on lipid profiles among patients with coronary artery disease: A systematic review and meta-analysis of randomized controlled trials. *Lipids Health Dis.* **2018**, *17*, 230. [CrossRef]

41. Lucas-Hourani, M.; Munier-Lehmann, H.; El Mazouni, F.; Malmquist, N.A.; Harpon, J.; Coutant, E.P.; Guillou, S.; Helynck, O.; Noel, A.; Scherf, A.; et al. Original 2-(3-alkoxy-1h-pyrazol-1-yl)azines inhibitors of human dihydroorotate dehydrogenase (dhodh). *J. Med. Chem.* **2015**, *58*, 5579–5598. [CrossRef]

42. Ziosi, M.; Di Meo, I.; Kleiner, G.; Gao, X.H.; Barca, E.; Sanchez-Quintero, M.J.; Tadesse, S.; Jiang, H.; Qiao, C.; Rodenburg, R.J.; et al. Coenzyme Q deficiency causes impairment of the sulfide oxidation pathway. *EMBO Mol. Med.* **2017**, *9*, 96–111. [CrossRef]

43. Salvi, F.; Gadda, G. Human choline dehydrogenase: Medical promises and biochemical challenges. *Arch. Biochem. Biophys.* **2013**, *537*, 243–252. [CrossRef] [PubMed]

44. Szabados, L.; Savoure, A. Proline: A multifunctional amino acid. *Trends Plant Sci.* **2010**, *15*, 89–97. [CrossRef]

45. Bentinger, M.; Tekle, M.; Dallner, G. Coenzyme Q–biosynthesis and functions. *Biochem. Biophys. Res. Commun.* **2010**, *396*, 74–79. [CrossRef] [PubMed]

46. Garrido-Maraver, J.; Cordero, M.D.; Oropesa-Avila, M.; Vega, A.F.; de la Mata, M.; Pavon, A.D.; Alcocer-Gomez, E.; Calero, C.P.; Paz, M.V.; Alanis, M.; et al. Clinical applications of coenzyme Q10. *Front. Biosci. (Landmark Ed)* **2014**, *19*, 619–633. [CrossRef]

47. Zozina, V.I.; Covantev, S.; Goroshko, O.A.; Krasnykh, L.M.; Kukes, V.G. Coenzyme Q10 in cardiovascular and metabolic diseases: Current state of the problem. *Curr. Cardiol. Rev.* **2018**, *14*, 164–174. [CrossRef] [PubMed]

48. Bhagavan, H.N.; Chopra, R.K. Plasma coenzyme Q10 response to oral ingestion of coenzyme Q10 formulations. *Mitochondrion* **2007**, *7*, S78–S88. [CrossRef] [PubMed]

49. Ochiai, A.; Itagaki, S.; Kurokawa, T.; Kobayashi, M.; Hirano, T.; Iseki, K. Improvement in intestinal coenzyme Q10 absorption by food intake. *Yakugaku zasshi: J. Pharm. Soc. Jpn.* **2007**, *127*, 1251–1254. [CrossRef]

50. Mohr, D.; Bowry, V.W.; Stocker, R. Dietary supplementation with coenzyme Q10 results in increased levels of ubiquinol-10 within circulating lipoproteins and increased resistance of human low-density lipoprotein to the initiation of lipid peroxidation. *Biochim. Biophys. Acta* **1992**, *1126*, 247–254. [CrossRef]

51. Hargreaves, I.P. Ubiquinone: Cholesterol's reclusive cousin. *Ann. Clin. Biochem.* **2003**, *40*, 207–218. [CrossRef] [PubMed]

52. Ogasahara, S.; Engel, A.G.; Frens, D.; Mack, D. Muscle coenzyme Q deficiency in familial mitochondrial encephalomyopathy. *Proc. Natl. Acad. Sci. USA* **1989**, *86*, 2379–2382. [CrossRef] [PubMed]

53. Miles, M.V. The uptake and distribution of coenzyme Q10. *Mitochondrion* **2007**, *7*, S72–S77. [CrossRef]

54. Kwong, L.K.; Kamzalov, S.; Rebrin, I.; Bayne, A.C.; Jana, C.K.; Morris, P.; Forster, M.J.; Sohal, R.S. Effects of coenzyme Q(10) administration on its tissue concentrations, mitochondrial oxidant generation, and oxidative stress in the rat. *Free Radic. Biol. Med.* **2002**, *33*, 627–638. [CrossRef]

55. Niklowitz, P.; Menke, T.; Wiesel, T.; Mayatepek, E.; Zschocke, J.; Okun, J.G.; Andler, W. Coenzyme Q10 in plasma and erythrocytes: Comparison of antioxidant levels in healthy probands after oral supplementation and in patients suffering from sickle cell anemia. *Clin. Chim. Acta* **2002**, *326*, 155–161. [CrossRef]

56. Duncan, A.J.; Heales, S.J.; Mills, K.; Eaton, S.; Land, J.M.; Hargreaves, I.P. Determination of coenzyme Q10 status in blood mononuclear cells, skeletal muscle, and plasma by HPLC with di-propoxy-coenzyme Q10 as an internal standard. *Clin. Chem.* **2005**, *51*, 2380–2382. [CrossRef]

57. Bhagavan, H.N.; Chopra, R.K. Coenzyme Q10: Absorption, tissue uptake, metabolism and pharmacokinetics. *Free Radic. Res.* **2006**, *40*, 445–453. [CrossRef] [PubMed]

58. Musumeci, O.; Naini, A.; Slonim, A.E.; Skavin, N.; Hadjigeorgiou, G.L.; Krawiecki, N.; Weissman, B.M.; Tsao, C.Y.; Mendell, J.R.; Shanske, S.; et al. Familial cerebellar ataxia with muscle coenzyme Q10 deficiency. *Neurology* **2001**, *56*, 849–855. [CrossRef]

59. Gempel, K.; Topaloglu, H.; Talim, B.; Schneiderat, P.; Schoser, B.G.; Hans, V.H.; Palmafy, B.; Kale, G.; Tokatli, A.; Quinzii, C.; et al. The myopathic form of coenzyme Q10 deficiency is caused by mutations in the electron-transferring-flavoprotein dehydrogenase (ETFDH) gene. *Brain* **2007**, *130*, 2037–2044. [CrossRef] [PubMed]

60. Quinzii, C.M.; Kattah, A.G.; Naini, A.; Akman, H.O.; Mootha, V.K.; DiMauro, S.; Hirano, M. Coenzyme Q deficiency and cerebellar ataxia associated with an aprataxin mutation. *Neurology* **2005**, *64*, 539–541. [CrossRef]

61. Ihara, Y.; Namba, R.; Kuroda, S.; Sato, T.; Shirabe, T. Mitochondrial encephalomyopathy (MELAS): Pathological study and successful therapy with coenzyme Q10 and idebenone. *J. Neurol. Sci.* **1989**, *90*, 263–271. [CrossRef]

62. Quinzii, C.M.; Hirano, M. Primary and secondary CoQ(10) deficiencies in humans. *BioFactors* **2011**, *37*, 361–365. [CrossRef]

63. Hathcock, J.N.; Shao, A. Risk assessment for coenzyme Q10 (ubiquinone). *Regul. Toxicol. Pharmacol.* **2006**, *45*, 282–288. [CrossRef] [PubMed]

64. Balreira, A.; Boczonadi, V.; Barca, E.; Pyle, A.; Bansagi, B.; Appleton, M.; Graham, C.; Hargreaves, I.P.; Rasic, V.M.; Lochmuller, H.; et al. Ano10 mutations cause ataxia and coenzyme Q(1)(0) deficiency. *J. Neurol.* **2014**, *261*, 2192–2198. [CrossRef]

65. Baruteau, J.; Hargreaves, I.; Krywawych, S.; Chalasani, A.; Land, J.M.; Davison, J.E.; Kwok, M.K.; Christov, G.; Karimova, A.; Ashworth, M.; et al. Successful reversal of propionic acidaemia associated cardiomyopathy: Evidence for low myocardial coenzyme Q10 status and secondary mitochondrial dysfunction as an underlying pathophysiological mechanism. *Mitochondrion* **2014**, *17*, 150–156. [CrossRef]

66. Yubero, D.; O'Callaghan, M.; Montero, R.; Ormazabal, A.; Armstrong, J.; Espinos, C.; Rodriguez, M.A.; Jou, C.; Castejon, E.; Aracil, M.A.; et al. Association between coenzyme Q10 and glucose transporter (GLUT1) deficiency. *BMC Pediatr.* **2014**, *14*, 284. [CrossRef] [PubMed]

67. Beal, M.F. Coenzyme Q10 administration and its potential for treatment of neurodegenerative diseases. *BioFactors* **1999**, *9*, 261–266. [CrossRef]

68. Baggio, E.; Gandini, R.; Plancher, A.C.; Passeri, M.; Carmosino, G. Italian multicenter study on the safety and efficacy of coenzyme Q10 as adjunctive therapy in heart failure. CoQ10 drug surveillance investigators. *Mol. Asp. Med.* **1994**, *15*, s287–s294. [CrossRef]

69. Wallace, D.C. A mitochondrial paradigm of metabolic and degenerative diseases, aging, and cancer: A dawn for evolutionary medicine. *Annu. Rev. Genet.* **2005**, *39*, 359–407. [CrossRef] [PubMed]

70. Schniertshauer, D.; Gebhard, D.; Bergemann, J. Age-dependent loss of mitochondrial function in epithelial tissue can be reversed by coenzyme Q10. *J. Aging Res.* **2018**, *2018*, 6354680. [CrossRef] [PubMed]

71. Harman, D. The biologic clock: The mitochondria? *J. Am. Geriatr. Soc.* **1972**, *20*, 145–147. [CrossRef]

72. Krutmann, J.; Schroeder, P. Role of mitochondria in photoaging of human skin: The defective powerhouse model. *J. Investig. Dermatol. Symp. Proc.* **2009**, *14*, 44–49. [CrossRef]

73. Brunk, U.T.; Terman, A. The mitochondrial-lysosomal axis theory of aging: Accumulation of damaged mitochondria as a result of imperfect autophagocytosis. *Eur. J. Biochem.* **2002**, *269*, 1996–2002. [CrossRef]

74. Clayton, D.A.; Doda, J.N.; Friedberg, E.C. The absence of a pyrimidine dimer repair mechanism in mammalian mitochondria. *Proc. Natl. Acad. Sci. USA* **1974**, *71*, 2777–2781. [CrossRef]

75. Demple, B.; Harrison, L. Repair of oxidative damage to DNA: Enzymology and biology. *Annu. Rev. Biochem.* **1994**, *63*, 915–948. [CrossRef]

76. Barja, G. Mitochondrial oxygen consumption and reactive oxygen species production are independently modulated: Implications for aging studies. *Rejuv. Res.* **2007**, *10*, 215–224. [CrossRef]

77. Miquel, J. An update on the oxygen stress-mitochondrial mutation theory of aging: Genetic and evolutionary implications. *Exp. Gerontol.* **1998**, *33*, 113–126. [CrossRef]

78. Sohal, R.S.; Mockett, R.J.; Orr, W.C. Mechanisms of aging: An appraisal of the oxidative stress hypothesis. *Free Radic. Biol. Med.* **2002**, *33*, 575–586. [CrossRef]

79. Maurya, P.K.; Noto, C.; Rizzo, L.B.; Rios, A.C.; Nunes, S.O.; Barbosa, D.S.; Sethi, S.; Zeni, M.; Mansur, R.B.; Maes, M.; et al. The role of oxidative and nitrosative stress in accelerated aging and major depressive disorder. *Prog. Neuro-Psychopharmacol. Biol. Psychiatry* **2016**, *65*, 134–144. [CrossRef] [PubMed]

80. Wallace, D.C.; Fan, W.; Procaccio, V. Mitochondrial energetics and therapeutics. *Annu. Rev. Pathol.* **2010**, *5*, 297–348. [CrossRef]

81. Elchuri, S.; Oberley, T.D.; Qi, W.; Eisenstein, R.S.; Jackson Roberts, L.; Van Remmen, H.; Epstein, C.J.; Huang, T.T. Cuznsod deficiency leads to persistent and widespread oxidative damage and hepatocarcinogenesis later in life. *Oncogene* **2005**, *24*, 367–380. [CrossRef]

82. Li, Y.; Huang, T.T.; Carlson, E.J.; Melov, S.; Ursell, P.C.; Olson, J.L.; Noble, L.J.; Yoshimura, M.P.; Berger, C.; Chan, P.H.; et al. Dilated cardiomyopathy and neonatal lethality in mutant mice lacking manganese superoxide dismutase. *Nat. Genet.* **1995**, *11*, 376–381. [CrossRef]

83. Ma, D.; Stokes, K.; Mahngar, K.; Domazet-Damjanov, D.; Sikorska, M.; Pandey, S. Inhibition of stress induced premature senescence in presenilin-1 mutated cells with water soluble coenzyme Q10. *Mitochondrion* **2014**, *17*, 106–115. [CrossRef]

84. Sohal, R.S.; Sohal, B.H. Hydrogen peroxide release by mitochondria increases during aging. *Mech. Ageing Dev.* **1991**, *57*, 187–202. [CrossRef]

85. Asensi, M.; Sastre, J.; Pallardo, F.V.; Lloret, A.; Lehner, M.; Garcia-de-la Asuncion, J.; Vina, J. Ratio of reduced to oxidized glutathione as indicator of oxidative stress status and DNA damage. *Methods Enzymol.* **1999**, *299*, 267–276.

86. Halliwell, B. The wanderings of a free radical. *Free Radic. Biol. Med.* **2009**, *46*, 531–542. [CrossRef]

87. Lambert, A.J.; Boysen, H.M.; Buckingham, J.A.; Yang, T.; Podlutsky, A.; Austad, S.N.; Kunz, T.H.; Buffenstein, R.; Brand, M.D. Low rates of hydrogen peroxide production by isolated heart mitochondria associate with long maximum lifespan in vertebrate homeotherms. *Aging Cell* **2007**, *6*, 607–618. [CrossRef]

88. Barja, G. Updating the mitochondrial free radical theory of aging: An integrated view, key aspects, and confounding concepts. *Antioxid. Redox Signal.* **2013**, *19*, 1420–1445. [CrossRef]

89. Hekimi, S.; Lapointe, J.; Wen, Y. Taking a "good" look at free radicals in the aging process. *Trends Cell Biol.* **2011**, *21*, 569–576. [CrossRef]

90. Wang, Y.; Hekimi, S. Mitochondrial dysfunction and longevity in animals: Untangling the knot. *Science* **2015**, *350*, 1204–1207. [CrossRef]

91. Feng, J.; Bussiere, F.; Hekimi, S. Mitochondrial electron transport is a key determinant of life span in caenorhabditis elegans. *Dev. Cell* **2001**, *1*, 633–644. [CrossRef]

92. Hekimi, S. Enhanced immunity in slowly aging mutant mice with high mitochondrial oxidative stress. *Oncoimmunology* **2013**, *2*, e23793. [CrossRef] [PubMed]

93. Wang, Y.; Oxer, D.; Hekimi, S. Mitochondrial function and lifespan of mice with controlled ubiquinone biosynthesis. *Nat. Commun.* **2015**, *6*, 6393. [CrossRef]

94. Van Remmen, H.; Ikeno, Y.; Hamilton, M.; Pahlavani, M.; Wolf, N.; Thorpe, S.R.; Alderson, N.L.; Baynes, J.W.; Epstein, C.J.; Huang, T.T.; et al. Life-long reduction in mnsod activity results in increased DNA damage and higher incidence of cancer but does not accelerate aging. *Physiol. Genom.* **2003**, *16*, 29–37. [CrossRef] [PubMed]

95. Hepple, R.T. Mitochondrial involvement and impact in aging skeletal muscle. *Front. Aging Neurosci.* **2014**, *6*, 211. [CrossRef]

96. Buffenstein, R.; Edrey, Y.H.; Yang, T.; Mele, J. The oxidative stress theory of aging: Embattled or invincible? Insights from non-traditional model organisms. *Age* **2008**, *30*, 99–109. [CrossRef] [PubMed]

97. Varela-Lopez, A.; Giampieri, F.; Battino, M.; Quiles, J.L. Coenzyme Q and its role in the dietary therapy against aging. *Molecules* **2016**, *21*, 373. [CrossRef]

98. Sohal, R.S.; Forster, M.J. Coenzyme Q, oxidative stress and aging. *Mitochondrion* **2007**, *7*, S103–S111. [CrossRef]

99. Jonassen, T.; Davis, D.E.; Larsen, P.L.; Clarke, C.F. Reproductive fitness and quinone content of caenorhabditis elegans clk-1 mutants fed coenzyme Q isoforms of varying length. *J. Biol. Chem.* **2003**, *278*, 51735–51742. [CrossRef] [PubMed]

100. Asencio, C.; Navas, P.; Cabello, J.; Schnabel, R.; Cypser, J.R.; Johnson, T.E.; Rodriguez-Aguilera, J.C. Coenzyme Q supports distinct developmental processes in caenorhabditis elegans. *Mech. Ageing Dev.* **2009**, *130*, 145–153. [CrossRef]

101. Gavilan, A.; Asencio, C.; Cabello, J.; Rodriguez-Aguilera, J.C.; Schnabel, R.; Navas, P.C. Elegans knockouts in ubiquinone biosynthesis genes result in different phenotypes during larval development. *BioFactors* **2005**, *25*, 21–29. [CrossRef]

102. Hihi, A.K.; Gao, Y.; Hekimi, S. Ubiquinone is necessary for caenorhabditis elegans development at mitochondrial and non-mitochondrial sites. *J. Biol. Chem.* **2002**, *277*, 2202–2206. [CrossRef] [PubMed]

103. Quinzii, C.M.; Lopez, L.C.; Von-Moltke, J.; Naini, A.; Krishna, S.; Schuelke, M.; Salviati, L.; Navas, P.; DiMauro, S.; Hirano, M. Respiratory chain dysfunction and oxidative stress correlate with severity of primary CoQ10 deficiency. *Faseb J.* **2008**, *22*, 1874–1885. [CrossRef] [PubMed]

104. Quinzii, C.M.; López, L.C.; Gilkerson, R.W.; Dorado, B.; Coku, J.; Naini, A.B.; Lagier-Tourenne, C.; Schuelke, M.; Salviati, L.; Carrozzo, R.; et al. Reactive oxygen species, oxidative stress, and cell death correlate with level of CoQ10 deficiency. *Faseb J.* **2010**, *24*, 3733–3743. [CrossRef] [PubMed]

105. Tian, G.; Sawashita, J.; Kubo, H.; Nishio, S.Y.; Hashimoto, S.; Suzuki, N.; Yoshimura, H.; Tsuruoka, M.; Wang, Y.; Liu, Y.; et al. Ubiquinol-10 supplementation activates mitochondria functions to decelerate senescence in senescence-accelerated mice. *Antioxid. Redox Signal.* **2014**, *20*, 2606–2620. [CrossRef] [PubMed]

106. Xu, Z.; Huo, J.; Ding, X.; Yang, M.; Li, L.; Dai, J.; Hosoe, K.; Kubo, H.; Mori, M.; Higuchi, K.; et al. Coenzyme Q10 improves lipid metabolism and ameliorates obesity by regulating camkii-mediated pde4 inhibition. *Sci. Rep.* **2017**, *7*, 8253. [CrossRef] [PubMed]

107. Liu, X.; Jiang, N.; Hughes, B.; Bigras, E.; Shoubridge, E.; Hekimi, S. Evolutionary conservation of the clk-1-dependent mechanism of longevity: Loss of mclk1 increases cellular fitness and lifespan in mice. *Genes Dev.* **2005**, *19*, 2424–2434. [CrossRef]

108. Ochoa, J.J.; Quiles, J.L.; Lopez-Frias, M.; Huertas, J.R.; Mataix, J. Effect of lifelong coenzyme Q10 supplementation on age-related oxidative stress and mitochondrial function in liver and skeletal muscle of rats fed on a polyunsaturated fatty acid (PUFA)-rich diet. *J. Gerontol. Ser. A Biol. Sci. Med. Sci.* **2007**, *62*, 1211–1218. [CrossRef]

109. Quiles, J.L.; Ochoa, J.J.; Battino, M.; Gutierrez-Rios, P.; Nepomuceno, E.A.; Frias, M.L.; Huertas, J.R.; Mataix, J. Life-long supplementation with a low dosage of coenzyme Q10 in the rat: Effects on antioxidant status and DNA damage. *BioFactors* **2005**, *25*, 73–86. [CrossRef]

110. Quiles, J.L.; Pamplona, R.; Ramirez-Tortosa, M.C.; Naudi, A.; Portero-Otin, M.; Araujo-Nepomuceno, E.; Lopez-Frias, M.; Battino, M.; Ochoa, J.J. Coenzyme Q addition to an n-6 PUFA-rich diet resembles benefits on age-related mitochondrial DNA deletion and oxidative stress of a MUFA-rich diet in rat heart. *Mech. Ageing Dev.* **2010**, *131*, 38–47. [CrossRef]

111. Schmelzer, C.; Kubo, H.; Mori, M.; Sawashita, J.; Kitano, M.; Hosoe, K.; Boomgaarden, I.; Doring, F.; Higuchi, K. Supplementation with the reduced form of Coenzyme Q10 decelerates phenotypic characteristics of senescence and induces a peroxisome proliferator-activated receptor-alpha gene expression signature in SAMP1 mice. *Mol. Nutr. Food Res.* **2010**, *54*, 805–815. [CrossRef]

112. Matthews, R.T.; Yang, L.; Browne, S.; Baik, M.; Beal, M.F. Coenzyme Q10 administration increases brain mitochondrial concentrations and exerts neuroprotective effects. *Proc. Natl. Acad. Sci. USA* **1998**, *95*, 8892–8897. [CrossRef]

113. Wolters, M.; Hahn, A. Plasma ubiquinone status and response to six-month supplementation combined with multivitamins in healthy elderly women–results of a randomized, double-blind, placebo-controlled study. *Int. J. Vitam. Nutr. Res.* **2003**, *73*, 207–214. [CrossRef] [PubMed]

114. Kalen, A.; Appelkvist, E.L.; Dallner, G. Age-related changes in the lipid compositions of rat and human tissues. *Lipids* **1989**, *24*, 579–584. [CrossRef]

115. Soderberg, M.; Edlund, C.; Kristensson, K.; Dallner, G. Lipid compositions of different regions of the human brain during aging. *J. Neurochem.* **1990**, *54*, 415–423. [CrossRef] [PubMed]

116. Edlund, C.; Soderberg, M.; Kristensson, K.; Dallner, G. Ubiquinone, dolichol, and cholesterol metabolism in aging and Alzheimer's disease. *Biochem. Cell Biol.* **1992**, *70*, 422–428. [CrossRef]

117. Nagase, M.; Yamamoto, Y.; Matsumoto, N.; Arai, Y.; Hirose, N. Increased oxidative stress and coenzyme Q10 deficiency in centenarians. *J. Clin. Biochem. Nutr.* **2018**, *63*, 129–136. [CrossRef]

118. Bentinger, M.; Brismar, K.; Dallner, G. The antioxidant role of coenzyme Q. *Mitochondrion* **2007**, *7*, S41–S50. [CrossRef] [PubMed]

119. Del Pozo-Cruz, J.; Rodriguez-Bies, E.; Ballesteros-Simarro, M.; Navas-Enamorado, I.; Tung, B.T.; Navas, P.; Lopez-Lluch, G. Physical activity affects plasma coenzyme Q10 levels differently in young and old humans. *Biogerontology* **2014**, *15*, 199–211. [CrossRef]

120. Del Pozo-Cruz, J.; Rodriguez-Bies, E.; Navas-Enamorado, I.; Del Pozo-Cruz, B.; Navas, P.; Lopez-Lluch, G. Relationship between functional capacity and body mass index with plasma coenzyme Q10 and oxidative damage in community-dwelling elderly-people. *Exp. Gerontol.* **2014**, *52*, 46–54. [CrossRef] [PubMed]

121. Johansson, P.; Dahlstrom, O.; Dahlstrom, U.; Alehagen, U. Improved health-related quality of life, and more days out of hospital with supplementation with selenium and coenzyme Q10 combined. Results from a double blind, placebo-controlled prospective study. *J. Nutr. Health Aging* **2015**, *19*, 870–877. [CrossRef]

122. Fischer, A.; Onur, S.; Niklowitz, P.; Menke, T.; Laudes, M.; Rimbach, G.; Doring, F. Coenzyme Q10 status as a determinant of muscular strength in two independent cohorts. *PLoS ONE* **2016**, *11*, e0167124. [CrossRef] [PubMed]

123. Liu, Z.X.; Artmann, C. Relative bioavailability comparison of different coenzyme Q10 formulations with a novel delivery system. *Altern. Ther. Health Med.* **2009**, *15*, 42–46.

124. Koroshetz, W.J.; Jenkins, B.G.; Rosen, B.R.; Beal, M.F. Energy metabolism defects in Huntington's disease and effects of coenzyme Q10. *Ann. Neurol.* **1997**, *41*, 160–165. [CrossRef] [PubMed]

125. Balaban, R.S.; Nemoto, S.; Finkel, T. Mitochondria, oxidants, and aging. *Cell* **2005**, *120*, 483–495. [CrossRef] [PubMed]

126. Liu, J.; Wang, L.N. Mitochondrial enhancement for neurodegenerative movement disorders: A systematic review of trials involving creatine, coenzyme Q10, idebenone and mitoquinone. *CNS Drugs* **2014**, *28*, 63–68. [CrossRef] [PubMed]

127. Molina, J.A.; de Bustos, F.; Ortiz, S.; Del Ser, T.; Seijo, M.; Benito-Leon, J.; Oliva, J.M.; Perez, S.; Manzanares, J. Serum levels of coenzyme Q in patients with Lewy body disease. *J. Neural Transm. (Vienna, Austria : 1996)* **2002**, *109*, 1195–1201. [CrossRef] [PubMed]

128. Isobe, C.; Abe, T.; Terayama, Y. Levels of reduced and oxidized coenzyme Q-10 and 8-hydroxy-2'-deoxyguanosine in the cerebrospinal fluid of patients with living Parkinson's disease demonstrate that mitochondrial oxidative damage and/or oxidative DNA damage contributes to the neurodegenerative process. *Neurosci. Lett.* **2010**, *469*, 159–163.

129. McGarry, A.; McDermott, M.; Kieburtz, K.; de Blieck, E.A.; Beal, F.; Marder, K.; Ross, C.; Shoulson, I.; Gilbert, P.; Mallonee, W.M.; et al. A randomized, double-blind, placebo-controlled trial of coenzyme Q10 in Huntington disease. *Neurology* **2017**, *88*, 152–159. [CrossRef]

130. Buhmann, C.; Arlt, S.; Kontush, A.; Moller-Bertram, T.; Sperber, S.; Oechsner, M.; Stuerenburg, H.J.; Beisiegel, U. Plasma and CSF markers of oxidative stress are increased in Parkinson's disease and influenced by antiparkinsonian medication. *Neurobiol. Dis.* **2004**, *15*, 160–170. [CrossRef] [PubMed]

131. Haas, R.H.; Nasirian, F.; Nakano, K.; Ward, D.; Pay, M.; Hill, R.; Shults, C.W. Low platelet mitochondrial complex I and complex II/III activity in early untreated Parkinson's disease. *Ann. Neurol.* **1995**, *37*, 714–722. [CrossRef]

132. Mischley, L.K.; Allen, J.; Bradley, R. Coenzyme Q10 deficiency in patients with Parkinson's disease. *J. Neurol. Sci.* **2012**, *318*, 72–75. [CrossRef] [PubMed]

133. Shults, C.W.; Oakes, D.; Kieburtz, K.; Beal, M.F.; Haas, R.; Plumb, S.; Juncos, J.L.; Nutt, J.; Shoulson, I.; Carter, J.; et al. Effects of coenzyme Q10 in early Parkinson disease: Evidence of slowing of the functional decline. *Arch. Neurol.* **2002**, *59*, 1541–1550. [CrossRef] [PubMed]

134. Negida, A.; Menshawy, A.; El Ashal, G.; Elfouly, Y.; Hani, Y.; Hegazy, Y.; El Ghonimy, S.; Fouda, S.; Rashad, Y. Coenzyme Q10 for patients with Parkinson's disease: A systematic review and meta-analysis. *CNS Neurol. Disord. Drug Targets* **2016**, *15*, 45–53. [CrossRef]

135. Shetty, R.A.; Forster, M.J.; Sumien, N. Coenzyme Q(10) supplementation reverses age-related impairments in spatial learning and lowers protein oxidation. *Age* **2013**, *35*, 1821–1834. [CrossRef]

136. Galasko, D.R.; Peskind, E.; Clark, C.M.; Quinn, J.F.; Ringman, J.M.; Jicha, G.A.; Cotman, C.; Cottrell, B.; Montine, T.J.; Thomas, R.G.; et al. Antioxidants for Alzheimer disease: A randomized clinical trial with cerebrospinal fluid biomarker measures. *Arch. Neurol.* **2012**, *69*, 836–841. [CrossRef]

137. Flowers, N.; Hartley, L.; Todkill, D.; Stranges, S.; Rees, K. Co-enzyme Q10 supplementation for the primary prevention of cardiovascular disease. *Cochrane Database Syst. Rev.* **2014**, *12*, Cd010405. [CrossRef]

138. Ho, M.J.; Li, E.C.; Wright, J.M. Blood pressure lowering efficacy of coenzyme Q10 for primary hypertension. *Cochrane Database Syst. Rev.* **2016**, *3*, Cd007435. [CrossRef] [PubMed]

139. Hosoe, K.; Kitano, M.; Kishida, H.; Kubo, H.; Fujii, K.; Kitahara, M. Study on safety and bioavailability of ubiquinol (Kaneka QH) after single and 4-week multiple oral administration to healthy volunteers. *Regul. Toxicol. Pharmacol.* **2007**, *47*, 19–28. [CrossRef] [PubMed]

140. Rundek, T.; Naini, A.; Sacco, R.; Coates, K.; DiMauro, S. Atorvastatin decreases the coenzyme Q10 level in the blood of patients at risk for cardiovascular disease and stroke. *Arch. Neurol.* **2004**, *61*, 889–892. [CrossRef] [PubMed]

141. Lamperti, C.; Naini, A.B.; Lucchini, V.; Prelle, A.; Bresolin, N.; Moggio, M.; Sciacco, M.; Kaufmann, P.; DiMauro, S. Muscle coenzyme Q10 levels in statin-related myopathy. *Arch. Neurol.* **2005**, *62*, 1709–1712. [CrossRef]

142. Caso, G.; Kelly, P.; McNurlan, M.A.; Lawson, W.E. Effect of coenzyme Q10 on myopathic symptoms in patients treated with statins. *Am. J. Cardiol.* **2007**, *99*, 1409–1412. [CrossRef]

143. Fedacko, J.; Pella, D.; Fedackova, P.; Hanninen, O.; Tuomainen, P.; Jarcuska, P.; Lopuchovsky, T.; Jedlickova, L.; Merkovska, L.; Littarru, G.P. Coenzyme Q(10) and selenium in statin-associated myopathy treatment. *Can. J. Physiol. Pharmacol.* **2013**, *91*, 165–170. [CrossRef]

144. Schirris, T.J.; Renkema, G.H.; Ritschel, T.; Voermans, N.C.; Bilos, A.; van Engelen, B.G.; Brandt, U.; Koopman, W.J.; Beyrath, J.D.; Rodenburg, R.J.; et al. Statin-induced myopathy is associated with mitochondrial complex III inhibition. *Cell Metab.* **2015**, *22*, 399–407. [CrossRef] [PubMed]

145. de Frutos, F.; Gea, A.; Hernandez-Estefania, R.; Rabago, G. Prophylactic treatment with coenzyme Q10 in patients undergoing cardiac surgery: Could an antioxidant reduce complications? A systematic review and meta-analysis. *Interact. Cardiovasc. Thorac. Surg.* **2015**, *20*, 254–259. [CrossRef] [PubMed]

146. Alehagen, U.; Aaseth, J.; Alexander, J.; Johansson, P. Still reduced cardiovascular mortality 12 years after supplementation with selenium and coenzyme Q10 for four years: A validation of previous 10-year follow-up results of a prospective randomized double-blind placebo-controlled trial in elderly. *PLoS ONE* **2018**, *13*, e0193120. [CrossRef] [PubMed]

147. Mortensen, S.A.; Rosenfeldt, F.; Kumar, A.; Dolliner, P.; Filipiak, K.J.; Pella, D.; Alehagen, U.; Steurer, G.; Littarru, G.P. The effect of coenzyme Q10 on morbidity and mortality in chronic heart failure: Results from Q-SYMBIO: A randomized double-blind trial. *JACC Heart Fail.* **2014**, *2*, 641–649. [CrossRef]

148. Yubero-Serrano, E.M.; Gonzalez-Guardia, L.; Rangel-Zuniga, O.; Delgado-Lista, J.; Gutierrez-Mariscal, F.M.; Perez-Martinez, P.; Delgado-Casado, N.; Cruz-Teno, C.; Tinahones, F.J.; Villalba, J.M.; et al. Mediterranean diet supplemented with coenzyme Q10 modifies the expression of proinflammatory and endoplasmic reticulum stress-related genes in elderly men and women. *J. Gerontol. Ser. A Biol. Sci. Med. Sci.* **2012**, *67*, 3–10. [CrossRef]

149. Tsai, H.Y.; Lin, C.P.; Huang, P.H.; Li, S.Y.; Chen, J.S.; Lin, F.Y.; Chen, J.W.; Lin, S.J. Coenzyme Q10 attenuates high glucose-induced endothelial progenitor cell dysfunction through AMP-activated protein kinase pathways. *J. Diabetes Res.* **2016**, *2016*, 6384759. [CrossRef] [PubMed]

150. Ishikawa, A.; Kawarazaki, H.; Ando, K.; Fujita, M.; Fujita, T.; Homma, Y. Renal preservation effect of ubiquinol, the reduced form of coenzyme Q10. *Clin. Exp. Nephrol.* **2011**, *15*, 30–33. [CrossRef] [PubMed]

151. Rivara, M.B.; Yeung, C.K.; Robinson-Cohen, C.; Phillips, B.R.; Ruzinski, J.; Rock, D.; Linke, L.; Shen, D.D.; Ikizler, T.A.; Himmelfarb, J. Effect of coenzyme Q10 on biomarkers of oxidative stress and cardiac function in hemodialysis patients: The CoQ10 biomarker trial. *Am. J. Kidney Dis.* **2017**, *69*, 389–399. [CrossRef] [PubMed]

152. Bolignano, D.; Cernaro, V.; Gembillo, G.; Baggetta, R.; Buemi, M.; D'Arrigo, G. Antioxidant agents for delaying diabetic kidney disease progression: A systematic review and meta-analysis. *PLoS ONE* **2017**, *12*, e0178699. [CrossRef]

153. Abdollahzad, H.; Aghdashi, M.A.; Asghari Jafarabadi, M.; Alipour, B. Effects of coenzyme Q10 supplementation on inflammatory cytokines (tnf-alpha, il-6) and oxidative stress in rheumatoid arthritis patients: A randomized controlled trial. *Arch. Med. Res.* **2015**, *46*, 527–533. [CrossRef] [PubMed]

154. Mazidi, M.; Kengne, A.P.; Banach, M. Effects of coenzyme Q10 supplementation on plasma c-reactive protein concentrations: A systematic review and meta-analysis of randomized controlled trials. *Pharmacol. Res.* **2018**, *128*, 130–136. [CrossRef] [PubMed]

155. Tiano, L.; Busciglio, J. Mitochondrial dysfunction and Down's syndrome: Is there a role for coenzyme Q(10)? *BioFactors* **2011**, *37*, 386–392. [CrossRef]

156. Zhang, X.X.; Qian, K.J.; Zhang, Y.; Wang, Z.J.; Yu, Y.B.; Liu, X.J.; Cao, X.T.; Liao, Y.H.; Zhang, D.Y. Efficacy of coenzyme Q10 in mitigating spinal cord injury-induced osteoporosis. *Mol. Med. Rep.* **2015**, *12*, 3909–3915. [CrossRef] [PubMed]

157. Moon, H.J.; Ko, W.K.; Jung, M.S.; Kim, J.H.; Lee, W.J.; Park, K.S.; Heo, J.K.; Bang, J.B.; Kwon, I.K. Coenzyme Q10 regulates osteoclast and osteoblast differentiation. *J. Food Sci.* **2013**, *78*, H785–H891. [CrossRef]

158. Zheng, D.; Cui, C.; Yu, M.; Li, X.; Wang, L.; Chen, X.; Lin, Y. Coenzyme Q10 promotes osteoblast proliferation and differentiation and protects against ovariectomy-induced osteoporosis. *Mol. Med. Rep.* **2018**, *17*, 400–407. [CrossRef]

159. Jolliet, P.; Simon, N.; Barre, J.; Pons, J.Y.; Boukef, M.; Paniel, B.J.; Tillement, J.P. Plasma coenzyme Q10 concentrations in breast cancer: Prognosis and therapeutic consequences. *Int. J. Clin. Pharmacol. Ther.* **1998**, *36*, 506–509.

160. Folkers, K.; Osterborg, A.; Nylander, M.; Morita, M.; Mellstedt, H. Activities of vitamin Q10 in animal models and a serious deficiency in patients with cancer. *Biochem. Biophys. Res. Commun.* **1997**, *234*, 296–299. [CrossRef]

161. Rusciani, L.; Proietti, I.; Paradisi, A.; Rusciani, A.; Guerriero, G.; Mammone, A.; De Gaetano, A.; Lippa, S. Recombinant interferon alpha-2b and coenzyme Q10 as a postsurgical adjuvant therapy for melanoma: A 3-year trial with recombinant interferon-alpha and 5-year follow-up. *Melanoma Res.* **2007**, *17*, 177–183. [CrossRef]

162. Mano, T.; Iwase, K.; Hayashi, R.; Hayakawa, N.; Uchimura, K.; Makino, M.; Nagata, M.; Sawai, Y.; Oda, N.; Hamada, M.; et al. Vitamin E and coenzyme Q concentrations in the thyroid tissues of patients with various thyroid disorders. *Am. J. Med. Sci.* **1998**, *315*, 230–232. [PubMed]

163. Quiles, J.L.; Farquharson, A.J.; Ramirez-Tortosa, M.C.; Grant, I.; Milne, L.; Huertas, J.R.; Battino, M.; Mataix, J.; Wahle, K.W. Coenzyme Q differentially modulates phospholipid hydroperoxide glutathione peroxidase gene expression and free radicals production in malignant and non-malignant prostate cells. *BioFactors* **2003**, *18*, 265–270. [CrossRef]

14

Vitamin D Deficiency: Effects on Oxidative Stress, Epigenetics, Gene Regulation and Aging

Sunil J. Wimalawansa

Professor of Medicine, Endocrinology & Nutrition, Cardio Metabolic and Endocrine Institute, NJ 08873, USA; suniljw@hotmail.com

Abstract: Recent advances in vitamin D research indicate that this vitamin, a secosteroid hormone, has beneficial effects on several body systems other than the musculoskeletal system. Both 25 dihydroxy vitamin D [25(OH)$_2$D] and its active hormonal form, 1,25-dihydroxyvitamin D [1,25(OH)$_2$D] are essential for human physiological functions, including damping down inflammation and the excessive intracellular oxidative stresses. Vitamin D is one of the key controllers of systemic inflammation, oxidative stress and mitochondrial respiratory function, and thus, the aging process in humans. In turn, molecular and cellular actions form 1,25(OH)$_2$D slow down oxidative stress, cell and tissue damage, and the aging process. On the other hand, hypovitaminosis D impairs mitochondrial functions, and enhances oxidative stress and systemic inflammation. The interaction of 1,25(OH)$_2$D with its intracellular receptors modulates vitamin D–dependent gene transcription and activation of vitamin D-responsive elements, which triggers multiple second messenger systems. Thus, it is not surprising that hypovitaminosis D increases the incidence and severity of several age-related common diseases, such as metabolic disorders that are linked to oxidative stress. These include obesity, insulin resistance, type 2 diabetes, hypertension, pregnancy complications, memory disorders, osteoporosis, autoimmune diseases, certain cancers, and systemic inflammatory diseases. Vitamin D adequacy leads to less oxidative stress and improves mitochondrial and endocrine functions, reducing the risks of disorders, such as autoimmunity, infections, metabolic derangements, and impairment of DNA repair; all of this aids a healthy, graceful aging process. Vitamin D is also a potent anti-oxidant that facilitates balanced mitochondrial activities, preventing oxidative stress-related protein oxidation, lipid peroxidation, and DNA damage. New understandings of vitamin D-related advances in metabolomics, transcriptomics, epigenetics, in relation to its ability to control oxidative stress in conjunction with micronutrients, vitamins, and antioxidants, following normalization of serum 25(OH)D and tissue 1,25(OH)$_2$D concentrations, likely to promise cost-effective better clinical outcomes in humans.

Keywords: 25(OH)D; 1,25(OH)$_2$D; aging; cytokines; inflammation; morbidity and mortality; prevention; reactive oxygen species; ultraviolet

1. Introduction

Vitamin D is a micronutrient that is metabolized into a multifunctional secosteroid hormone that is essential for human health. Globally, its deficiency is a major public health problem affecting all ages and ethnic groups; it has surpassed iron deficiency as the most common nutritional deficiency in the world. The increasing prevalence of vitamin D deficiency and its associated complications are prominent in countries furthest from the equator. However, incidence is also high among those who live within 1,000 km of the equator (e.g., in Sri Lanka, India, and Far Eastern, Middle Eastern, Central American, and Persian Gulf countries) because of a combination of climatic conditions, ethnic and cultural habits, and having darker skin color [1–4].

Most of the vitamin D the human body requires can be generated by an individual's exposure to summer-like sunlight, with dietary sources playing a supporting role when sunlight exposure is limited or ineffective for vitamin D production. Despite the above, more than 50% of the population in the group of countries mentioned has vitamin D deficiency [5,6]. If effective public health guidelines are implemented, vitamin D deficiency can be easily and cost-effectively treated and prevented, saving millions of dollars and lives. Although excessive sun exposure does not cause hypervitaminosis D, it can cause other harm because of dermal cell DNA damage [7–9]. Thus, guidelines for safe sun exposure are needed for each country.

During the past decade, many advances in the understanding of the physiology and biology of vitamin D and its receptor ecology have emerged [10]. Vitamin D metabolism and functions are modulated by many factors. Accumulating evidence supports biological associations of vitamin D with disease risk reduction and improved physical and mental functions. The field is rapidly advancing, including the knowledge of the physiology of vitamin D-vitamin D receptor (VDR) interactions and the biology and metabolism of vitamin D and their effects on vitamin D axis and gene polymorphisms [11]. Together these data have facilitated our understanding of new pathways to intervene to prevent and treat human diseases.

However, what is lacking is the adequately powered, conducted for sufficient duration, well-designed randomized controlled clinical studies (RCTs) conducted in an unbiased manner with the nutrient vitamin D as the key intervention and having predefined hard endpoints/primary outcomes [12]. Moreover, such studies must recruit persons with vitamin D deficiency [i.e., serum 25(OH)D concentrations less than 20 ng/mL (50 nmol/L)] and achieve a pre-determined target serum 25(OH)D concentration through daily oral administration and/or safe exposure to ultraviolet rays; not merely by relying on oral administered doses. The goal of this review is to explore the effects from vitamin D-modulated gene interactions and the effects of hypovitaminosis-induced, mitochondria-based oxidative stress on aging.

1.1. Extrarenal Generation of 1,25(OH)$_2$D

The active form of vitamin D, 1,25-dihydroxyvitamin D [1,25(OH)$_2$D], is generated not only in renal tubular cells (endocrine functions as a hormone) but also in extrarenal target tissue cells, providing autocrine and paracrine functions. However, because it remains within the target tissue cells, the intra-cellular concentrations achieved are unclear. In addition, the catabolic activity of 24-hydroxylase in target tissues plays an important part in regulating both 25-hydroxy vitamin D [25(OH)D; calcidiol], and 1,25(OH)$_2$D (calcitriol) concentrations and their availability.

The amounts of 1,25(OH)$_2$D generated in renal tubules and target cells can vary from person to person and day to day and are hard to quantify. Although the calcitriol in the circulation is modulated by parathyroid hormone (PTH) and serum ionized calcium concentrations [13], the intracellular content is regulated largely through serum 25(OH)D availability and calcidiol and calcitriol catabolism through hydroxylation at the molecular positions C-24 and C-23 by a specific 24-hydroxylase (CYP24A1) [14].

1.2. Excess Sun Exposure Does Not Cause Hypervitaminosis D

After exposure to ultraviolet B (UVB) rays, dermal cells actively synthesize vitamin D. As a feedback mechanism, excess precursors produced are catabolized within the dermal cells by the same UVB rays. In addition, skin also contains the inactivating enzyme 24-hydroxylase, which also prevents over-production of vitamin D by 24-hydroxylation of vitamin D [15]. This process of homeostasis is regulated by UVB, PTH, and serum ionized calcium concentrations [16]. When an individual is overexposed to ultraviolet rays, the mentioned built-in protective mechanism prevents excessive retention of vitamin D in the skin. Therefore, sun exposure does not raise serum 25(OH)D to pathological levels, cause hypervitaminosis D or its complications, such as hypercalcemia.

In addition, vitamin D synthesized in the skin from UVB exposure in excess of need is catabolized in part through 20-hydroxylation by the cholesterol side chain cleavage enzyme CYP11A1 [17]. Thus, there are multiple intrinsic mechanisms present to prevent excess vitamin D from reaching the circulation. The efficiency of vitamin D synthesis in the skin is affected by many factors, including the density of melanin pigment, condition of the skin and age, and the use of sunscreen and UV-blocking makeup, creams, and ointments and clothing. In addition, older age or scarred skin, as well as time of day or year and the duration of sun exposure affect vitamin D synthesis in the skin [18–21].

Although solar radiation is the source of vitamin D generation in the skin, excessive exposure, particularly in those who are genetically vulnerable, may cause skin cancers [22–24]. On the other hand, optimal vitamin D status protects against several types of internal cancers, melanoma, and several other diseases. Therefore, one needs to balance sun exposure in favor of benefits while avoiding potential harmful effects [25–27].

2. Vitamin D and Gene Regulation

$1,25(OH)_2D$ regulates many genes within the human genome [28]. Tissue vitamin D concentrations and its receptor gene polymorphisms, not only influence mechanism of actions and modulate second messenger systems, but also modulate the ability of the ligand-bound VDR to bind to vitamin D response elements (VDREs) on promoter regions in genes and initiate second messenger systems [29]. The National Human Genome Research Institute (NHGRI) launched a public research consortium, ENCODE [Encyclopedia of DNA Elements; http://www.genome.gov/10005107] to answer pertinent questions [30].

ENCODE has demonstrated the genome-wide actions of $1,25(OH)_2D_3$ on the formation rates of proteins, such as the insulator protein CTCF (transcriptional repressor CTCF; 11-zinc finger protein, CCCTC-binding factor, etc.) and the VDR [31,32]. These findings suggest the presence of numerous functional VDRE regions across the human genome [29,33]. In addition, it has been suggested that the expression of these genes could be used as biomarkers for different actions of vitamin D in varied tissues and cells and assessment of vulnerabilities [34].

Hormone, $1,25(OH)_2D$ modulates cell proliferation through direct and indirect pathways. For example, vitamin D inhibits the pathways related to transcription factor NF-κB [35]. People with chronic non-communicable diseases, such as cardiovascular disease, type 2 diabetes, autoimmune diseases, arthritis, and osteoporosis are reported to have chronically elevated NF-κB [36]. NF-κB enhances the oxidative stress and cellular responses to inflammation and injury; including following head injury [37]. Whereas, $1,25(OH)_2D$ (calcitriol) suppresses NF-κB and thereby reduces chronic diffuse somatic inflammation [38,39]. In addition, calcitriol also reduce cell proliferation and enhance cell differentiation—key anti-cancer effects of vitamin D [40].

2.1. Epigenetic Mechanisms Influence Cancer Genesis

Epigenetic mechanisms influence cancer genesis, growth, dissemination, and aging phenomena [41–44]. For example, the epigenetic modifications of VDR–$1,25(OH)_2D$ effects can be mediated through complex processes involving CYP27A1 and CYP27B1 and via the vitamin D-catabolizing enzyme CYP24 [14,44]. These actions can be favorably influenced by modifications of VDREs across the genome modulated by both histone acetylases and deacetylases [28,29,45].

Epigenetic regulation of vitamin D metabolism influences several physiological mechanisms and modulate outcomes of some human diseases. Example of diseases include adenocarcinoma of the lung [44], specific gene mutations in Asians with advanced non-small cell lung cancer [41], and genetic alterations in the effectiveness of systemic therapy for lung cancer induced by cigarette smoking [42]. In severely obese children, low 25(OH)D concentrations are associated with increased markers of oxidative and nitrosative stress, inflammation, and endothelial over-activation [46].

CYP27B1-mediated target tissue production of 1,25(OH)D is critically important for the paracrine and autocrine functions of calcitriol to obtain the full biological potential of vitamin D. Taken together, the benefits of having adequate serum 25(OH)D concentrations and maintaining vitamin D repletion in the long run and considering the overall health benefits of vitamin D, there is an urgent need to create national policies to combat hypovitaminosis D. The savings derived from reducing the risks and severity of infectious and parasitic diseases alone would pay-off the cost of this public health approach. This can be achieved through targeting to raise the population serum 25(OH)D concentration, leading to a tangible positive impact on humans and on the economy.

2.2. Epigenetics and Molecular Genetics of Vitamin D

Molecular and genetic studies confirm that vitamin D also modulates risks of several other human diseases, including autoimmune disorders such as multiple sclerosis [47]. Although the predominant cause of cancer is modulation of the underlying metabolic abnormalities through genes, such as p53 and c-myc modifying the metastatic risks, the responsiveness to therapy is in part determined by epigenetic modifications of genes.

Tumor-related key metabolic abnormalities include imbalance between glucose fermentation and oxidative phosphorylation (under aerobic and anaerobic conditions—the Warburg effect); dysregulation of metabolic enzymes, such as pyruvate kinase, fumarate hydratase, and succinate dehydrogenase; isocitrate dehydrogenase mutations; and alterations of gene expression levels linked to tumorigenesis that are influenced by the vitamin D status [48].

Examples related to activity of the vitamin D axis include epigenetic changes that affect the expression of the CYP24A1 gene and VDR polymorphisms. Although epigenetic enhancement can occur through methylation and repression by histone-modifications of DNA, vitamin D markedly influences the regulation of cell replication [42,44]. This substantiates targeting of CYP24A1 to optimize the antiproliferative effects of 1,25(OH)$_2$D in a target-specific manner [49].

In addition, gene activation following the interaction of 1,25(OH)$_2$D with VDR is important for mitochondrial integrity and respiration, and many other physiological activities. Moreover, the vitamin D signaling pathway plays a central role in protecting cells from elevated mitochondrial respiration and associated damage and overproduction of reactive oxygen species (ROS), which can lead to cellular and DNA damage [50].

3. Vitamin D–Oxidative Stress

1,25(OH)$_2$D is involved in many intracellular genomic activities and biochemical and enzymatic reactions, whereas 25(OH)D concentrations are important in overcoming inflammation, the destruction of invading microbes and parasites, the minimization of oxidative stress following the day-to-day exposure to toxic agents, and controlling the aging process [51,52].

For example, the presence of a physiologic 25(OH)D concentration enhances the expression of the nuclear factor, erythroid-2(Nf-E2)-related factor 2(Nrf2) [53–55] and enhances Klotho, a phosphate regulating hormone and also an antiaging protein [56,57]. It also facilitates protein stabilization [11]. Klotho also regulates cellular signaling systems, including the formation of antioxidants [58]. Consequently, in mice, functional abnormalities of the Klotho gene or removal of it through gene knock-out procedures induce premature aging syndrome [59]. In animal studies, inefficient FGF23 and/or Klotho expression have shown to cause premature aging. Figure 1 is a schematic representation of various key factors and their interactions that influence aging and death.

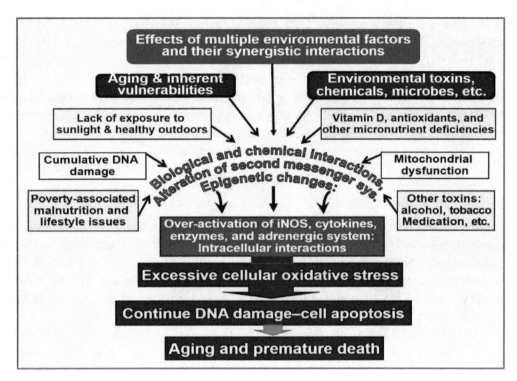

Figure 1. Environmental, microbial, biological and chemical interactions that modify the DNA and mitochondrial functions and epigenetics, which modifies the aging process. Vitamin D deficiency is one of the factors that enhances this oxidative-stress cycle and accelerating premature cell death [abbreviations used: DNA = deoxyribonucleic acid; iNOS = inducible nitric oxide enzyme].

Influences of Vitamin D on Oxidative Stress

When vitamin D status is adequate, many of the intracellular oxidative stress-related activities are downregulated. Having suboptimal concentrations of serum 25(OH)D fails to subdue oxidative stress conditions, augment intracellular oxidative damage and the rate of apoptosis. The intracellular Nrf2 level is inversely correlated with the accumulation of mitochondrial ROS [51,60] and the consequent escalation of oxidative stress. Thus, Nrf2 plays a key role in protecting cells against oxidative stress; this is modulated by vitamin D [61,62].

In addition, vitamin D supports cellular oxidation and reduction (redox) control by maintaining normal mitochondrial functions [63–65]. Loss in the redox control of the cell cycle may lead to aberrant cell proliferation, cell death, the development of neurodegenerative diseases, and accelerated aging [65–68]. Peroxisome proliferator-activated receptor-coactivator 1α (PGC-1α) is bound to mitochondrial deacetylase (SIRT3). PGC-1α directly couples to the oxidative stress cycle [69] and interacts with Nrf2. This complex regulates the expression of SIRT3; this process is influenced by vitamin D metabolites [70]. In addition, the activation of the mitochondrial Nrf2/PGC-1α-SIRT3 path is dependent on intracellular calcitriol concentrations.

Calcitriol has overarching beneficial effects in upregulating the expression of certain antioxidants and anti-inflammatory cytokines [71], thereby protecting the tissues from toxins, micronutrient deficiency-related abnormalities, and parasitic and intracellular microbe-induced harm [72]. It regulates ROS levels through its anti-inflammatory effects and mitochondrial-based expression of antioxidants through cell-signaling pathways [67,73].

4. Role of Vitamin D in Neutralization of Toxins and Aging-Related Compounds

Following 1,25(OH)$_2$D—VDR interaction, the transcription factor Nrf2 translocates from the cytoplasm to the nucleus. Nrf2 activates the expression of several genes that have antioxidant activity [52,54,67]. When Nrf2 activity is insufficient, risks from oxidative stress-related tissue damage increases [61,74]. The resultant excessive ROS formation by dysregulated mitochondria leads to a pathologic oxidative stress cycle, a key cause of toxin-induced and age-related cell death [68,75,76].

Meanwhile, the Nrf2 activity in part is controlled by the cytosolic protein Keap1 [77], another transcription factor and a negative regulator of Nrf2 [55,61]. Keap1 also controls the subcellular distribution of Nrf2 that correlates with its antioxidant activity [53,54]. When confronted with intracellular oxidative and/or electrophilic stresses, as a protective mechanism, the Nrf2-antioxidant response path is activated. This response enhances gene transcription and translation of protein products that are necessary to eliminate and/or neutralize toxins, ROS, and cumulating aging-related products through conjugation [78,79].

4.1. The Concept and the Process of Aging

Aging generally refers to the biological process of growing older, also known as cellular senescence, and is a complex process. Advancing age is, especially after adulthood, is associated with a gradual decline of physiological functions and capacities [80]. Aging has also been quantified from mortality curves using mathematical modeling; for example, by using Gompertz equation $m(t) = Ae^{Gt}$, for which, $m(t)$ = the mortality rate as a function of time or age (t); A = extrapolated constant to birth or maturity; G = the exponential (Gompertz) mortality rate coefficient] [79].

Moreover, efficiency and the functions of the body decline after sexual maturity, suggesting a connection between the aging process after fulfilling the procreation needs. Most age-related functions are irreversible, in part due to accumulation of oxidative stress-related toxic products, methylation of DNA, and mitochondrial damage, leading to reduced viability of cells and consequent accelerated cell death [81]. There is also a parallel decline in the immune system functions (i.e., immune-senescence) and an increase in inflammation, demonstrable with increased circulating pro-inflammatory cytokines [82,83]. These are likely to contribute to several age-related disorders, such as Alzheimer's disease, cardiovascular and pulmonary diseases, and susceptibility to autoimmunity and infections [82,83].

Many bodily functions slow with aging, including response and reaction time; access to and the capacity of memory; pulmonary, gastrointestinal, and cardiovascular capacities; and even the ability to generate vitamin D in the skin. While age is perhaps the strongest risk factors for death, age-related disorders are the number one cause of death among the adults. This scenario is aggravated in the presence of vitamin D deficiency.

Chronic hypovitaminosis D is associated with cardiovascular and metabolic dysfunctions and premature deaths [84], even among children [85]. Overall data suggest that vitamin D deficiency could be considered an important comorbidity or a risk factor for premature death [84–87]. In fact, inverse relationships have been reported with vitamin D adequacy, with reduced all-cause mortality [88–90], and cancer [90–93].

4.2. Effects of Vitamin D on Apoptosis and Aging

The generalized inflammatory process is known to cause cellular damage and increase apoptosis [94], as in the case of interstitial tubular cell damage in chronic kidney disease, and thus is a part of the aging process [52,55,95]. In addition, hypovitaminosis D and dysfunctional mitochondrial activity increase inflammation [73,96,97]. Thus, the anti-inflammatory effects from having adequate, physiological vitamin D concentrations are important [95,98]. Hypovitaminosis D increases the expression of inflammatory cytokines [71,99] such as tumor necrosis factor-α (TNF-α), increasing the expression of the InsP3Rs and resulting in increased intracellular Ca^{2+} and accelerating cellular damage, apoptosis, and aging [66,75].

Many of the genes in the Klotho–Nrf2 regulatory system have multiple functions that are regulated by calcitriol [57,62,65]. These include, increasing intracellular antioxidant concentration, maintaining the redox homeostasis and, normal intracellular-reduced environment by removing excess ROS, and thereby down-regulating the oxidative stress [100]. In addition, the vitamin D-dependent expression of γ-glutamyl transpeptidase, glutamate cysteine ligase, and glutathione reductase contribute to the synthesis of the key redox agent glutathione (an essential antioxidant of low–molecular-weight thiol) [99,101].

Vitamin D also upregulates the expression of glutathione peroxidase that converts the ROS molecule H_2O_2 to water [101]. Vitamin D also effect the formation of glutathione through activation of the enzyme glucose-6-phosphate dehydrogenase [101]—which downregulates nitrogen oxide (NOx), a potent precursor for generating ROS that converts O_2^- to H_2O_2 and upregulating superoxide dismutase (SOD). These vitamin D-related actions collectively reduce the burden of intracellular ROS.

Telomeres are repetitive DNA sequences that caps end of linear chromosomes protecting DNA molecules [102]. Aging is associated with shortening of telomeres, including in stem cells. The amount of telomerase present is gradually become too short to maintain its protective effects on DNA during cell division, and thus cell apoptosis. While vitamin D deficiency increases inflammation and the intracellular oxidative stress, the latter enhances the rate of telomere shortening during cell proliferation, resulting in genomic instability [36].

4.3. Hypovitaminosis D Leads to Deranged Mitochondrial Respiration

Activated vitamin D is an essential component for maintaining physiological respiratory chain activity in mitochondria, facilitating the generation of energy [103,104]. In addition, 25(OH)D regulates the expression of the uncoupling protein that is attached to the inner membrane of mitochondria that regulates thermogenesis [105–107]. Chronic vitamin D deficiency reduces the capacity of mitochondrial respiration through modulating nuclear mRNA [108–110]. The latter also downregulates the expression of complex I of the electron transport chain and thus reduces the formation of adenosine triphosphate (ATP) [67,75], another mechanism that increases cancer risks. Consequently, a low level of electron transport chain increases the formation of ROS and oxidative stress, a common phenomenon following acute and chronic exposure to toxins and many chronic diseases and seen in aging [66,111,112].

The accumulation of intracellular toxins and/or age-related products disrupts signaling pathways, including the G protein–coupled systems, caspases, mitochondria, and the death receptor-linked mechanisms, triggering cell apoptosis and causing premature cell death [113,114]. The process is aggravated by stimulating G proteins, leading to activation of downstream pathways, including protein kinase A and C (PKA and PKC), phosphatidylinositol 3 kinase (PI3-kinase), Ca^{2+} and MAP kinase-dependent systems, tyrosine phosphorylation [75,114], and work additively, aiding cancer genesis [93] and accelerating the aging process.

4.4. Calcitriol Protects Mitochondrial Functions

Toxins, chronic metabolic abnormalities, and the aging process are known to cause mitochondrial dysfunction [66,106–108,115]. Abnormal mitochondria produce suboptimal amounts of ATP while generating excess ROS, creating a vicious cycle of enhanced and persisting the effects from excessive oxidative stress [106,107,116]. These events cause DNA damage (and impair DNA repair systems), premature cell death, and accelerated aging [62,66]. Data are accumulating that suggest that mitochondrial dysfunction is likely fueled by sustained intracellular inflammation, as in the case with vitamin D deficiency [79,95,97,117].

Based on animal studies, researchers have reported that mitochondrial decay, a part of the aging process, can be slowed by micronutrient supplementation (e.g., by lipoic acid, acetyl carnitine, vitamin K, and vitamin D) and by boosting coenzyme levels through high doses of vitamin B, such as pantothenic acid [118]. The NAD^+-dependent protein deacetylases sirtuins function as antiaging proteins that also neutralize excess ROS [11]. For example, sirtuin 1 (SIRT) is essential to maintaining normal mitochondrial functions; meanwhile, calcitriol and SIRT1 work synergistically to regenerate mitochondria [119,120]. Their actions facilitate the removal and neutralization of toxins and thereby reduce the rate and the effects of aging [121,122].

Dysfunctional mitochondria also have reduced intracellular Ca^{2+} buffering capacity, resulting in increased (and fluctuating) intracellular Ca^{2+} levels, which are cytotoxic and contribute to sustenance of several chronic diseases [108,115]. Sub physiological concentrations of calcitriol, at least in part, enhance and maintain oxidative stress, autophagy, inflammation, mitochondrial dysfunction, epigenetic changes, DNA damage, intracellular Ca^{2+}, and generation and signaling of ROS. Therefore, sustained, adequate serum 25(OH)D concentrations should allow target tissues to keep many of these harmful processes under control [68,71,73]. Multiple benefits of controlling excessive oxidative stress are illustrated in Figure 2.

Figure 2. Oxidative stress is harmful to cells. Controlling oxidative stresses through vitamin D adequacy leads to cellular and organ protection and reduces the effects of aging [abbreviations used: CNS = central nervous system; DNA = deoxyribonucleic acid; MI = myocardial infarction; PVD = peripheral vascular diseases].

5. Discussion

The proper functioning of the vitamin D endocrine, paracrine, and autocrine systems is essential for many human physiological functions. Vitamin D deficiency, as determined by serum 25(OH)D concentrations of less than 30 ng/mL, is associated with increased risks of illnesses and disorders and increased all-cause mortality even among apparently healthy individuals, including those with normal serum 1,25(OH)$_2$D. Some of the key functions of vitamin D include subduing oxidative stress and chronic inflammation and maintaining mitochondrial respiratory functions. Through its targeted mitochondrial activity and subduing of ROS through multiple mechanisms, vitamin D has key beneficial effects on controlling oxidative stress, inflammation, and energy metabolism.

Normal serum concentrations of both 25(OH)D and 1,25(OH)$_2$D are essential for optimal cellular function and protect from the excessive oxidative stress-related DNA damage. However, increased risk for illnesses and reduced longevity can occur despite the presence of physiologic concentrations of calcitriol because this is not the only mechanism protecting cells from oxidative stress. Physiologic serum 25(OH)D and 1,25(OH)$_2$D levels in target tissues allow exertion of the homeostatic modulatory effects on enzymatic reactions, mitochondrial activities, and functioning of optimal second messenger systems. These are essential parts of the actions of vitamin D mediated through the mentioned mechanisms.

Vitamin D metabolism and functions are modulated by many factors, including physical activities and lifestyles, certain medications, environmental pollutants, and epigenetics, all of which also modify the balance between energy intake and expenditure through mitochondrial metabolic control [123]. For reductions in the incidence of diseases, longer-term maintenance of a steady state of the serum 25(OH)D concentration is necessary [124]. The minimal level is considered to be 30 ng/mL (50 nmol/L).

After correction of vitamin D deficiency through loading doses of oral vitamin D (or safe sun exposure), adequate maintenance doses of vitamin D_3 are needed. This can be achieved in approximately 90% of the adult population with vitamin D supplementation between 1000 to 4000 IU/day, 10,000 IU twice a week, or 50,000 IU twice a month [10,125]. On a population basis, such doses would allow approximately 97% of people to maintain their serum 25(OH)D concentrations above 30 ng/mL [19,126]. Others, such as persons with obesity, those with gastrointestinal disorders, and during pregnancy and lactation, are likely to require doses of 6,000 IU/day [127,128].

Acknowledgments: The author greatly appreciates the helpful comments of Eugene L. Heyden.

Abbreviations

1,25(OH)$_2$D	1,25-dihydroxyvitamin D
25(OH)D	25-hydroxy vitamin D
Nrf2	Nuclear factor erythroid 2 (Nf-E2)-related factor 2
PTH	Parathyroid hormone
ROS	Reactive oxygen species
UVB	Ultraviolet B
VDR	Vitamin D receptor
VDRE	Vitamin D response element

References

1. Van Schoor, N.M.; Lips, P. Worldwide vitamin D status. *Best Pract. Res. Clin. Endocrinol. Metab.* **2011**, *25*, 671–680. [CrossRef] [PubMed]

2. Eggemoen, A.R.; Knutsen, K.V.; Dalen, I.; Jenum, A.K. Vitamin D status in recently arrived immigrants from Africa and Asia: A cross-sectional study from Norway of children, adolescents and adults. *BMJ Open* **2013**, *3*, e003293. [CrossRef] [PubMed]

3. Garland, C.F.; Gorham, E.D.; Mohr, S.B.; Garland, F.C. Vitamin D for cancer prevention: Global perspective. *Ann. Epidemiol.* **2009**, *19*, 468–483. [CrossRef]

4. Hilger, J.; Friedel, A.; Herr, R.; Rausch, T.; Roos, F.; Wahl, D.A.; Pierroz, D.D.; Weber, P.; Hoffmann, K. A systematic review of vitamin D status in populations worldwide. *Br. J. Nutr.* **2014**, *111*, 23–45. [CrossRef]

5. Haq, A.; Wimalawansa, S.J.; Carlberg, C. Highlights from the 5th International Conference on Vitamin D Deficiency, Nutrition and Human Health, Abu Dhabi, United Arab Emirates, March 24-25, 2016. *J. Steroid Biochem. Mol. Biol.* **2018**, *175*, 1–3. [CrossRef]

6. Pludowski, P.; Holick, M.F.; Grant, W.B.; Konstantynowicz, J.; Mascarenhas, M.R.; Haq, A.; Povoroznyuk, V.; Balatska, N.; Barbosa, A.P.; Karonova, T.; et al. Vitamin D supplementation guidelines. *J. Steroid Biochem. Mol. Biol.* **2018**, *175*, 125–135. [CrossRef]

7. Felton, S.J.; Cooke, M.S.; Kift, R.; Berry, J.L.; Webb, A.R.; Lam, P.M.; de Gruijl, F.R.; Vail, A.; Rhodes, L.E. Concurrent beneficial (vitamin D production) and hazardous (cutaneous DNA damage) impact of repeated low-level summer sunlight exposures. *Br. J. Dermatol.* **2016**, *175*, 1320–1328. [CrossRef] [PubMed]

8. Gordon-Thomson, C.; Tongkao-on, W.; Song, E.J.; Carter, S.E.; Dixon, K.M.; Mason, R.S. Protection from ultraviolet damage and photocarcinogenesis by vitamin D compounds. *Adv. Exp. Med. Biol.* **2014**, *810*, 303–328. [PubMed]

9. Petersen, B.; Wulf, H.C.; Triguero-Mas, M.; Philipsen, P.A.; Thieden, E.; Olsen, P.; Heydenreich, J.; Dadvand, P.; Basagana, X.; Liljendahl, T.S.; et al. Sun and ski holidays improve vitamin D status, but are associated with high levels of DNA damage. *J. Investig. Dermatol.* **2014**, *134*, 2806–2813. [CrossRef] [PubMed]

10. Wimalawansa, S.J. Vitamin D. What clinicians would like to know. *Sri Lanka Journal of Diabetes, Endocrinology and Metabolism* **2012**, *1*, 73–88. [CrossRef]

11. Mark, K.A.; Dumas, K.J.; Bhaumik, D.; Schilling, B.; Davis, S.; Oron, T.R.; Sorensen, D.J.; Lucanic, M.; Brem, R.B.; Melov, S.; et al. Vitamin D Promotes Protein Homeostasis and Longevity via the Stress Response Pathway Genes skn-1, ire-1, and xbp-1. *Cell Rep.* **2016**, *17*, 1227–1237. [CrossRef] [PubMed]

12. Grant, W.B.; Boucher, B.J.; Bhattoa, H.P.; Lahore, H. Why vitamin D clinical trials should be based on 25-hydroxyvitamin D concentrations. *J. Steroid Biochem. Mol. Biol.* **2018**, *177*, 266–269. [CrossRef] [PubMed]

13. Kroll, M.H.; Bi, C.; Garber, C.C.; Kaufman, H.W.; Liu, D.; Caston-Balderrama, A.; Zhang, K.; Clarke, N.; Xie, M.; Reitz, R.E.; et al. Temporal relationship between vitamin D status and parathyroid hormone in the United States. *PLoS ONE* **2015**, *10*, e0118108. [CrossRef] [PubMed]

14. Jones, G.; Prosser, D.E.; Kaufmann, M. 25-Hydroxyvitamin D-24-hydroxylase (CYP24A1): Its important role in the degradation of vitamin D. *Arch. Biochem. Biophys.* **2012**, *523*, 9–18. [CrossRef] [PubMed]

15. Webb, A.R.; DeCosta, B.R.; Holick, M.F. Sunlight regulates the cutaneous production of vitamin D3 by causing its photodegradation. *J. Clin. Endocrinol. Metab.* **1989**, *68*, 882–887. [CrossRef]

16. Armbrecht, H.J.; Hodam, T.L.; Boltz, M.A.; Partridge, N.C.; Brown, A.J.; Kumar, V.B. Induction of the vitamin D 24-hydroxylase (CYP24) by 1,25-dihydroxyvitamin D3 is regulated by parathyroid hormone in UMR106 osteoblastic cells. *Endocrinology* **1998**, *139*, 3375–3381. [CrossRef]

17. Miller, W.L. Genetic disorders of Vitamin D biosynthesis and degradation. *J. Steroid Biochem. Mol. Biol.* **2017**, *165*, 101–108. [CrossRef]

18. Mithal, A.; Wahl, D.A.; Bonjour, J.P.; Burckhardt, P.; Dawson-Hughes, B.; Eisman, J.A.; El-Hajj Fuleihan, G.; Josse, R.G.; Lips, P.; Morales-Torres, J. Global vitamin D status and determinants of hypovitaminosis D. *Osteoporos. Int.* **2009**, *20*, 1807–1820. [CrossRef]

19. Wimalawansa, S.J. Vitamin D in the new millennium. *Curr. Osteoporos. Rep.* **2012**, *10*, 4–15. [CrossRef]

20. Grant, W.B.; Wimalawansa, S.J.; Holick, M.F. Vitamin D supplements and reasonable solar UVB should be recommended to prevent escalating incidence of chronic diseases. *Br. Med. J.* **2015**, *350*, h321.

21. Holick, M.F. High prevalence of vitamin D inadequacy and implications for health. *Mayo Clin. Proc.* **2006**, *81*, 353–373. [CrossRef]

22. Calzavara-Pinton, P.; Ortel, B.; Venturini, M. Non-melanoma skin cancer, sun exposure and sun protection. *Giornale Italiano di Dermatologia e Venereologia* **2015**, *150*, 369–378.

23. Cascinelli, N.; Krutmann, J.; MacKie, R.; Pierotti, M.; Prota, G.; Rosso, S.; Young, A. European School of Oncology advisory report. Sun exposure, UVA lamps and risk of skin cancer. *Eur. J. Cancer* **1994**, *30A*, 548–560. [PubMed]

24. Moan, J.; Porojnicu, A.C.; Dahlback, A.; Setlow, R.B. Addressing the health benefits and risks, involving vitamin D or skin cancer, of increased sun exposure. *Proc. Natl. Acad. Sci. USA* **2008**, *105*, 668–673. [CrossRef]

25. Omura, Y. Clinical Significance of Human Papillomavirus Type 16 for Breast Cancer & Adenocarcinomas of Various Internal Organs and Alzheimer's Brain with Increased beta-amyloid (1-42); Combined Use of Optimal Doses of Vitamin D3 and Taurine 3 times/day Has Significant Beneficial Effects of Anti-Cancer, Anti-Ischemic Heart, and Memory & Other Brain Problems By Significant Urinary Excretion of Viruses, Bacteria, and Toxic Metals & Substances. *Acupunct. Electro-Ther. Res.* **2016**, *41*, 127–134.

26. Gilad, L.A.; Bresler, T.; Gnainsky, J.; Smirnoff, P.; Schwartz, B. Regulation of vitamin D receptor expression via estrogen-induced activation of the ERK 1/2 signaling pathway in colon and breast cancer cells. *J. Endocrinol.* **2005**, *185*, 577–592. [CrossRef] [PubMed]

27. Robsahm, T.E.; Tretli, S.; Dahlback, A.; Moan, J. Vitamin D3 from sunlight may improve the prognosis of breast-, colon- and prostate cancer (Norway). *Cancer Causes Control* **2004**, *15*, 149–158. [CrossRef] [PubMed]

28. Jeon, S.M.; Shin, E.A. Exploring vitamin D metabolism and function in cancer. *Exp. Mol. Med.* **2018**, *50*, 20. [CrossRef] [PubMed]

29. Valdivielso, J.M. The physiology of vitamin D receptor activation. *Contrib. Nephrol.* **2009**, *163*, 206–212. [PubMed]

30. Farnham, P.J. Thematic minireview series on results from the ENCODE Project: Integrative global analyses of regulatory regions in the human genome. *J. Biol. Chem.* **2012**, *287*, 30885–30887. [CrossRef]

31. Washington, S.D.; Edenfield, S.I.; Lieux, C.; Watson, Z.L.; Taasan, S.M.; Dhummakupt, A.; Bloom, D.C.; Neumann, D.M. Depletion of the insulator protein CTCF results in HSV-1 reactivation in vivo. *J. Virol.* **2018**. [CrossRef]

32. MacPherson, M.J.; Sadowski, P.D. The CTCF insulator protein forms an unusual DNA structure. *BMC Mol. Biol.* **2010**, *11*, 101. [CrossRef] [PubMed]

33. Carlberg, C. Genome-wide (over)view on the actions of vitamin D. *Front. Physiol.* **2014**, *5*, 167. [CrossRef]

34. Narvaez, C.J.; Matthews, D.; LaPorta, E.; Simmons, K.M.; Beaudin, S.; Welsh, J. The impact of vitamin D in breast cancer: Genomics, pathways, metabolism. *Front. Physiol.* **2014**, *5*, 213. [CrossRef]

35. Tilstra, J.S.; Robinson, A.R.; Wang, J.; Gregg, S.Q.; Clauson, C.L.; Reay, D.P.; Nasto, L.A.; St Croix, C.M.; Usas, A.; Vo, N.; et al. NF-kappaB inhibition delays DNA damage-induced senescence and aging in mice. *J. Clin. Investig.* **2012**, *122*, 2601–2612. [CrossRef]

36. Pusceddu, I.; Farrell, C.J.; Di Pierro, A.M.; Jani, E.; Herrmann, W.; Herrmann, M. The role of telomeres and vitamin D in cellular aging and age-related diseases. *Clin. Chem. Lab. Med.* **2015**, *53*, 1661–1678. [CrossRef] [PubMed]

37. Tang, H.; Hua, F.; Wang, J.; Sayeed, I.; Wang, X.; Chen, Z.; Yousuf, S.; Atif, F.; Stein, D.G. Progesterone and vitamin D: Improvement after traumatic brain injury in middle-aged rats. *Horm. Behav.* **2013**, *64*, 527–538. [CrossRef] [PubMed]

38. Wang, Q.; He, Y.; Shen, Y.; Zhang, Q.; Chen, D.; Zuo, C.; Qin, J.; Wang, H.; Wang, J.; Yu, Y. Vitamin D inhibits COX-2 expression and inflammatory response by targeting thioesterase superfamily member 4. *J. Biol. Chem.* **2014**, *289*, 11681–11694. [CrossRef] [PubMed]

39. Myszka, M.; Klinger, M. The immunomodulatory role of Vitamin D. *Postepy Hig. Med. Dosw.* **2014**, *68*, 865–878. [CrossRef]

40. Watanabe, R.; Inoue, D. Current Topics on Vitamin D. Anti-cancer effects of vitamin D. *Clin. Calcium* **2015**, *25*, 373–380.

41. Shi, Y.; Au, J.S.; Thongprasert, S.; Srinivasan, S.; Tsai, C.M.; Khoa, M.T.; Heeroma, K.; Itoh, Y.; Cornelio, G.; Yang, P.C. A prospective, molecular epidemiology study of EGFR mutations in Asian patients with advanced non-small-cell lung cancer of adenocarcinoma histology (PIONEER). *J. Thorac. Oncol.* **2014**, *9*, 154–162. [CrossRef]

42. O'Malley, M.; King, A.N.; Conte, M.; Ellingrod, V.L.; Ramnath, N. Effects of cigarette smoking on metabolism and effectiveness of systemic therapy for lung cancer. *J. Thorac. Oncol.* **2014**, *9*, 917–926. [CrossRef] [PubMed]

43. Iswariya, G.T.; Paital, B.; Padma, P.R.; Nirmaladevi, R. MicroRNAs: Epigenetic players in cancer and aging. *Front. Biosci. (Schol Ed)* **2019**, *11*, 29–55.

44. Ramnath, N.; Nadal, E.; Jeon, C.K.; Sandoval, J.; Colacino, J.; Rozek, L.S.; Christensen, P.J.; Esteller, M.; Beer, D.G.; Kim, S.H. Epigenetic regulation of vitamin D metabolism in human lung adenocarcinoma. *J. Thorac. Oncol.* **2014**, *9*, 473–482. [CrossRef]

45. Karlic, H.; Varga, F. Impact of vitamin D metabolism on clinical epigenetics. *Clin. Epigenet.* **2011**, *2*, 55–61. [CrossRef] [PubMed]

46. Codoner-Franch, P.; Tavarez-Alonso, S.; Simo-Jorda, R.; Laporta-Martin, P.; Carratala-Calvo, A.; Alonso-Iglesias, E. Vitamin D status is linked to biomarkers of oxidative stress, inflammation, and endothelial activation in obese children. *J. Pediatr.* **2012**, *161*, 848–854. [CrossRef]

47. Zeitelhofer, M.; Adzemovic, M.Z.; Gomez-Cabrero, D.; Bergman, P.; Hochmeister, S.; N'Diaye, M.; Paulson, A.; Ruhrmann, S.; Almgren, M.; Tegner, J.N.; et al. Functional genomics analysis of vitamin D effects on CD4+ T cells in vivo in experimental autoimmune encephalomyelitis. *Proc. Natl. Acad. Sci. USA* **2017**, *114*, E1678–E1687. [CrossRef] [PubMed]

48. Wu, W.; Zhao, S. Metabolic changes in cancer: Beyond the Warburg effect. *Acta Biochim. Biophys. Sin.* **2013**, *45*, 18–26. [CrossRef]

49. Garcia-Quiroz, J.; Garcia-Becerra, R.; Barrera, D.; Santos, N.; Avila, E.; Ordaz-Rosado, D.; Rivas-Suarez, M.; Halhali, A.; Rodriguez, P.; Gamboa-Dominguez, A.; et al. Astemizole synergizes calcitriol antiproliferative activity by inhibiting CYP24A1 and upregulating VDR: A novel approach for breast cancer therapy. *PLoS ONE* **2012**, *7*, e45063. [CrossRef]

50. Ricca, C.; Aillon, A.; Bergandi, L.; Alotto, D.; Castagnoli, C.; Silvagno, F. Vitamin D Receptor Is Necessary for Mitochondrial Function and Cell Health. *Int. J. Mol. Sci.* **2018**, *19*, 1672. [CrossRef]

51. Holmes, S.; Abbassi, B.; Su, C.; Singh, M.; Cunningham, R.L. Oxidative stress defines the neuroprotective or neurotoxic properties of androgens in immortalized female rat dopaminergic neuronal cells. *Endocrinology* **2013**, *154*, 4281–4292. [CrossRef]

52. Petersen, K.S.; Smith, C. Ageing-Associated Oxidative Stress and Inflammation Are Alleviated by Products from Grapes. *Oxid. Med. Cell. Longev.* **2016**, *2016*, 6236309. [CrossRef]

53. Nakai, K.; Fujii, H.; Kono, K.; Goto, S.; Kitazawa, R.; Kitazawa, S.; Hirata, M.; Shinohara, M.; Fukagawa, M.; Nishi, S. Vitamin D activates the Nrf2-Keap1 antioxidant pathway and ameliorates nephropathy in diabetic rats. *Am. J. Hypertens.* **2014**, *27*, 586–595. [CrossRef] [PubMed]

54. Lewis, K.N.; Mele, J.; Hayes, J.D.; Buffenstein, R. Nrf2, a guardian of healthspan and gatekeeper of species longevity. *Integr. Comp. Biol.* **2010**, *50*, 829–843. [CrossRef] [PubMed]

55. Tullet, J.M.A.; Green, J.W.; Au, C.; Benedetto, A.; Thompson, M.A.; Clark, E.; Gilliat, A.F.; Young, A.; Schmeisser, K.; Gems, D. The SKN-1/Nrf2 transcription factor can protect against oxidative stress and increase lifespan in C. elegans by distinct mechanisms. *Aging Cell* **2017**, *16*, 1191–1194. [CrossRef] [PubMed]

56. Forster, R.E.; Jurutka, P.W.; Hsieh, J.C.; Haussler, C.A.; Lowmiller, C.L.; Kaneko, I.; Haussler, M.R.; Kerr Whitfield, G. Vitamin D receptor controls expression of the anti-aging klotho gene in mouse and human renal cells. *Biochem. Biophys. Res. Commun.* **2011**, *414*, 557–562. [CrossRef]

57. Berridge, M.J. Vitamin D: A custodian of cell signalling stability in health and disease. *Biochem. Soc. Trans.* **2015**, *43*, 349–358. [CrossRef]

58. Razzaque, M.S. FGF23, klotho and vitamin D interactions: What have we learned from in vivo mouse genetics studies? *Adv. Exp. Med. Biol.* **2012**, *728*, 84–91.

59. Kuro-o, M. Klotho and aging. *Biochim. Biophys. Acta* **2009**, *1790*, 1049–1058. [CrossRef]

60. Tseng, A.H.; Shieh, S.S.; Wang, D.L. SIRT3 deacetylates FOXO3 to protect mitochondria against oxidative damage. *Free Radic. Biol. Med.* **2013**, *63*, 222–234. [CrossRef]

61. Wang, L.; Lewis, T.; Zhang, Y.L.; Khodier, C.; Magesh, S.; Chen, L.; Inoyama, D.; Chen, Y.; Zhen, J.; Hu, L.; et al. The identification and characterization of non-reactive inhibitor of Keap1-Nrf2 interaction through HTS using a fluorescence polarization assay. In *Probe Reports from the NIH Molecular Libraries Program*; National Center for Biotechnology Information (US): Bethesda, MD, USA, 2010.

62. Berridge, M.J. Vitamin D deficiency: Infertility and neurodevelopmental diseases (attention deficit hyperactivity disorder, autism, and schizophrenia). *Am. J. Physiol. Cell Physiol.* **2018**, *314*, C135–C151. [CrossRef]

63. Ryan, Z.C.; Craig, T.A.; Folmes, C.D.; Wang, X.; Lanza, I.R.; Schaible, N.S.; Salisbury, J.L.; Nair, K.S.; Terzic, A.; Sieck, G.C.; et al. 1alpha,25-Dihydroxyvitamin D3 Regulates Mitochondrial Oxygen Consumption and Dynamics in Human Skeletal Muscle Cells. *J. Biol. Chem.* **2016**, *291*, 1514–1528. [CrossRef]

64. Bouillon, R.; Verstuyf, A. Vitamin D, mitochondria, and muscle. *J. Clin. Endocrinol. Metab.* **2013**, *98*, 961–963. [CrossRef]

65. Sarsour, E.H.; Kumar, M.G.; Chaudhuri, L.; Kalen, A.L.; Goswami, P.C. Redox control of the cell cycle in health and disease. *Antioxid. Redox Signal.* **2009**, *11*, 2985–3011. [CrossRef]

66. Lin, M.T.; Beal, M.F. Mitochondrial dysfunction and oxidative stress in neurodegenerative diseases. *Nature* **2006**, *443*, 787–795. [CrossRef]

67. Berridge, M.J. Vitamin D cell signalling in health and disease. *Biochem. Biophys. Res. Commun.* **2015**, *460*, 53–71. [CrossRef]

68. Ureshino, R.P.; Rocha, K.K.; Lopes, G.S.; Bincoletto, C.; Smaili, S.S. Calcium signaling alterations, oxidative stress, and autophagy in aging. *Antioxid. Redox Signal.* **2014**, *21*, 123–137. [CrossRef]

69. Chen, Y.; Zhang, J.; Lin, Y.; Lei, Q.; Guan, K.L.; Zhao, S.; Xiong, Y. Tumour suppressor SIRT3 deacetylates and activates manganese superoxide dismutase to scavenge ROS. *EMBO Rep.* **2011**, *12*, 534–541. [CrossRef]

70. Song, C.; Fu, B.; Zhang, J.; Zhao, J.; Yuan, M.; Peng, W.; Zhang, Y.; Wu, H. Sodium fluoride induces nephrotoxicity via oxidative stress-regulated mitochondrial SIRT3 signaling pathway. *Sci. Rep.* **2017**, *7*, 672. [CrossRef]

71. Wei, R.; Christakos, S. Mechanisms Underlying the Regulation of Innate and Adaptive Immunity by Vitamin D. *Nutrients* **2015**, *7*, 8251–8260. [CrossRef]

72. George, N.; Kumar, T.P.; Antony, S.; Jayanarayanan, S.; Paulose, C.S. Effect of vitamin D3 in reducing metabolic and oxidative stress in the liver of streptozotocin-induced diabetic rats. *Br. J. Nutr.* **2012**, *108*, 1410–1418. [CrossRef]

73. Shelton, R.C.; Claiborne, J.; Sidoryk-Wegrzynowicz, M.; Reddy, R.; Aschner, M.; Lewis, D.A.; Mirnics, K. Altered expression of genes involved in inflammation and apoptosis in frontal cortex in major depression. *Mol. Psychiatry* **2011**, *16*, 751–762. [CrossRef]

74. Ramsey, C.P.; Glass, C.A.; Montgomery, M.B.; Lindl, K.A.; Ritson, G.P.; Chia, L.A.; Hamilton, R.L.; Chu, C.T.; Jordan-Sciutto, K.L. Expression of Nrf2 in neurodegenerative diseases. *J. Neuropathol. Exp. Neurol.* **2007**, *66*, 75–85. [CrossRef] [PubMed]

75. Petersen, O.H.; Verkhratsky, A. Calcium and ATP control multiple vital functions. *Philos. Trans. R. Soc. Lond. B Biol. Sci.* **2016**, *371*, 20150418. [CrossRef]

76. Petrosillo, G.; Di Venosa, N.; Moro, N.; Colantuono, G.; Paradies, V.; Tiravanti, E.; Federici, A.; Ruggiero, F.M.; Paradies, G. In vivo hyperoxic preconditioning protects against rat-heart ischemia/reperfusion injury by inhibiting mitochondrial permeability transition pore opening and cytochrome c release. *Free Radic. Biol. Med.* **2011**, *50*, 477–483. [CrossRef]

77. McMahon, M.; Itoh, K.; Yamamoto, M.; Hayes, J.D. Keap1-dependent proteasomal degradation of transcription factor Nrf2 contributes to the negative regulation of antioxidant response element-driven gene expression. *J. Biol. Chem.* **2003**, *278*, 21592–21600. [CrossRef] [PubMed]

78. Nguyen, T.; Nioi, P.; Pickett, C.B. The Nrf2-antioxidant response element signaling pathway and its activation by oxidative stress. *J. Biol. Chem.* **2009**, *284*, 13291–13295. [CrossRef]

79. Finch, C.E.; Pike, M.C. Maximum life span predictions from the Gompertz mortality model. *J. Gerontol. A Biol. Sci. Med. Sci.* **1996**, *51*, B183–B194. [CrossRef]

80. Macedo, J.C.; Vaz, S.; Logarinho, E. Mitotic Dysfunction Associated with Aging Hallmarks. *Adv. Exp. Med. Biol.* **2017**, *1002*, 153–188.

81. Jallali, N.; Ridha, H.; Thrasivoulou, C.; Underwood, C.; Butler, P.E.; Cowen, T. Vulnerability to ROS-induced cell death in ageing articular cartilage: The role of antioxidant enzyme activity. *Osteoarthr. Cartil.* **2005**, *13*, 614–622. [CrossRef]

82. Fulop, T.; Larbi, A.; Dupuis, G.; Le Page, A.; Frost, E.H.; Cohen, A.A.; Witkowski, J.M.; Franceschi, C. Immunosenescence and Inflamm-Aging As Two Sides of the Same Coin: Friends or Foes? *Front. Immunol.* **2017**, *8*, 1960. [CrossRef]

83. Franceschi, C.; Bonafe, M.; Valensin, S.; Olivieri, F.; De Luca, M.; Ottaviani, E.; De Benedictis, G. Inflamm-aging. An evolutionary perspective on immunosenescence. *Ann. N. Y. Acad. Sci.* **2000**, *908*, 244–254. [CrossRef]

84. Pilz, S.; Marz, W.; Wellnitz, B.; Seelhorst, U.; Fahrleitner-Pammer, A.; Dimai, H.P.; Boehm, B.O.; Dobnig, H. Association of vitamin D deficiency with heart failure and sudden cardiac death in a large cross-sectional study of patients referred for coronary angiography. *J. Clin. Endocrinol. Metab.* **2008**, *93*, 3927–3935. [CrossRef] [PubMed]

85. Cohen, M.C.; Offiah, A.; Sprigg, A.; Al-Adnani, M. Vitamin D deficiency and sudden unexpected death in infancy and childhood: A cohort study. *Pediatr. Dev. Pathol.* **2013**, *16*, 292–300. [CrossRef] [PubMed]

86. Grant, W.B. Vitamin D Deficiency May Explain Comorbidity as an Independent Risk Factor for Death Associated with Cancer in Taiwan. *Asia Pac. J. Public Health* **2015**, *27*, 572–573. [CrossRef] [PubMed]

87. Scorza, F.A.; Albuquerque, M.; Arida, R.M.; Terra, V.C.; Machado, H.R.; Cavalheiro, E.A. Benefits of sunlight: Vitamin D deficiency might increase the risk of sudden unexpected death in epilepsy. *Med. Hypotheses* **2010**, *74*, 158–161. [CrossRef]

88. Autier, P.; Mullie, P.; Macacu, A.; Dragomir, M.; Boniol, M.; Coppens, K.; Pizot, C.; Boniol, M. Effect of vitamin D supplementation on non-skeletal disorders: A systematic review of meta-analyses and randomised trials. *Lancet Diabetes Endocrinol.* **2017**, *5*, 986–1004. [CrossRef]

89. Brenner, H.; Jansen, L.; Saum, K.U.; Holleczek, B.; Schottker, B. Vitamin D Supplementation Trials Aimed at Reducing Mortality Have Much Higher Power When Focusing on People with Low Serum 25-Hydroxyvitamin D Concentrations. *J. Nutr.* **2017**, *147*, 1325–1333. [CrossRef]

90. Autier, P.; Boniol, M.; Pizot, C.; Mullie, P. Vitamin D status and ill health: A systematic review. *Lancet Diabetes Endocrinol.* **2014**, *2*, 76–89. [CrossRef]

91. Bjelakovic, G.; Gluud, L.L.; Nikolova, D.; Whitfield, K.; Krstic, G.; Wetterslev, J.; Gluud, C. Vitamin D supplementation for prevention of cancer in adults. *Cochrane Database Syst. Rev.* **2014**. [CrossRef] [PubMed]

92. Pilz, S.; Tomaschitz, A.; Marz, W.; Drechsler, C.; Ritz, E.; Zittermann, A.; Cavalier, E.; Pieber, T.R.; Lappe, J.M.; Grant, W.B.; et al. Vitamin D, cardiovascular disease and mortality. *Clin. Endocrinol.* **2011**, *75*, 575–584. [CrossRef]

93. Van der Reest, J.; Gottlieb, E. Anti-cancer effects of vitamin C revisited. *Cell Res.* **2016**, *26*, 269–270. [CrossRef]

94. Da Luz Dias, R.; Basso, B.; Donadio, M.V.F.; Pujol, F.V.; Bartrons, R.; Haute, G.V.; Gassen, R.B.; Bregolin, H.D.; Krause, G.; Viau, C.; et al. Leucine reduces the proliferation of MC3T3-E1 cells through DNA damage and cell senescence. *Toxicol. In Vitro* **2018**, *48*, 1–10. [CrossRef]

95. Cevenini, E.; Caruso, C.; Candore, G.; Capri, M.; Nuzzo, D.; Duro, G.; Rizzo, C.; Colonna-Romano, G.; Lio, D.; Di Carlo, D.; et al. Age-related inflammation: The contribution of different organs, tissues and systems. How to face it for therapeutic approaches. *Curr. Pharm. Des.* **2010**, *16*, 609–618. [CrossRef]

96. Talmor, Y.; Bernheim, J.; Klein, O.; Green, J.; Rashid, G. Calcitriol blunts pro-atherosclerotic parameters through NFkappaB and p38 in vitro. *Eur. J. Clin. Investig.* **2008**, *38*, 548–554. [CrossRef]

97. Morris, G.; Maes, M. Mitochondrial dysfunctions in myalgic encephalomyelitis/chronic fatigue syndrome explained by activated immuno-inflammatory, oxidative and nitrosative stress pathways. *Metab. Brain Dis.* **2014**, *29*, 19–36. [CrossRef]

98. Berk, M.; Williams, L.J.; Jacka, F.N.; O'Neil, A.; Pasco, J.A.; Moylan, S.; Allen, N.B.; Stuart, A.L.; Hayley, A.C.; Byrne, M.L.; et al. So depression is an inflammatory disease, but where does the inflammation come from? *BMC Med.* **2013**, *11*, 200. [CrossRef]

99. Beilfuss, J.; Berg, V.; Sneve, M.; Jorde, R.; Kamycheva, E. Effects of a 1-year supplementation with cholecalciferol on interleukin-6, tumor necrosis factor-alpha and insulin resistance in overweight and obese subjects. *Cytokine* **2012**, *60*, 870–874. [CrossRef]

100. Calton, E.K.; Keane, K.N.; Soares, M.J.; Rowlands, J.; Newsholme, P. Prevailing vitamin D status influences mitochondrial and glycolytic bioenergetics in peripheral blood mononuclear cells obtained from adults. *Redox Biol.* **2016**, *10*, 243–250. [CrossRef]

101. Liu, Y.; Hyde, A.S.; Simpson, M.A.; Barycki, J.J. Emerging regulatory paradigms in glutathione metabolism. *Adv. Cancer Res.* **2014**, *122*, 69–101.

102. Weipoltshammer, K.; Schofer, C.; Almeder, M.; Philimonenko, V.V.; Frei, K.; Wachtler, F.; Hozak, P. Intranuclear anchoring of repetitive DNA sequences: Centromeres, telomeres, and ribosomal DNA. *J. Cell Biol.* **1999**, *147*, 1409–1418. [CrossRef] [PubMed]

103. Consiglio, M.; Viano, M.; Casarin, S.; Castagnoli, C.; Pescarmona, G.; Silvagno, F. Mitochondrial and lipogenic effects of vitamin D on differentiating and proliferating human keratinocytes. *Exp. Dermatol.* **2015**, *24*, 748–753. [CrossRef] [PubMed]

104. Wyckelsma, V.L.; Levinger, I.; McKenna, M.J.; Formosa, L.E.; Ryan, M.T.; Petersen, A.C.; Anderson, M.J.; Murphy, R.M. Preservation of skeletal muscle mitochondrial content in older adults: Relationship between mitochondria, fibre type and high-intensity exercise training. *J. Physiol.* **2017**, *595*, 3345–3359. [CrossRef] [PubMed]

105. Constantinescu, A.A.; Abbas, M.; Kassem, M.; Gleizes, C.; Kreutter, G.; Schini-Kerth, V.; Mitrea, I.L.; Toti, F.; Kessler, L. Differential influence of tacrolimus and sirolimus on mitochondrial-dependent signaling for apoptosis in pancreatic cells. *Mol. Cell. Biochem.* **2016**, *418*, 91–102. [CrossRef] [PubMed]

106. Petrosillo, G.; Matera, M.; Casanova, G.; Ruggiero, F.M.; Paradies, G. Mitochondrial dysfunction in rat brain with aging Involvement of complex I, reactive oxygen species and cardiolipin. *Neurochem. Int.* **2008**, *53*, 126–131. [CrossRef] [PubMed]

107. Petrosillo, G.; Matera, M.; Moro, N.; Ruggiero, F.M.; Paradies, G. Mitochondrial complex I dysfunction in rat heart with aging: Critical role of reactive oxygen species and cardiolipin. *Free Radic. Biol. Med.* **2009**, *46*, 88–94. [CrossRef] [PubMed]

108. Yin, F.; Sancheti, H.; Patil, I.; Cadenas, E. Energy metabolism and inflammation in brain aging and Alzheimer's disease. *Free Radic. Biol. Med.* **2016**, *100*, 108–122. [CrossRef] [PubMed]

109. Prior, S.; Kim, A.; Yoshihara, T.; Tobita, S.; Takeuchi, T.; Higuchi, M. Mitochondrial respiratory function induces endogenous hypoxia. *PLoS ONE* **2014**, *9*, e88911. [CrossRef] [PubMed]

110. Scaini, G.; Rezin, G.T.; Carvalho, A.F.; Streck, E.L.; Berk, M.; Quevedo, J. Mitochondrial dysfunction in bipolar disorder: Evidence, pathophysiology and translational implications. *Neurosci. Biobehav. Rev.* **2016**, *68*, 694–713. [CrossRef] [PubMed]

111. Zhu, Q.S.; Xia, L.; Mills, G.B.; Lowell, C.A.; Touw, I.P.; Corey, S.J. G-CSF induced reactive oxygen species involves Lyn-PI3-kinase-Akt and contributes to myeloid cell growth. *Blood* **2006**, *107*, 1847–1856. [CrossRef] [PubMed]

112. Lin, Y.; Berg, A.H.; Iyengar, P.; Lam, T.K.; Giacca, A.; Combs, T.P.; Rajala, M.W.; Du, X.; Rollman, B.; Li, W.; et al. The hyperglycemia-induced inflammatory response in adipocytes: The role of reactive oxygen species. *J. Biol. Chem.* **2005**, *280*, 4617–4626. [CrossRef] [PubMed]

113. Agalakova, A.A.; Gusev, G.P. Molecular mechanisms of cytotoxicity and apoptosis induced by inorganic fluoride. *ISRN Cell Biol.* **2012**, *2012*, 403835. [CrossRef]

114. Agalakova, N.I.; Gusev, G.P. Fluoride induces oxidative stress and ATP depletion in the rat erythrocytes in vitro. *Environ. Toxicol. Pharmacol.* **2012**, *34*, 334–337. [CrossRef]

115. Yin, F.; Sancheti, H.; Liu, Z.; Cadenas, E. Mitochondrial function in ageing: Coordination with signalling and transcriptional pathways. *J. Physiol.* **2016**, *594*, 2025–2042. [CrossRef] [PubMed]

116. Marzetti, E.; Calvani, R.; Cesari, M.; Buford, T.W.; Lorenzi, M.; Behnke, B.J.; Leeuwenburgh, C. Mitochondrial dysfunction and sarcopenia of aging: From signaling pathways to clinical trials. *Int. J. Biochem. Cell Biol.* **2013**, *45*, 2288–2301. [CrossRef]

117. Morris, G.; Berk, M. The many roads to mitochondrial dysfunction in neuroimmune and neuropsychiatric disorders. *BMC Med.* **2015**, *13*, 68. [CrossRef]

118. Ames, B.N. Optimal micronutrients delay mitochondrial decay and age-associated diseases. *Mech. Ageing Dev.* **2010**, *131*, 473–479. [CrossRef]

119. Manna, P.; Achari, A.E.; Jain, S.K. Vitamin D supplementation inhibits oxidative stress and upregulate SIRT1/AMPK/GLUT4 cascade in high glucose-treated 3T3L1 adipocytes and in adipose tissue of high fat diet-fed diabetic mice. *Arch. Biochem. Biophys.* **2017**, *615*, 22–34. [CrossRef]

120. Marampon, F.; Gravina, G.L.; Festuccia, C.; Popov, V.M.; Colapietro, E.A.; Sanita, P.; Musio, D.; De Felice, F.; Lenzi, A.; Jannini, E.A.; et al. Vitamin D protects endothelial cells from irradiation-induced senescence and apoptosis by modulating MAPK/SirT1 axis. *J. Endocrinol. Investig.* **2016**, *39*, 411–422. [CrossRef]

121. Grabowska, W.; Sikora, E.; Bielak-Zmijewska, A. Sirtuins, a promising target in slowing down the ageing process. *Biogerontology* **2017**, *18*, 447–476. [CrossRef]

122. Imai, S.; Guarente, L. Ten years of NAD-dependent SIR2 family deacetylases: Implications for metabolic diseases. *Trends Pharmacol. Sci.* **2010**, *31*, 212–220. [CrossRef] [PubMed]

123. Binkley, N.; Ramamurthy, R.; Krueger, D. Low vitamin D status: Definition, prevalence, consequences, and correction. *Rheum. Dis. Clin. N. Am.* **2012**, *38*, 45–59. [CrossRef] [PubMed]

124. Hollis, B.W.; Wagner, C.L. Clinical review: The role of the parent compound vitamin D with respect to metabolism and function: Why clinical dose intervals can affect clinical outcomes. *J. Clin. Endocrinol. Metab.* **2013**, *98*, 4619–4628. [CrossRef] [PubMed]

125. Holick, M.F.; Binkley, N.C.; Bischoff-Ferrari, H.A.; Gordon, C.M.; Hanley, D.A.; Heaney, R.P.; Murad, M.H.; Weaver, C.M.; Endocrine, S. Evaluation, treatment, and prevention of vitamin D deficiency: An Endocrine Society clinical practice guideline. *J. Clin. Endocrinol. Metab.* **2011**, *96*, 1911–1930. [CrossRef] [PubMed]

126. Wimalawansa, S.J. *Vitamin D: Everything You Need to Know*; Karunaratne & Sons: Homagama, Sri Lanka, 2012; ISBN 978-955-9098-94-2.

127. Heyden, E.L.; Wimalawansa, S.J. Vitamin D: Effects on human reproduction, pregnancy, and fetal well-being. *J. Steroid Biochem. Mol. Biol.* **2018**, *180*, 41–50. [CrossRef] [PubMed]

128. Hewison, M.; Wagner, C.L.; Hollis, B.W. Vitamin D Supplementation in Pregnancy and Lactation and Infant Growth. *N. Engl. J. Med.* **2018**, *379*, 1880–1881.

Permissions

The contributors of this book come from diverse backgrounds, making this book a truly international effort. This book will bring forth new frontiers with its revolutionizing research information and detailed analysis of the nascent developments around the world.

We would like to thank all the contributing authors for lending their expertise to make the book truly unique. They have played a crucial role in the development of this book. Without their invaluable contributions this book wouldn't have been possible. They have made vital efforts to compile up to date information on the varied aspects of this subject to make this book a valuable addition to the collection of many professionals and students.

This book was conceptualized with the vision of imparting up-to-date information and advanced data in this field. To ensure the same, a matchless editorial board was set up. Every individual on the board went through rigorous rounds of assessment to prove their worth. After which they invested a large part of their time researching and compiling the most relevant data for our readers.

The editorial board has been involved in producing this book since its inception. They have spent rigorous hours researching and exploring the diverse topics which have resulted in the successful publishing of this book. They have passed on their knowledge of decades through this book. To expedite this challenging task, the publisher supported the team at every step. A small team of assistant editors was also appointed to further simplify the editing procedure and attain best results for the readers.

Apart from the editorial board, the designing team has also invested a significant amount of their time in understanding the subject and creating the most relevant covers. They scrutinized every image to scout for the most suitable representation of the subject and create an appropriate cover for the book.

The publishing team has been an ardent support to the editorial, designing and production team. Their endless efforts to recruit the best for this project, has resulted in the accomplishment of this book. They are a veteran in the field of academics and their pool of knowledge is as vast as their experience in printing. Their expertise and guidance has proved useful at every step. Their uncompromising quality standards have made this book an exceptional effort. Their encouragement from time to time has been an inspiration for everyone.

The publisher and the editorial board hope that this book will prove to be a valuable piece of knowledge for researchers, students, practitioners and scholars across the globe.

List of Contributors

David C. Geary
Department of Psychological Sciences, Interdisciplinary Neuroscience, University of Missouri, Columbia, MO 65211-2500, USA

Marisol Fernández-Ortiz, José Fernández-Martínez, Antonia Cionfrini and Paula Aranda-Martínez
Centro de Investigación Biomédica, Departamento de Fisiología, Facultad de Medicina, Instituto de Biotecnología, Parque Tecnológico de Ciencias de la Salud, Universidad de Granada, 18016 Granada, Spain

Ramy K. A. Sayed
Centro de Investigación Biomédica, Departamento de Fisiología, Facultad de Medicina, Instituto de Biotecnología, Parque Tecnológico de Ciencias de la Salud, Universidad de Granada, 18016 Granada, Spain
Department of Anatomy and Embryology, Faculty of Veterinary Medicine, Sohag University, Sohag 82524, Egypt

Germaine Escames
Centro de Investigación Biomédica, Departamento de Fisiología, Facultad de Medicina, Instituto de Biotecnología, Parque Tecnológico de Ciencias de la Salud, Universidad de Granada, 18016 Granada, Spain
CIBERfes, Ibs. Granada, 18016 Granada, Spain

Tomás de Haro
UGC de Laboratorios Clínicos, Hospital Universitario San Cecilio, 18016 Granada, Spain

Darío Acuña-Castroviejo
Centro de Investigación Biomédica, Departamento de Fisiología, Facultad de Medicina, Instituto de Biotecnología, Parque Tecnológico de Ciencias de la Salud, Universidad de Granada, 18016 Granada, Spain
CIBERfes, Ibs. Granada, 18016 Granada, Spain
UGC de Laboratorios Clínicos, Hospital Universitario San Cecilio, 18016 Granada, Spain

Magdalene K Montgomery
Department of Physiology, School of Biomedical Sciences, University of Melbourne, Melbourne 3010, Australia

Veronica Granatiero and Giovanni Manfredi
Feil Family Brain and Mind Research Institute, Weill Cornell Medicine, 407 East 61st Street, New York, NY 10065, USA

Janis T. Eells
Department of Biomedical Sciences, University of Wisconsin-Milwaukee, Milwaukee, WI 53211, USA

Peter J. McGuire
Metabolism, Infection and Immunity Section, National Human Genome Research Institute, National Institutes of Health, Bethesda, MD 20892, USA

Nima B. Fakouri
Laboratory of Molecular Gerontology, National Institute on Aging, National Institutes of Health, Baltimore, MD 21224, USA

Thomas Lau Hansen, Claus Desler, Sharath Anugula and Lene Juel Rasmussen
Center for Healthy Aging, Department of Cellular and Molecular Medicine, University of Copenhagen, 2200 Copenhagen, Denmark

Yvonne Will and Jefry E. Shields
SCIENTIA LLC, Ledyard, CT 06339, USA

Kendall B. Wallace
Department of Biomedical Sciences, University of Minnesota Medical School, Duluth, MN 55455, USA

Robert K. Naviaux
The Mitochondrial and Metabolic Disease Center, Departments of Medicine, Pediatrics, Pathology, University of California, San Diego School of Medicine, San Diego, CA 92103, USA

Jason Duran, Armando Martinez and Eric Adler
Department of Cardiology, University of California San Diego Medical Center, La Jolla, CA 92037, USA

Roisin Stout and Mark Birch-Machin
Dermatological Sciences, Institute of Cellular Medicine, Medical School, Newcastle University, Newcastle upon Tyne NE2 4HH, UK

Chun Chen, Doug M. Turnbull and Amy K. Reeve
Wellcome Centre for Mitochondrial Research, Institute for Neuroscience, Newcastle University Institute for Ageing, Newcastle University, Newcastle upon Tyne, NE2 4HH, UK
Newcastle University LLHW Centre for Ageing and Vitality, Newcastle University, Newcastle upon Tyne, NE2 4HH, UK

Isabella Peixoto de Barcelos
Department of Neurosciences, University of California
San Diego, San Diego, CA 92093-0935, USA

Richard H. Haas
Department of Neurosciences, University of California
San Diego, San Diego, CA 92093-0935, USA

Department of Pediatrics, University of California San
Diego, San Diego, CA 92093-0935, USA

Sunil J. Wimalawansa
Professor of Medicine, Endocrinology & Nutrition,
Cardio Metabolic and Endocrine Institute, NJ 08873, USA

Index

Printed in the USA
CPSIA information can be obtained
at www.ICGtesting.com
JSHW051626061123
51533JS00005B/121